GOODMAN'S NEUROSURGERY ORAL BOARD REVIEW

GOODMAN'S NEUROSURGERY ORAL BOARD REVIEW

A PRIMER

SECOND EDITION

EDITED BY

Allan D. Levi, MD, PhD, FAANS

PROFESSOR AND CHAIRMAN DEPARTMENT OF NEUROLOGICAL SURGERY

UNIVERSITY OF MIAMI MILLER SCHOOL OF MEDICINE

MIAMI, FLORIDA

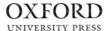

OXFORD
UNIVERSITY PRESS

OXFORD
UNIVERSITY PRESS

Oxford University Press is a department of the University of Oxford. It furthers
the University's objective of excellence in research, scholarship, and education
by publishing worldwide. Oxford is a registered trade mark of Oxford University
Press in the UK and certain other countries.

Published in the United States of America by Oxford University Press
198 Madison Avenue, New York, NY 10016, United States of America.

© Oxford University Press 2020

First Edition published in 2016
Second Edition published in 2020

Library of Congress Cataloging-in-Publication Data
Names: Levi, Allan D., 1961– editor.
Title: Goodman's neurosurgery oral board review : a primer / edited by Allan D. Levi.
Other titles: Neurosurgery oral board review : a primer |
Medical specialty board review.
Description: Second edition. | New York, NY : Oxford University Press, [2020] |
Series: Medical specialty board review |
Includes bibliographical references and index. |
Identifiers: LCCN 2019048673 (print) | LCCN 2019048674 (ebook) |
ISBN 9780190055189 (paperback) | ISBN 9780190055202 (epub) |
Subjects: MESH: Neurosurgical Procedures | Certification | Problems and Exercises
Classification: LCC RD593 (print) | LCC RD593 (ebook) |
NLM WL 18.2 | DDC 617.4/80076—dc23
LC record available at https://lccn.loc.gov/2019048673
LC ebook record available at https://lccn.loc.gov/2019048674

This material is not intended to be, and should not be considered, a substitute for medical or other professional
advice. Treatment for the conditions described in this material is highly dependent on the individual
circumstances. And, while this material is designed to offer accurate information with respect to the subject
matter covered and to be current as of the time it was written, research and knowledge about medical and health
issues is constantly evolving and dose schedules for medications are being revised continually, with new side
effects recognized and accounted for regularly. Readers must therefore always check the product information
and clinical procedures with the most up-to-date published product information and data sheets provided by
the manufacturers and the most recent codes of conduct and safety regulation. The publisher and the authors
make no representations or warranties to readers, express or implied, as to the accuracy or completeness of this
material. Without limiting the foregoing, the publisher and the authors make no representations or warranties as
to the accuracy or efficacy of the drug dosages mentioned in the material. The authors and the publisher do not
accept, and expressly disclaim, any responsibility for any liability, loss, or risk that may be claimed or incurred as a
consequence of the use and/or application of any of the contents of this material

Printed by Marquis, Canada

CONTENTS

ACKNOWLEDGMENT AND DEDICATION TO DR. JULIUS GOODMAN

Dr. Julius Goodman was an eminent neurosurgeon who was completely dedicated to the education and teaching of medical students, residents, fellows, and faculty, and as such, he influenced the careers of numerous neurosurgeons.

Julius completed his BA (1957) and MD (1960) degrees at George Washington University, his internship at UCLA, and his neurosurgical training at Indiana University (1968). He spent his entire neurosurgical career in Indianapolis, working primarily at Methodist Hospital, which is currently run by Clarian Health, part of Indiana University School of Medicine. He served as Clinical Professor of Neurosurgery from 1986 onward.

Dr. Goodman served as a co-founder of the Indiana Neurosurgery Group (ING), one of the largest private practice groups in North American neurosurgery. His colleague and contemporary, Dr. Robert Campbell, former Chairman of Neurosurgery at Indiana University, practiced neurosurgery for more than 32 years. These two men mentored and inspired generations of neurosurgeons and paved the way in creating the Goodman–Campbell Brain and Spine group. Dr. Goodman was completely dedicated to his profession and never married. He was very close to his immediate family including his siblings, nieces, and nephews. He was generous to his family and partners, and in the 15 years running the ING, he never lost a partner. He was truly a great administrator. When he was not practicing neurosurgery or teaching, he loved to travel and to recount his adventures across the world. His home was filled with beautiful artwork and cars that he purchased locally along his travels.

While performing as a brilliant neurosurgeon, Julius's knowledge base extended far beyond his own surgical discipline and included neurology, internal medicine, and general surgery. It was not uncommon to see him with the latest issue of *Annals of Internal Medicine* or the *New England Journal of Medicine* under his arm. There were frequent consults between him and his long-time friend and colleague, Dr. Robert Alonso. His areas of interest in neurosurgery included pituitary surgery, neuro-ophthalmology, trigeminal neuralgia, neurotrauma, and critical care, as well as brain tumors. Julius published more than 50 peer-reviewed papers on topics including pituitary tumors, the natural history of skull base meningiomas, and tic douloureux. One of his most influential papers was published in the *Journal of the American Medical Association*,[1] which discussed the determination of brain death using noninvasive isotope angiography.

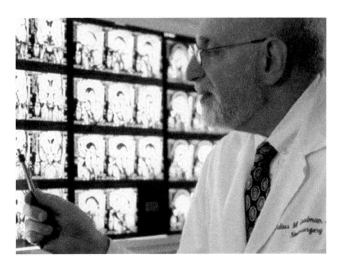

Figure P.1. Dr. Goodman reviewing MRI images.

Julius's true passion was medical and neuroscience education, and he received numerous teaching awards during his career, including Teacher of the Year, Methodist Hospital, 1971, 1972, and 1979; Teacher of the Year, St. Vincent Hospital, 1976; and a Life Time Teaching Award, Department of Emergency Medicine, Indiana University School of Medicine, 2001.

Helping neurosurgeons attain the milestone of board certification was near and dear to the heart of Dr. Goodman (Figure P.1).

Recognizing the stress associated with the Oral Board Examination, which forms part of the American Board of Neurological Surgery (ABNS) board certification process, Julius developed the course curriculum that still exists and forms part of this American Association of Neurological Surgeons (AANS) Oral Board course offering. The course is highly interactive and covers the entire practice of neurosurgery by reviewing cases and their management in all of the neurosurgical subspecialties including neurological disorders that may mimic neurosurgical conditions. In 2006, in honor of Julius M. Goodman, the AANS officially renamed the oral boards course *Goodman Oral Board Preparation: Neurosurgery Review by Case Management* (see Chapter 3 of this volume for a full description). In expected fashion, Dr. Goodman was "speechless" and "astonished" following the announcement of the AANS board course title change to recognize his contribution. After 10 years of directing the course, Dr. Goodman was presented with a plaque commemorating the occasion (Figure P.2). Julius was incredibly humble and almost painfully shy, not your typical neurosurgeon, despite all of his major accomplishments. Unfortunately, after arriving home from a 3-week trip in India, Julius was diagnosed with a large butterfly glioblastoma. After the diagnosis, he preferred not to have adjuvant therapy, and he passed peacefully in January 2008. Julius suggested that he wanted his own case shown at the board course. He felt that the management of a 72-year-old man with a malignant glioma was fair game. The case was never presented, but what we really can learn from this, is that Julius Goodman was a man who had education at the forefront of his mind to the very last minute.

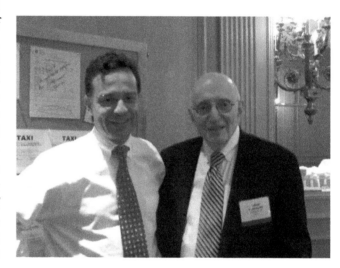

Figure P.2. Dr. Allan, D. Levi, and Dr. Julius Goodman at the American Association of Neurological Surgery (AANS) oral board course.

REFERENCE

1. Goodman J, Mishkin F, Dyken M. Determination of brain death by isotope angiography. *JAMA.* 1969;209:1869–1872.

PREFACE

Why a second edition of the text book—Goodman's Neurosurgery Oral Board Review?

The American Board of Neurological Surgery Oral Examination is the important final step in the certification process of a neurosurgeon. The examination has been in a constant state of evolution over the last 75 years. A major change in the examination process occurred in 2017, and the details of this transition are nicely outlined in Chapter 1 of the book. In keeping with this significant change in the Oral Board Examination format, I felt that the Goodman course needed to change to keep up with the examination (see Chapter 3 of this volume). The second edition of the book now also reflects these updates with an emphasis on how to prepare for the current exam format.

ACKNOWLEDGMENTS

I dedicate this book to my loving wife, Teresa, and to our nuclear family—David, Jessica, Julian, and Victor. Dr. Julius Goodman is the creator and inspiration for the American Association of Neurological Surgeons Oral Board course. His confidence and mentorship will never be forgotten.

I sincerely thank Linda Alberga for her editorial assistance with the book chapters and Roberto Suazo for his assistance with the book's figures.

Finally, I am indebted to my long-time neurosurgical and neurology colleagues and contributors to *Goodman's Neurosurgery Oral Board Review: A Primer*. Sharing their expertise in the course and now in the second edition of the text is an incredible repayment to the neurosurgical profession as a whole.

CONTRIBUTORS

Angela M. Bohnen, MD
Department of Neurological Surgery
Mayo Clinic
Jacksonville, FL

Kaisorn L. Chaichana, MD
Department of Neurological Surgery
Mayo Clinic
Jacksonville, FL

Roberto C. Heros, MD
Department of Neurological Surgery
University of Miami Miller School of Medicine
Miami, FL

Pascal Jabbour, MD
Division of Neurovascular Surgery and Endovascular
    Neurosurgery
Thomas Jefferson University Hospital
Philadelphia, PA

Douglas Kondziolka, MD, MSc
Department of Neurosurgery
New York University
New York, NY

Thomas Leipzig, MD
Goodman Campbell Brain and Spine
Indianapolis, IN

Allan D. Levi, MD, PhD
Department of Neurological Surgery
University of Miami Miller School of Medicine
Miami, FL

Kristine O'Phelan, MD
Department of Neurology
University of Miami Miller School of Medicine
Miami, FL

Alfredo Quinones-Hinojosa, MD
Department of Neurological Surgery
Mayo Clinic
Jacksonville, FL

Gary Simonds, MD
Virginia Tech School of Neuroscience
Virginia Tech Carilion School of Medicine
Roanoke, VA

Konstantin V. Slavin, MD
Department of Neurosurgery
University of Illinois at Chicago
Chicago, IL

Jodi L. Smith, MD, PhD
Department of Neurosurgery
Indiana University School of Medicine
Indianapolis, IN

Robert J. Spinner, MD
Department of Neurosurgery
Mayo Clinic
Rochester, MN

Robert M. Starke, MD, MSc
Department of Neurological Surgery and Radiology
University of Miami Miller School of Medicine
Miami, FL

Ahmad Sweid, MD
Department of Neurological Surgery
Thomas Jefferson University Hospital
Philadelphia, PA

Nitin Tandon, MD
The Vivian L. Smith Department of Neurosurgery
Memorial Hermann Texas Medical Center
Houston, TX

1.

THE ABNS ORAL BOARD EXAMINATION

Douglas Kondziolka

The American Board of Neurological Surgery (ABNS) is a member organization of the American Board of Medical Specialties. It is important to recognize that the ABNS represents both the specialty of neurosurgery and the public that it serves. It offers an oral examination that serves as the final step in the board certification process. The examination has evolved over the last 78 years. The current structure of the examination including content, scoring, and conduct are described in this chapter. The examination aims to evaluate neurosurgeons on a mix of their broad knowledge and actual practice, with the belief that this increases public safety, by evaluating practice realities while also recognizing that most neurosurgeons take call and must be well versed in the full spectrum of neurosurgery. Details of the Oral Board Examination application and case-base submission process, as well as exam specifics are available at https://www.abns.org/oral-examination/.

The ABNS Oral Board Examination is the final step in the certification process of an individual neurosurgeon by the ABNS. The application should be submitted within 3½ years of neurosurgical residency graduation. The oral exam is typically conducted within 5 years of completion of residency or postgraduate fellowship training. The Oral Board Examination currently is administered twice yearly (May and November) by the ABNS in Scottsdale, Arizona. At each examination, approximately 120 to 150 candidates are examined.

CANDIDATE SELECTION AND CREDENTIALING: REQUIREMENTS FOR ELIGIBILITY FOR THE ORAL EXAMINATION

To be allowed to take the examination, a candidate must have successfully completed a neurosurgical residency program approved by the Neurosurgery Residency Review Committee of the Accreditation Council for Graduate Medical Education. The candidate must have already passed, for credit, the ABNS Primary Examination (i.e., the written exam). The candidate must then submit an application and be scheduled to take the examination within 5 years of completing the residency or have prior approval of the ABNS if this has not been possible for personal reasons (such as military duty, health issues, or other concerns).

The candidate must also log and submit 125 consecutive, major cases in which he or she was the attending surgeon of record. There should be no fewer than 100 individual patient encounters. Cases are submitted using the POST (Practice and Outcomes of Surgical Therapies) software platform created by the ABNS, which collects both text and imaging information together with immediate and longer-term outcomes. Staged procedures count as individual cases toward the 125 but take-backs (e.g., for a complication) do not. Each case must have a minimum of 3 months follow-up. Cases during residency or fellowships are not to be included. If tracking for American Board Pediatric Neurological Surgery/ ABNS (i.e. pediatric certification) dual credential, 95 of the 125 must be cases performed on patients 21 years or younger. Diagnostic angiograms are currently considered a major case.

The POST submission process is divided into the following categories:

- Overview: Patient and Site of Service

- Medical History and Medications

- Neurological Diagnoses

- Surgical Management: description of procedure(s), surgical adjunct used, surgical role, and Current Procedural Terminology (CPT) code entry

- Clinical Summary: history and presentation and physical examination

- Imaging and Testing: include up to 8 images—preoperative, intraoperative, and/or postoperative

- Nonsurgical Management

- Surgical Outcomes: objectives of surgery, immediate postoperative outcomes (during hospital stay), intermediate postoperative outcomes (discharge to 3 months), and late outcomes (3–12 months)

These cases are reviewed by a current ABNS director. Any concerns regarding management or outcomes must be addressed adequately to be approved to sit for the oral examination.

Required letters of recommendation, evidence of medical licensure, and current hospital appointments are other data elements reviewed by the ABNS staff and credentialing committee directors before approval is granted to take the oral examination.

THE NEW ORAL EXAMINATION FORMAT

The examination consists of three 45-minute sessions. Examinations are typically given on a Saturday or a Sunday. There are three pairs of examiners for each candidate, a different pair each hour. One of the examiners is a current ABNS director (directors serve a 6-year term), a former director, or an experienced surgeon who has participated in numerous examinations and has committed their time to this process, called an ABNS examiner. The lead examiner is paired with a guest neurosurgeon who is an invited, senior, well-established neurosurgeon with a history of training residents.

The change in the oral board exam process started in the spring session of 2017 and is outlined in Table 1.1.

Table 1.1 SUMMARY OF CHANGES TO THE ORAL BOARD EXAM PROCESS

PRIOR EXAM	CURRENT EXAM
3 × 60-minute sessions	3 × 45-minute sessions
Cranial – Spine – "Other"	General – Focus – Own Practice
50% standard questions	100% standard questions
Typically 6 cases per session	5 cases per session
2 examiners per session Director/former director + guest	2 examiners per session Director/former director/ABNS examiner + guest
Located in Houston, TX	Located in Scottsdale, AZ

There were several driving forces that led to the change in the exam format and include but are not limited to increasing the relevance of the oral exam to actual practice, as we are testing neurosurgeons on what they actually do on a day-to-day basis. This process also increases public safety by evaluating practice realities. There are already several specialties including orthopedic surgery who test candidates on their own cases. Finally, starting your career acquiring prospective outcome data helps the ABNS better understand the training product and how neurosurgical practice actually exists. At the same time, early neurosurgical practitioners will appreciate the importance of data acquisition to improve their own outcome quality.

During each session, the candidates are examined on 5 clinical cases (average of 9 minutes per vignette). The sessions are divided into the following and may be administered in any order.

1. General neurosurgery

2. Focused practice

3. Candidate cases

General neurosurgery includes the broad range of conditions that neurosurgeons may see during the course of practice (including while on call or in consultation). The ABNS website provides a list of topics. The ABNS now uses only standard questions reviewed and edited in advance by ABNS directors.

The *focused practice* session allows the candidate to focus on a particular area of interest that may be a core component of their actual practice. Thus, a neurosurgeon who is predominantly doing spinal procedures can choose to have this session focus on spinal neurosurgery. However, a neurosurgeon who performs a broad array of procedures and considers himself or herself to be a generalist can choose to have this next session focus additionally on general neurosurgery. For the focused practice session, the candidate must choose in advance 1 of the following: general neurosurgery, spinal neurosurgery, vascular, tumor, functional, trauma and critical care, or pediatric neurosurgery. If a neurosurgical practitioner does primarily (80%–90%) spine cases but limits his practice to simply spine, such as decompression or limited fusions primarily in the cervical and lumbar spine, the candidate may be best suited to take the general session in session 2. The focused spine practice will consist of higher-level spine cases including spinal deformity.

The session on *candidate cases* include 10 cases selected by a director from the candidate's own data submitted through the POST platform. Ten cases will have been selected (the PowerPoint slides are automatically created by the software for use in the examination), and 5 will be chosen by the examiners on the day of the examination for discussion and grading.

It is imperative that all 5 cases be completed so that 5 scores can be granted. Thus, the examiner may move the candidate along to the next case if one is simply taking too much time. In each case scenario, the safety of the approach and management described by the candidate is judged by the examiners, who again will keep the session moving to explore the candidate's breadth of knowledge across all vignettes. During each case, an actual clinical encounter is simulated. The history, background information, and physical examination are provided usually followed by pertinent imaging. Candidates are free to ask for data needed to solve the problems that are presented. In some instances, nonimaging-based data such as laboratory or neurophysiologic testing may be relevant. The candidate is typically asked what diagnoses and/or management elements they may be considering. They may be asked about the natural history of the disorder or about both nonoperative and operative strategies. Several physical models are available for use with the candidate, including models of the head and spine, which can be used to draw incisions or surgical exposures or to describe surgical techniques. The candidate may also be presented with perioperative or intraoperative complications for which he or she should be able to provide an explanation and/or care plan. Postoperative management is commonly discussed. A postoperative complication or management scenario such as a follow-up plan may also be presented for discussion. The examiners are instructed to be open to alternative solutions that are reasonable and can be justified by the candidate. The examination is comprehensive, and the candidate should be able to answer all questions regarding the entire spectrum of neurosurgical diseases presented, notwithstanding subspecialization of their practice.

EXAMINATION GRADING

For the purposes of grading, each case is given a comprehensive score that is based on elements of knowledge, safety, and professionalism. This composite score is based on different subsets of the case discussed, including diagnosis and management of the patient, relevant problem, and the handling of complications and/or aftercare. If no treatment is rendered, the candidate would be expected to describe in detail the natural history of the disorder.

At the end of the session, a grade is given for each of the 5 questions. Since the maximum score per question is 4, the maximum grade from each examiner is 20.

Each candidate is graded on a 4-point scale. Grades 3 and 4 are passing grades.

For the General and Focused Practice Sessions

Grade 4: Provides knowledgeable and safe answers

Grade 3: Provides acceptable answers; has some knowledge gaps that would not affect patient safety

Grade 2: Provides answers that demonstrate knowledge gaps that compromise safe care

Grade 1: Provides dangerous and unsafe answers possibly owing to carelessness, a profound lack of knowledge, or a lack of professionalism

For the Candidate Cases Session

Grade 4: Strong knowledge base, excellent indications for surgery, superior management of case and complications

Grade 3: Adequate knowledge base, satisfactory indications for surgery, supports care decisions, satisfactory management of case and complications

Grade 2: Weak knowledge base, marginal indications for surgery, care not supported, marginal management of case and complications

Grade 1: Inadequate knowledge base, poor indications for surgery, major safety or ethical/professional concerns, unacceptable management of case and complications

A grade of 1 or 2 is considered a failing score for any particular case. A grade of 2 by either or both examiners could result in an overall failing grade for the session if the total score is low enough. A candidate with multiple scores of 2 will have a higher likelihood of failing. Each examiner in each session grades independently of the other examiner and is blind to the score that the other examiner gives.

To pass the ABNS Oral Examination, each candidate must pass *each* of the 3 sessions.

POSTEXAMINATION ANALYTICS AND PASS/FAIL

Following the examination, scores are provided to an outside consultant psychometrician. The ultimate pass/fail grade (pass point) is determined by a detailed analysis of all of the data derived from the examination and examiners. This takes approximately 2 weeks after the examination to complete. The final grades are adjusted for the severity of examiner (level of difficulty based on comparison with other examiners using similar case questions), the difficulty of the questions, and the three sessions. It is important to note that the ABNS seeks to be as fair as possible from one examination to the next, so that one examination is not more difficult than another. A *fair average score* is used for the pass point that is calculated and is consistent between examinations. Following the examination, the results are reviewed by the directors to maintain fairness and quality of the process.

OUTCOME OF THE EXAMINATION

Candidates are notified of the outcome of the examination 2 to 3 weeks after the examination date. A successful completion of the examination will complete the ABNS certification process. If the candidate fails to pass the examination, he or she will be eligible to retake it at a subsequent administration. Many candidates will choose to retake it at the next available opportunity. Because the examination will require another session of candidate cases, the candidate has the option of providing a set of 75 new cases or using 10 cases from the prior submission. Some candidates who have changed their practice pattern may choose to submit new cases using the POST system. A candidate who fails the examination twice may not use his or her initial case

submission for the third attempt. This process is detailed on the ABNS website.

A candidate who fails the oral examination three times (or fails to complete the entire process within 7 years of completing residency, unless an extension has been granted) will have fallen out of the process and must begin the process anew first by passing the primary (written) exam and then begin to collect a new set of 125 cases. Candidates who must begin anew are forever precluded from referring to themselves as "board eligible" or words to that effect since they did not complete the process within the initial timeframe mandated by the ABNS.

SUMMARY

The oral examination process is an important final element in the certification process of a neurosurgeon by the ABNS. The examination has evolved over the many decades of the ABNS. The format as described was developed and implemented for relevant candidate practice, with the design and implementation under constant review by the ABNS Directors. The goal is to provide a formal, rigorous, and fair assessment of candidate knowledge and practice on behalf of the public they serve.

ACKNOWLEDGMENT

The author acknowledges the contributions of ABNS directors, former directors, guest examiners, and staff.

2.

GETTING TO THE ABNS ORAL BOARD EXAMINATION

Robert M. Starke

The American Board of Neurological Surgery (ABNS) and its members are responsible for ensuring that the neurosurgery community provides safe, effective, quality-based, patient-centered, and appropriate care. The oral examination is the final step in the board certification process. The examination has changed significantly over the last 78 years. Details of the oral board examination application and case-base submission process, as well as specifics of the examination are available on the ABNS website www.abns.org/oral-examination/.

Starting in 2017, applicants will have 3½ years from the completion of residency to submit their application for the ABNS Oral Board Examination (Table 2.1). Following submission for application to the ABNS Oral Board Examination, every candidate preparing to take the oral examination must prepare and submit a log of 125 consecutive cases for review. These cases are loaded into and submitted through the Practice and Outcomes Surgical Therapies (POST) online portal. Once candidates have finished logging practice data, they submit an application for oral examination and certification. The online application provides candidates with a centralized application portal where they can submit all their required elements for assessment of eligibility for the examination.

Upon receipt of an application, the board takes appropriate steps to verify the submitted information. The application process generally takes about 18 months between submission of an application (including practice data) and sitting for oral examination, but this duration has also been decreasing significantly in recent years. The Oral Board Examination is offered twice yearly, in the spring and fall. After the applicant is offered a date for the examination, 10 cases will be selected by the ABNS board as potential cases for assessment during the Oral Board Examination. The POST system will create a PowerPoint of these cases and examiners will ultimately select 5 cases for review during the examination. Following completion of training, it is recommended that an applicant begin preparation and studying for the Oral Boards Examination. There is currently a wealth of further resources that can help prepare applicants for the examination. This process undergoes yearly updates, and it is optimal to stay up to date with the recommendations on the ABNS website.

TIMING OF APPLICATION

Oral Board Examination candidates who complete their residency on or after June 30, 2017 must submit a completed application (including completed practice data, references, and all other application materials required by the board) no later than December 31 of the calendar year (Table 2.1). Extensions may be granted by the ABNS under specific circumstances. Candidates are urged to be diligent and to submit their completed application (with all elements, including case data) as soon as possible after the completion of residency. For most candidates, it should be possible to submit completed applications within 24 to 30 months following residency.

The oral examination is typically conducted within 5 years of completion of residency, but more recently there is a movement to have applicants take the Oral Board Examination earlier to ensure they are conducting a safe clinical practice. Further information regarding timing of the application for the oral examination is available at the ABNS website: https://www.abns.org/deadlines-for-submission/. These rules and processes for the Oral Board Examination are subject to continued modifications. Candidates are advised to periodically check the ABNS website for updates and information.

GUIDELINES FOR CASE ACCRUAL AND SUBMISSION

It is recommended that residency and fellowship graduates obtain access to the ABNS POST system following completion of their training. Prior to 2018, the NeuroLog system was required to submit cases, which is no longer available. POST is available through the ABNS website: https://www.abns.org/abns-post/.

POST is an online platform that allows for the submission, analysis, and presentation of clinical cases. The goal of the POST system is uniform data submission to allow for objective and fair review and to decrease the chances for omission of relevant clinical information.

Cases from the first 3 months of practice are now admissible. Each case must have a minimum of 3 months follow-up. Cases during residency or fellowships are not to be included. If there is any concern by reviewers about the validity of practice data, an audit may be performed. In addition, 5% of POST submissions will be audited. Failure to follow the instructions outlined may result in a delay getting through the application process. Effective September 22, 2018, requirements for case log submission include the following.

- 125 consecutive cases

- All cases must have been performed over a period of 18 months or less.

- All cases must have three months follow-up.

- Follow-up may be performed outside the 18-month window.

- "Staged procedures" will count toward the total of 125.

- Complication management or revision ("take-back" surgery) is considered an extension of the original operation and will not be counted toward the 125 total cases.

- Clinical data must be from at least 100 unique patient encounters.

- No case older than 24 months from the date of submission

- Cases during residency or fellowships should not be included.

- If tracking for American Board Pediatric Neurological Surgery and ABNS dual credential (pediatric certification), 95 of the 125 must be cases performed on patients 21 years or younger.

- The total number of submitted surgical procedures may exceed 125 cases due to take-back surgeries.

A recent significant change is that diagnostic angiograms now count as major cases and should be entered into the POST. No more than 25 consecutive diagnostic angiograms can be counted as major cases. After 25 diagnostic angiograms have been entered into the POST, no more should be added. The only exception is that any patients having major complications related to angiography must be included, even if they occur after the first 25 angiograms. Without further exception, all other types of major cases must be entered consecutively.

SUBMISSION OF YOUR CASES TO THE POST SYSTEM

It is recommended that you log your cases into the POST system in a prospective fashion as you perform a surgery. This will allow for easier and more accurate collection of data and follow-up. When loading cases into the POST system, the ABNS recommends that applicants "consider the minimum amount of data you would require to adequately explain your surgical decision making *and* the observed clinical outcomes to a neurosurgical colleague."

When an applicant first logs into the POST system, they will encounter 4 main sections:

- Dashboard: project overview, system updates and links to important supplementary information

- Case Logs: a listing of all your case logs in the system. If you have only one case log, it opens it.

- My Practice: includes individual physician profile and practice details.

- My Cases: the POST clinical data entry system allows for adding new cases and editing existing ones. This

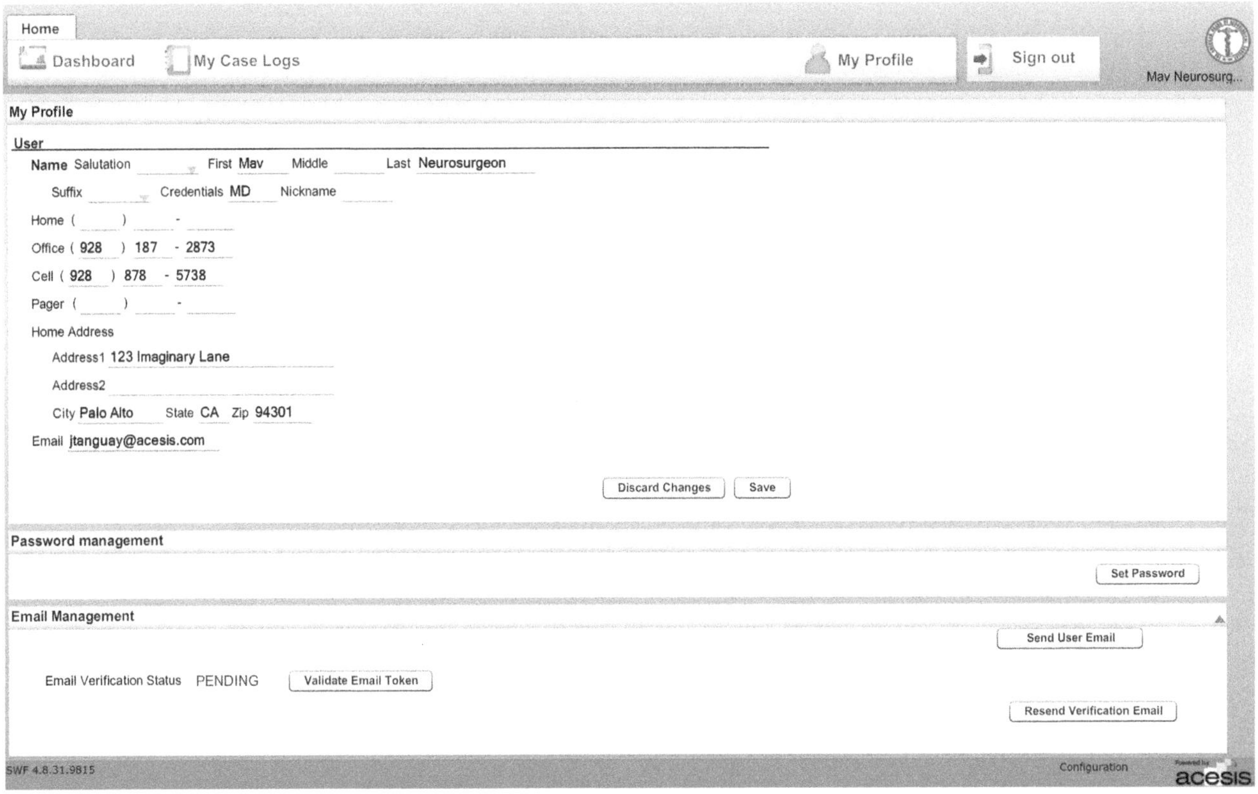

Figure 2.1 The "My Profile" tab is encountered after logging into the POST system, and applicants should ensure their contact information is up to date. Printed with permission from the ABNS. The images are the intellectual property of the ABNS, and may not be copied or disseminated without the express written permission of the ABNS. All rights to the images are reserved by the ABNS.

section is being modified to allow for generation of PowerPoint presentations to support the ABNS oral examination.

After logging into the POST system, an applicant should first direct their attention to the "My Profile" tab (Figure 2.1). Contact information should be up to date, and the email address should be verified. This will be the primary means by which the ABNS can contact you regarding the oral examination. Once completed, the applicant will be directed to the "My Cases" screen. Before logging your cases, you will need to go to the "My Practice" window and update your information (Figure 2.2). The "My Practice" screen contains updated information about your ABNS status and the required number of cases (Figure 2.3). Once completed, the applicant can begin to log cases.

Under "My Cases" the relevant categories include the following.

- Overview: Patient and Site of Service

- Medical History and Medications

- Neurological Diagnoses

- Surgical Management: description of procedure(s), surgical adjunct used, surgical role, and Current Procedural Terminology (CPT) code entry. It is recommended that an applicant include all relevant CPT codes for a given surgery.

- Clinical Summary: history and presentation and physical examination

- Imaging and Testing: include up to 8 images—preoperative, intraoperative, and/or postoperative

- Nonsurgical Management

- Surgical Outcomes: objectives of surgery, immediate postoperative outcomes (during hospital stay), intermediate postoperative outcomes (discharge to 3 months), and late outcomes (3–12 months)

Each case submission begins with the "New Case" tab (Figure 2.4). This will initiate the "Overview" (Figure 2.5), and the applicant can then move through the previously noted relevant categories to log each case.

The inclusion of relevant imaging is a significant element of case submission. Analysis of imaging data are critical to

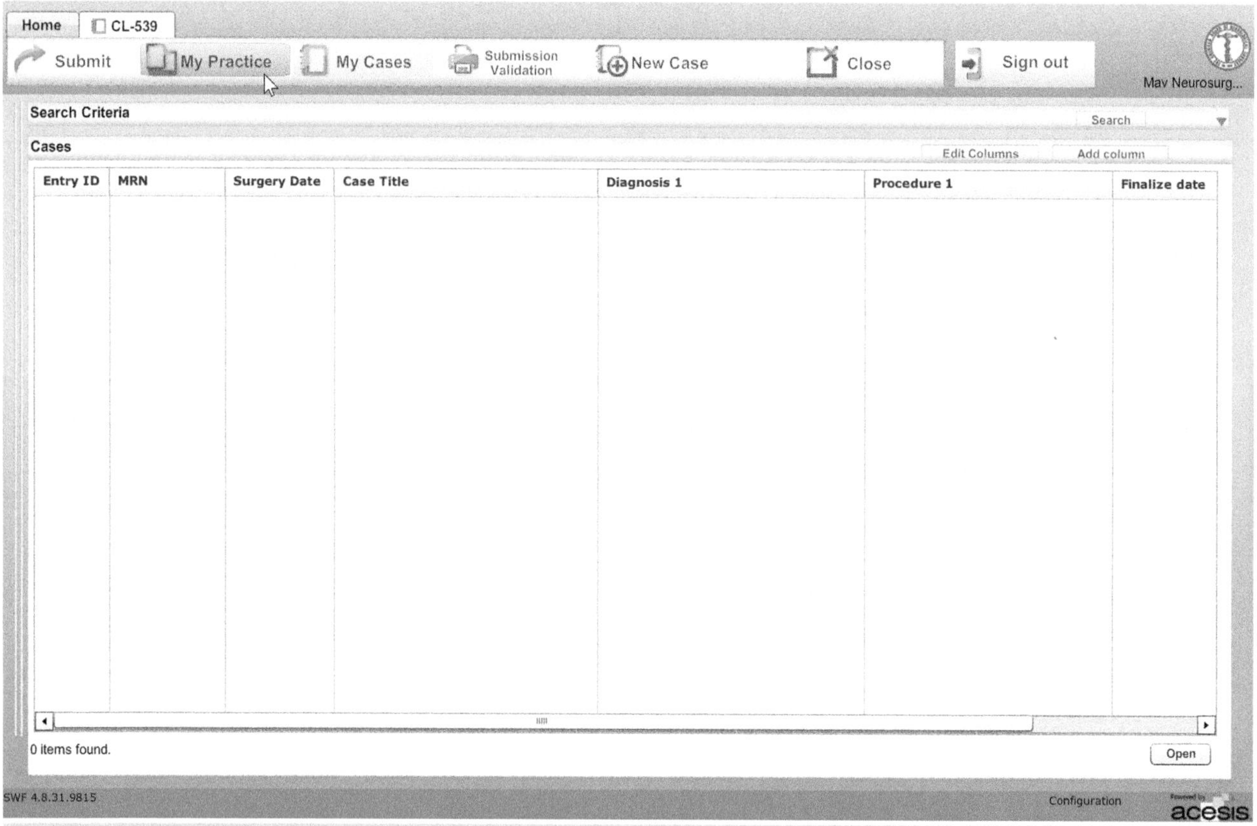

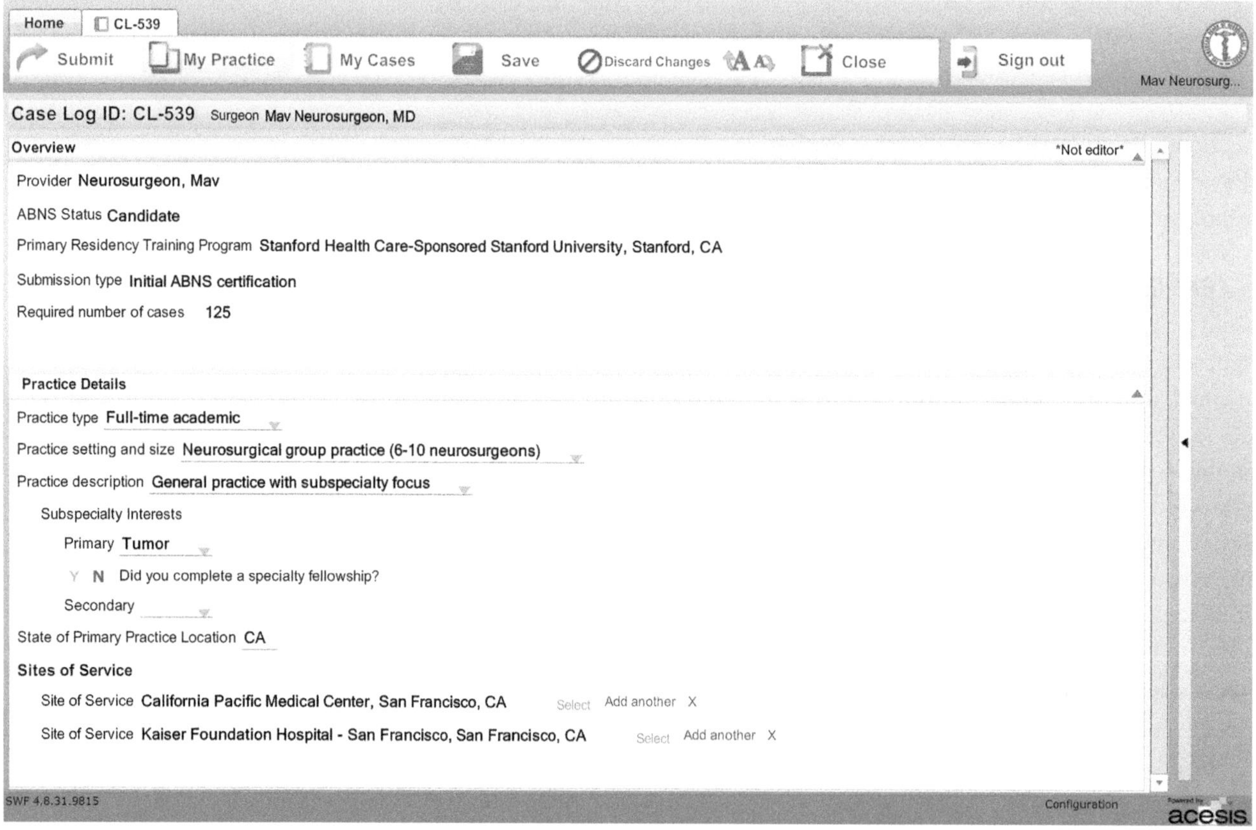

Home | CL-539

Submit | My Practice | My Cases | Submission Validation | New Case | Close | Sign out

Mav Neurosurg...

Search Criteria — Search ▼

Cases — Edit Columns | Add column

Entry ID	MRN	Surgery Date	Case Title	Diagnosis 1	Procedure 1	Finalize date

0 items found. — Open

SWF 4.8.31.9815 — Configuration — Powered by acesis

Home | CL-539

Submit | My Practice | My Cases | Save | Discard Changes | Close | Sign out

Mav Neurosurg...

Case Log ID: CL-539 Surgeon Mav Neurosurgeon, MD

Overview *Not editor*

Provider **Neurosurgeon, Mav**

ABNS Status **Candidate**

Primary Residency Training Program **Stanford Health Care-Sponsored Stanford University, Stanford, CA**

Submission type **Initial ABNS certification**

Required number of cases **125**

Practice Details

Practice type **Full-time academic**

Practice setting and size **Neurosurgical group practice (6-10 neurosurgeons)**

Practice description **General practice with subspecialty focus**

Subspecialty Interests

Primary **Tumor**

Y N Did you complete a specialty fellowship?

Secondary

State of Primary Practice Location **CA**

Sites of Service

Site of Service **California Pacific Medical Center, San Francisco, CA** Select Add another X

Site of Service **Kaiser Foundation Hospital - San Francisco, San Francisco, CA** Select Add another X

SWF 4.8.31.9815 — Configuration — Powered by acesis

Figures 2.2 and 2.3 Under the "My Practice" window and all relevant fields of an applicants' neurosurgery practice must be included prior to case entry. Printed with permission from the ABNS. The images are the intellectual property of the ABNS, and may not be copied or disseminated without the express written permission of the ABNS. All rights to the images are reserved by the ABNS.

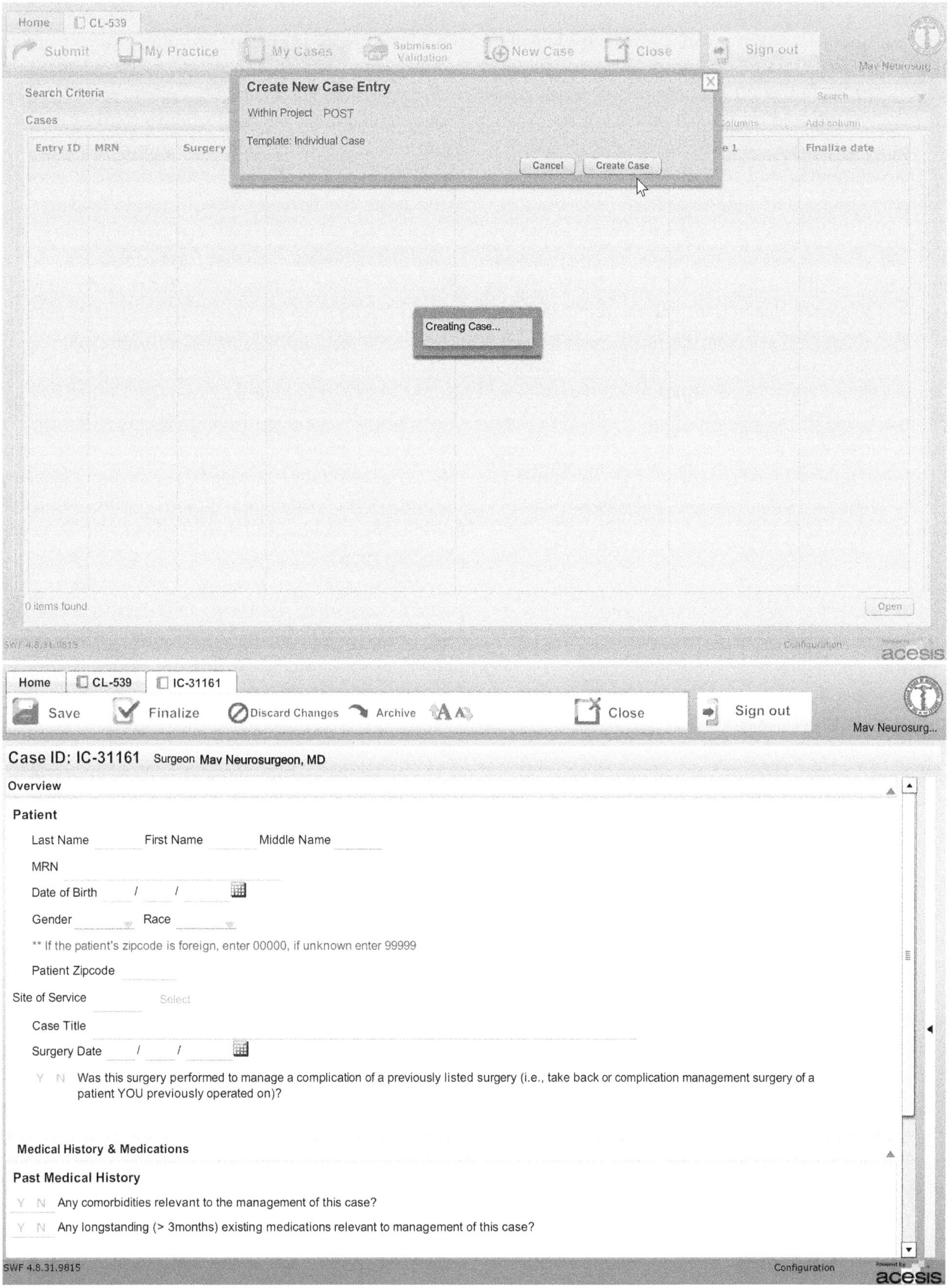

Home | CL-539

Submit | My Practice | My Cases | Submission Validation | New Case | Close | Sign out

Mav Neurosurg

Search Criteria

Cases

Search

Columns | Add column

Entry ID	MRN	Surgery		1	Finalize date

Create New Case Entry

Within Project   POST

Template: Individual Case

Cancel | Create Case

Creating Case...

0 items found.

Open

SWF 4.8.31.9815

Configuration

acesis

Home | CL-539 | IC-31161

Save | Finalize | Discard Changes | Archive | A A | Close | Sign out

Mav Neurosurg...

Case ID: IC-31161   Surgeon **Mav Neurosurgeon, MD**

Overview

Patient

Last Name _____   First Name _____   Middle Name _____

MRN _____

Date of Birth   /   /

Gender _____ ▾   Race _____ ▾

** If the patient's zipcode is foreign, enter 00000, if unknown enter 99999

Patient Zipcode _____

Site of Service   Select

Case Title _____

Surgery Date   /   /

Y N   Was this surgery performed to manage a complication of a previously listed surgery (i.e., take back or complication management surgery of a patient YOU previously operated on)?

Medical History & Medications

Past Medical History

Y N   Any comorbidities relevant to the management of this case?

Y N   Any longstanding (> 3months) existing medications relevant to management of this case?

SWF 4.8.31.9815

Configuration

acesis

Figures 2.4 and 2.5 Under "My Cases," applicants can begin to enter consecutive cases.   Printed with permission from the ABNS. The images are the intellectual property of the ABNS, and may not be copied or disseminated without the express written permission of the ABNS. All rights to the images are reserved by the ABNS.

understanding clinical outcomes and decision-making in neurological surgery. Review of imaging data is a key component of the oral examination format. When imaging is a standard part of the clinical decision-making process, candidates will be required to submit 1 to 8 case images (pre-, intra-, or postoperative). The acquisition of imaging data is very time consuming, and acquiring this information in a prospective fashion is strongly encouraged.

The amount of data input required will vary between submitted cases. In sections that allow for entry of variable amounts of information (e.g., medical history, imaging data), it is suggested that you include the minimum (i.e., essential) information you would require to explain *your* clinical decision-making and justify the clinical outcome(s) to another clinical colleague regarding the specific case being described. Examples of cases loaded into the POST system can be found on the ABNS website: https://www.abns.org/wp-content/uploads/2019/01/ABNSPOSTsamplecases.pdf. This provides further successful and appropriate input of sample cases.

APPLICATION FOR ORAL EXAMINATION AND CERTIFICATION

Once candidates have finished logging practice data, they should submit it to the ABNS board and begin work on the application for oral examination and certification. These documents can be found on the ABNS website: https://www.abns.org/. The online application provides candidates with an application portal where they can submit their application, upload supporting materials, make the appropriate payment, request reference letters, and check on the status of their application at any time. The new online system allows for expedited ABNS credential committee review. These cases are reviewed by a current ABNS director. Any concerns regarding management or outcomes must be addressed adequately to be approved to sit for the oral examination.

ABNS ASSESSMENT OF CANDIDATE'S ELIGIBILITY FOR ORAL EXAMINATION AND POTENTIAL CERTIFICATION

Upon receipt of an application, the ABNS board takes appropriate steps to verify the submitted documents. Prior to accepting a candidate into the certification process, the board requires a statement from the program director to the effect that he or she has met the minimum training requirements, performed in a satisfactory manner, and is well prepared to enter the independent practice of neurosurgery. Inquiries may be made from other references about training, practice, and hospital privileges. The board also searches each applicants' licenses to practice medicine through the Federation of State Medical Boards. In addition, at its discretion, the board may send representatives to review the candidate's practice. After considering all available information pertaining to the entire certification process, ABNS directors decide on the candidate's eligibility for oral examination and potential certification.

Candidates should be scheduled for oral examination, the final step in the certification process. Compliance with this regulation requires early submission of all information. If the 5-year limit lapses, the individual is no longer considered to be within the certification process and must repass the primary examination to return to tracking toward certification. The candidate will then be allowed 3 years to complete the process.

After an applicant receives a date to take the Oral Board Examination, the ABNS will select 10 of the applicants' cases to potentially review during the examination. These cases will be disclosed to the applicant and a PowerPoint will be generated from the POST system for assessment during the examination. This is another significant update, as applicants will no longer be able to generate or edit PowerPoint presentations based on ABNS selected cases. Therefore, it is advised that you review all of your cases before submission to ensure they are recorded accurately.

STUDY TECHNIQUES FOR BOARDS PREPARATION

Preparation for the oral board examination begins during residency and continues during an applicants' practice years. Studying should be outlined and broken down according to the updated guidelines of the ABNS available on its website: https://www.abns.org/oral-examination/. This includes relevant categories within neurosurgery. This is a substantial update to the Oral Boards Examination as an applicant is not responsible for "all areas" of neurosurgery but specific areas of both general neurosurgery and potentially their specific subspecialty category if they designate one. There are numerous neurosurgical textbooks that may help an applicant review the general knowledge required to be proficient during the examination.

As neurosurgeons, we are quite familiar with various written examinations starting before the SATs, through standardized examinations in college, medical school, and residency. The Oral Board Examination provides an entirely different structure that requires not only learning the necessary material, but also acquiring the ability to communicate this in an appropriate fashion during an oral examination. Aside from primary books, "case base" books are necessary to practice the ability to review a case based on the 3 Oral Board Examination scoring domains: Interpretation and Diagnosis, Management Strategy, and Assessment and Plan for Complications.

Aside from studying, verbal practice of case reviews is required to become proficient for the Oral Board Examination. In addition to the Goodman Oral Boards Course, the American Association of Neurological Surgeons and Congress of Neurological Surgeons provide courses and Web-based training sessions for examination preparation. It is imperative that applicants also review neurosurgical cases with their peers and mentors. Applicants at academic institutions often chose to review cases with faculty from multiple specialties. Many applicants also chose to travel to the location of their residency and/or fellowship to undergo case-based testing with prior faculty.

Once the ABNS provides a list of 10 potential cases, it is imperative that the applicant review these cases to know all relevant potential details of each case. While the ABNS discourages reviewing your own 10 cases selected by the board for defense with any oral board course faculty, it is recommended that an applicant review these cases with their peers and mentors. This should include practice presenting the cases in a fluid and proficient fashion.

The components of the cases on which the examinee is tested include knowledge, safety, surgical indications, care decision supported, and case management. The POST version 1 has been in use for about 9 months at the time of writing this chapter, and to date, over 30,000 cases have been logged. This has provided the ABNS with extensive data on the outcome of early neurosurgical practice and will form a baseline for which future generations can be compared. As with all components of the examination, future versions of POST may be anticipated.

SUMMARY

The Oral Board Examination has been significantly updated in an attempt to provide a fair and objective review of an applicants' practice of neurosurgery. Applicants are required to adhere to the relevant chronological deadlines for preparation of the necessary documents and case submission. Although most of the knowledge required for the oral boards is learned during residency and or fellowships, the Oral Board examination requires specific preparation and practice.

3.

THE GOODMAN ORAL BOARD COURSE

Allan D. Levi

Achievement of the American Board of Neurological Surgery (ABNS) certification, a key milestone on the path to a career in neurosurgery in the United States, is no easy feat, as those of us who have already been through the process well know. It represents the culmination of years of education and training in mastery of a knowledge base that is the foundation on which neurosurgeons rely as they provide the best care for patients throughout their careers.

The American Association of Neurological Surgery (AANS) Oral Board course recently marked 25 years of preparing attendees for success in the ABNS. "The success of the course is based in part on experienced, board-certified faculty members who produce an interactive, hands-on curriculum that provides participants with insights on what to expect on the rigorous oral board exam." The ever-evolving curriculum parallels the advances in the field and the clinical challenges being faced by neurosurgeons in practice.

In keeping with significant recent changes in the oral board exam format in 2017 there have been concurrent, significant changes in the course structure. While the basic division of course sessions into plenary and breakout sessions (see the following discussion) remains, there has been modifications of the course to address the following changes in the exam.

1. Plenary sessions typify hour # 1 of general exam and present more basic types of neurosurgery cases that you would see if you were on call for the emergency room, doing a locum, or maintained a very general practice.

2. Break out sessions typify hour # 2 and present more challenging and complicated cases that include general, spine, vascular, tumor, pediatrics, functional, and trauma/critical care

3. Pleanary sessions dedicated to the defense of your own cases - hour # 3

The changes in the course over the last 2 years included dropping the neurology evening session, 1 spine session, 1 pediatrics session, and the functional session that included a discussion of epilepsy, pain, and movement disorders. The majority of the cases presented in the general session are common, straightforward cases that are representative of the subspecialty session. We try to avoid esoteric or incredibly complex cases that might represent the most difficult cases seen by that subspecialty. In the breakout sessions that are assigned to the participants, we make sure that a minimum of 4 of 6 half-hour sessions are in that individual's subspecialty and that the faculty are experts in the same field, so that this part of the course will emulate hour 2 of their exam. The cases presented in the breakout sessions are more difficult than the general sessions; for example, the spine general session may address a large lumbar disc herniation with radiculopathy whereas the spine breakout session may consider a complex sagittal deformity case in an elderly patient.

Finally, in the afternoon of the last day of the course we have our faculty who have recently taken the exam defend their own cases in the general session and provide feedback to the participants on what they have learned in preparing their cases, submitting them through the POST system, and defending them in the oral board exam. We have a separate general session of case defense with 4 participants from the course who have submitted their cases, but have yet to take their oral exam. There are no concurrent breakout sessions during this part of the course. The cases presented cannot be actual cases that were used or will be used in the oral board exam. The ABNS and AANS are separate entities and instruction of a case defense case is not advised and represents a conflict of interest for the two organizations.

Dr. Goodman proposed the idea of the Neurosurgery Review by Case Management Oral Board Preparation Course. The first course was held on May 3–5, 1997, in San Diego with 32 registrants and 11 faculty members. The popularity of this course soon led to 2 course offerings per year, and the course over time has expanded to more than

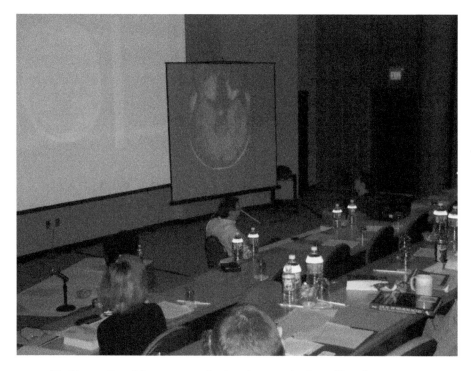

Figure 3.1 The "hot seat" candidate is presented a clinical vignette by the oral board course examiner while the large group learns from the content and style of the response. The examiner provides the correct answer and suggestions at the end of the case.

150 registrants per course taught by over 30 faculty members. Currently, the courses are offered in Phoenix, Arizona, just before the ABNS oral examination. Moving the course location from Houston to Phoenix parallels the move of the ABNS oral exam to that location.

The course is highly interactive and attempts to simulate the examination given by ABNS. The course features plenary sessions wherein an examiner interviews a participant in the "hot seat" while the larger group (150 participants) observes (Figure 3.1). Although this format is initially somewhat intimidating to participants, the opportunity for colleagues to "listen in" during the plenary sessions constitutes an invaluable learning experience. Each 2- or 2½-hour session is divided according to neurosurgical subspecialties, including vascular, endovascular, spine, brain tumors, pediatrics, peripheral nerve, head trauma, and neurocritical care. The examiners are experts in their respective fields and try to emulate the examination process and provide feedback to the examinee at the end of each case.

Concurrently, 30-minute breakout sessions are run in adjoining private rooms to the main session and allow 1-on-1 interaction between the participant and the examiner (Figure 3.2). Full-course registrants receive a minimum of 3 hours (six 1-on-1 breakout sessions) of direct face to face instruction. Plenary cases are posted after each subspecialty presentation on an outside computer or projector for the

duration of the course. Participants in these breakout sessions are able to develop techniques for answering questions pertaining to the clinical scenarios in a structured fashion, and they are able to practice rapidly responding to multiple clinical scenarios across numerous subspecialties. One of the advantages of these 1-on-1 sessions is that direct feedback can be given to the participant in relative anonymity. Although answer content is important, feedback on answering style is also given. This includes the flow and order of questioning

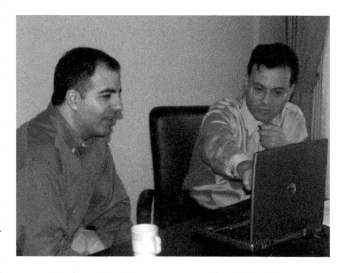

Figure 3.2 Breakout 1:1 sessions run concurrently with the plenary sessions.

when moving from diagnosis to management of complications (see chapter 4 regarding scoring of the ABNS examination). Maximizing points for each subsection is critical.

The learning objectives of the course include the following:

- Discuss contemporary neurosurgery topics, including trauma, cerebrovascular disease, tumors, pain, pediatrics, skull base, spine, and peripheral nerves.

- Comprehend the format of the ABNS Oral Board Examination.

- Compare your approach to standard and complex neurosurgical problems with those of your contemporaries.

- Review specific neurological disorders that might mimic conditions referred to a neurosurgeon.

- Identify those areas of neurosurgery in which further study would be beneficial in preparation for the ABNS Oral Board Examination.

The course has two purposes.

- First, participants are exposed to the format of the ABNS Oral Board Examination and have the opportunity to practice answering questions under pressure.

- Second, more than 200 case scenarios are presented, which will provide a broad review of pertinent topics in clinical neurosurgery. There are no lectures. The sessions are intense, comprehensive, and enjoyable. Experienced neurosurgical faculty will critique your patient management response and your ability to organize responses to simulated oral board exam questions.

The course spans the 3-day period immediately preceding the Oral Board Examination. Currently, examinations are held in May and November in Phoenix, Arizona. The lengths of each day of teaching at the course are approximately 10½ hours, not including food breaks. Neurology-type questions are sprinkled throughout the course to remind the participant that patients with primarily neurological disorders can present to the neurosurgeon, and they must be able to recognize and differentiate them from cases that require surgery. A complex spinal surgery breakout session occurs concurrently with the pediatric session in the afternoon of the first day of the course. This session is dedicated to participants who are taking a spine-focused exam in hour 2. The session is more didactic and includes an in-depth discussion of spinal deformity and its correction. More than 90% of people taking the Oral Board Examination take the course, and 60% of neurosurgeons take the course more than twice.

During the 3-day course, more than 200 cases are answered directly or observed by participants attending the course. A complimentary copy of Mark S. Greenberg, *Handbook of Neurosurgery* or this textbook is given. In each session, thoughts on techniques for answering questions, approach, and approach to new technologies in neurosurgery are covered. As part of the continuing medical education process, participants can obtain continuing medical education credits for the 3-day, 32-hour course. Evaluations are seriously considered, and significant changes have been made to the course curriculum based on prior suggestions.

What is the measure of a successful course? Soaring numbers of course participants is one obvious measure. The most dramatic testaments to course success, however, are the accolades voiced by the neurosurgeons who have participated. Their comments include the following:

- "This course is by far the most important thing you can do . . . to pass the exam."

- "Your course was an invaluable part of my success on the exam."

- "The AANS oral board course is indispensable in helping one prepare for the boards."

4.

THOUGHTS ON TECHNIQUES IN ANSWERING ORAL BOARD QUESTIONS

Allan D. Levi

WHO ARE YOUR EXAMINERS?

American Board of Neurological Surgery (ABNS) board membership is an elected official position that is extremely important in helping to regulate our profession, and one of the main purposes is to conduct examinations of candidates who voluntarily seek certification, as well as to issue certificates to those who meet the requirements of the board, and satisfactorily complete its examinations. The examiners are either board members of the ABNS or guest examiners. Most examiners are chairs, program directors, or division chiefs and are in the 45- to 65-year age group. Each is likely to be an academic neurosurgeon and is highly specialized. There are standardized questions provided by the ABNS that each examiner will give each candidate. If the examiner "knows you"—that is, you were a former resident or fellow in their program—they will recuse themselves from examining you.

BREAKING DOWN YOUR APPROACH

The discussion of answering techniques in case-based questions can be divided into two major areas: *content* and *style*. If an individual is excellent in one area and has not at least mastered the other area, problems can ensue. An example would be a neurosurgeon who has a large clinical experience as a resident, fellow, and new attending and is well read and has prepared whole heartedly for the examination but is simply incapable of a logical thought process in stringing together the results of diagnostic studies, surgical plan, and management of complications.

CONTENT

The oral board is a test of your knowledge in all areas of neurosurgery, and you are responsible for each area even if you have subspecialized in a certain area. For example, if you are a fellowship-trained spine surgeon, it may be 8 or 9 years since you have treated a lateral ventricular tumor, but you are still clearly responsible for handling this type of case on your oral board. Because you have already submitted your cases to the board, they know your practice pattern; therefore, there is no need to preface your answers with a statement such as, "I don't do this kind of case." In the past, the 3 hours of the examination were divided into Spine, Cranial, and Other, with neurological cases sprinkled in between. Currently, the examination is divided into general, focused practice, and a review of your submitted cases over the 3 sessions, and you must pass each session to pass the examination.

Gaining the experience and knowledge in neurosurgery starts when you are a medical student demonstrating your initial interest in neurosurgery and continues to the day of your examination. For all examinees, this represents thousands of cases that you participated in during your training and in your own practice. Cramming the night before your oral board session simply does not make sense.

In preparation for the examination, a general neurosurgical text, like Mark S. Greenberg's *Handbook of Neurosurgery*, can provide a broad overview of all neurosurgery. Selected readings from a specialty text may also be of value in covering areas in which you may be less versed. Receiving practice questions from a senior partner or colleague is helpful and, of course, attending the Goodman prep course is also very valuable.

STYLE

Remember strategically that your responses need to be divided into the following categories:

A.   Diagnosis

B.   Management

C.   Complications

DIAGNOSIS

The examiners will present you with clinical vignettes that are short and to the point, possibly only a line or two. The absolute key is to proceed diagnostically in a logical fashion, starting with a history, past medical history, or family history as appropriate. It can be advantageous to ask a few directed questions that demonstrate your understanding of the case and that can win you points. For example, in a patient with a cystic tumor of the spinal cord with an intensely enhancing mural nodule, you may ask whether the patient has a family history of von Hippel–Lindau disease; this immediately suggests that you are "on course," but asking for a family history of disease for each case may just waste valuable time.

Next is the physical and neurological examination. In a trauma case, you may need to know more about the vitals, including airway, breathing, and circulation (ABCs) and about the level of consciousness, including the Glasgow Coma Scale score. The neurological examination presented will also be short, but asking questions that help to localize the lesion in the neuraxis will be helpful.

Finally, additional imaging tests to the ones already presented may be needed, such as an angiogram, positron emission tomography, computed tomography, and/or a metastatic workup, may be required. Ideally, we always want to review all the radiologic studies and have excellent quality films, but only a certain number of films can be presented for any specific case. You can ask for more, but almost always, the next slide is the next slide. Ask, but you may not receive. There are no trick slides, and it would be unlikely that the area of interest would be a small structure in the very corner of the film.

Avoiding long periods of silence as you are gathering your thoughts is important. A lengthy pause may in fact annoy your examiner. Instead of silence, viewing the films and describing what you see can help win you points. This would include looking at a magnetic resonance image of the brain or spine, describing the imaging sequence, noting whether gadolinium was given, and describing the location of the lesion. Even if you do not know the exact diagnosis or surgical plan, you can make headway.

MANAGEMENT

With respect to management, do not necessarily jump to surgery. Think wisely about the natural history. A lumbar disk without a significant neurological deficit will need adequate conservative treatment, including pain medications, anti-inflammatory drugs, physical therapy, and possibly epidural injections. Jumping to surgery without having described conservative care will not be viewed well. On the other hand, the examiners may ultimately want you to do surgery after an appropriate trial of conservative care, so do not be afraid to move forward with a surgical plan—after all, this is a neurosurgical examination. Continually sending a patient back to physical therapy with a very large L4–L5 disk herniation, for example, may likewise disturb the examiner.

When proceeding with surgery, also proceed logically. Think about anesthetic considerations, antibiotics, positioning, skin preparations, additional equipment, precordial Doppler if you are operating in the sitting position, and so forth. Intraoperative electrophysiologic monitoring, including somatosensory evoked potentials (SSEPs) and motor evoked potentials (MEPs), may also serve as an important adjunct. SSEPs and MEPs are not considered standard of care in every spine surgery. Proponents against their use cite that if changes occur from a true intraoperative neurological problem, it will be too late to do anything about it. I recommend their use in high-risk cases, including intramedullary tumors, calcified thoracic disks, and cervical ossification of the posterior longitudinal ligament. Changes in MEPs as opposed to SSEPs are more specific in predicting a postoperative neurological deficit. Changes in latency as opposed to amplitude in SSEPS are more predictive of a postoperative neurological problem. Remember that there are many reasons for changes in the evoked potential monitoring, including but not limited to technical problems—leads that become detached, anesthetic agents, hypotension, and hypothermia, which can particularly effect SSEPs. Make sure to problem-solve technical issues before attributing the changes to a true neurological problem.

If you are being examined on a spine case, make sure to localize the area of the incision with fluoroscopy and be sure you are on the correct side for an asymmetrical spinal disease process.

COMPLICATIONS

When complications ensue, and they will, be ready to jump in. Come in and see the patient, lay hands on, express your concern. Do not send your resident or nurse practitioner or delay the visit until Monday if the problems are occurring on the weekend.

Also, make a well-defined plan for some of the following common complications that can be seen in neurosurgery. This way you can easily respond without generating too much stress.

- Postoperative wound infection
- Cerebrospinal fluid leak
- Postoperative neuropathic pain
- C5 nerve palsy
- Changes in electrophysiological monitoring
- Status epilepticus
- Postoperative cranial or spinal hematoma
- Hyponatremia
- Vasospasm
- Intraoperative aneurysm rupture—open or endovascular
- Uncontrolled intracranial pressure
- Brain swelling during operative exposure
- Esophageal injury

STYLE PITFALLS

A style pitfall is a burning desire of some candidates to demonstrate how "smart" they are to the examiner. This would include bringing in extraneous clinical information or citing articles that may not be relevant to the case at hand. This pressure of speech may lead the examiners to eventually pick up on something you say and take you down a direction you do not want to go, without getting you additional points.

CITING PAPERS OR REFERENCES

There are only a very few articles that you would want to cite during your oral examination in any particular sub-specialty. Some examples might include the STASCIS, ARUBA, NASCET, and ISUA trials. The purpose of citing

any references would be to help rationalize your management strategy.

TIMING

Neurosurgical residency may last 7 years, with countless nights on call, and you may be working in a neurosurgical practice for 3 to 5 years before you take the Oral Board Examination. But you have only three 45-minutes sessions to be able to show your knowledge in all areas of neurosurgery to the examiners.

Timing is everything. In general, you need to get through at least 5 questions in each 45- minute session. This translates to approximately 9 minutes per question. Answering only 4 questions in an hour will clearly put you at a major disadvantage in obtaining an overall passing score.

DISAGREEING WITH THE EXAMINER

Disagreeing with your examiner is not a good idea. Your examiner is always "correct." In a famous case, an examinee detailed how the examiner had not read his seminal paper on the topic on which the presented case was centered. The examiners are there to help you, so listen carefully to their questions. Do not argue with them. Also, remember that there is often more than one correct answer for a particular case example—for example, anterior versus posterior decompression of the cervical spine. As long as you have a reasonable explanation for your approach, it too can be the correct answer. Resist the temptation to be dogmatic about a certain answer because you may see the opposite approach on the next slide the examiner shows you. There is more than one way to skin a cat—and you will want to give your rat.

THOUGHTS ON NEW TECHNOLOGIES

Neurosurgery is in a constant process of evolution. I have been involved in teaching the Oral Board Examination course at the time of writing this textbook for 22 years. Over that period of time, there has been a dramatic change in the way we practice neurosurgery. Areas of growth that essentially did not exist 20 years ago include endovascular techniques for aneurysmal flow diversion and coiling, embolization of tumors and arteriovenous malformations, endovascular treatment of vasospasm, clot retrieval for stroke, carotid stenting, focused radiation for tumors and arteriovenous malformations, endoscopic techniques for skull base tumors, endoscopic third ventriculostomy, deep brain stimulation for Parkinson's disease, complex spinal instrumentation, and minimally invasive and lateral approaches to the spine. Many of these procedures have been around for more than 5 years and are fair game to discuss. You may not have been trained specifically to coil aneurysms, for example, but you should know the indications and principles for the procedure, if not the detailed techniques. Oral board examiners tend to be a little slower to adopt new technologies, so avoid discussing a technique that has been around for a very short time and for which long-term follow-up data have not been published. Also, note that some procedures are much less frequently performed, for example, open aneurysm clipping—particularly basilar artery aneurysms, percutaneous cordotomy for cancer pain, and brachytherapy.

DON'T LOOK BACK—KEEP LOOKING FORWARD

You are the master of your own destiny. You will make mistakes during your Oral Board Examination. Some examinees will come up with the desired response from the last case at the beginning of the next case. Don't think about the prior case response, because it will distract you from being on task with your current case.

OCCASIONALLY CHANGING YOUR APPROACH IN THE MIDDLE OF A CASE IS OK

While you are answering a case, the examiners may appear to be steering you away from a particular trajectory. Sometimes, it is acceptable to back out of your proposed approach. An example would be if you were evaluating and treating a "brain tumor," and while in the middle of surgery to resect the "tumor," you begin to understand that the lesion is likely tumefactive multiple sclerosis. You can indicate your further thoughts on the case and that you would instead recommend steroids and interferon and obtain follow-up magnetic resonance imaging in 3 months. If you are correct, the examiners will just move on to the next case.

DEFENDING YOUR OWN CASES

The addition of this session to the Oral Board Examination has been a game changer. The impetus for such a change includes increasing the relevance of the examination to actual practice and thus reducing failures by avoiding testing on cases that candidates are unlikely to do. There is certainly a precedent in other specialties to include this form of testing such as orthopedic surgery. Finally, this form of data collection and outcomes allow the ABNS to better understand the training product and how neurosurgical practice actually exists.

Successful defense of your cases begin well before the cases are even managed or operated upon. It should be abundantly clear to the candidate that case selection is key and that a careful analysis of this factor should form the backbone of your practice for the remainder of your career. Taking on a surgical case that does not adhere to sound neurosurgical principles with respect to indications will be very difficult to defend, particularly several years later when you are distilling the case in front of your examiners. Some very worrisome cases that I have seen over the years include a small (2 mm) aneurysm or convexity meningioma (1 cm) in an asymptomatic elderly patient and a thoracolumbar fusion for degenerative disc disease presenting as low back pain without sagittal imbalance. It is a great idea to bounce cases off a colleague, who you have a great respect for his or her clinical judgement. It is important to accrue the case data in real time, including the relevant imaging, and place the data in POST. Keep notes that can remind you of the nuances of the case, which might not be intrinsically obvious to the examiner who is reviewing the case. There is also an opportunity in POST to add these notes, so that the examiner may further understand your line of thinking.

What are the factors that lead the ABNS to select the 10 cases from the 125 cases that you submit? The two most common are images that do not justify the level of care and complications related to the management and operative procedure. Other reasons include common practice cases, problems with professionalism, unusual cases or an abundance of a certain case type, poor outcomes, coding concerns, and consistent lack of follow-up.

Fast forward to the actual examination date, and you are in front of the examiners defending your cases. First and foremost, know every aspect of each of these cases intimately. Review them with your colleagues or mentors several times before the examination. Be prepared to defend each step of your management from degree of conservative care, all the way to surgical treatment, and the various forms of surgical care offered (see https://youtu.be/Q6s5cbIZF2M for a video of Dr. Starke defending his cases on a mock Oral Board Examination). At the time of the examination, you may have learned through experience that the approach used was not likely the best way to proceed. Be prepared to acknowledge this, as part of the learning process. Trying to defend a position "to the death," particularly if it clearly has issues, is not a good approach. While I normally would not advocate citing the literature at your oral boards, there may be a role for citing a major study, specifically if it is a prospective, randomized study or provides level I evidence that supports your position. Acknowledge when appropriate that there are many surgical approaches to a given problem. Surgical techniques that may be considered unique or unusual that were learned during training or suggested by your partners should also be recognized.

THOUGHTS ON ATTIRE

A conservative dress code is likely the best policy: dark suits for men and conservative dresses or pant suits for women. Do not distinguish yourself by wearing jeans and a sweater to your Oral Board Examination. Keeping in mind religious or ethnic considerations, which are perfectly appropriate, it would be wise to show up clean shaven. Wearing flashy jewelry, such as large gold watches or flashy necklaces, will separate you from the pack, but not in a good way.

DOS AND DON'TS ON EXAMINATION DAY

- Do think of neurological diseases that might mimic the condition you are reviewing.

- Do "be safe."

- Do think of potential complications and their management.

- Don't suggest procedures that you have never heard of.

- Don't try to pass the case to another colleague or service.

- Don't short-change yourself with time on your flight into Phoenix for the examination.

5.

BRAIN TUMORS

Angela M. Bohnen, Kaisorn L. Chaichana, and Alfredo Quinones-Hinojosa

Angela M. Bohnen, Kaisorn L. Chaichana, and Alfredo Quinones-Hinojosa

CASE 1

HISTORY AND PHYSICAL EXAMINATION

A 72-year-old male, prior smoker and a history of melanoma presented to the emergency room with acute onset of nausea, dizziness, ataxia, and confusion. On examination, he was found to have normal mentation and 5/5 strength but suffered from right-sided dysmetria, dysdiadochokinesia, and gait ataxia. His medical history is complicated by coronary artery disease, multiple cardiac stents, and diabetes that is moderately controlled with an insulin pump. His systemic melanoma is controlled with Nivolumab (OPDIVO) treatment.

IMAGING STUDIES

An initial computed tomography (CT) scan revealed an area of right cerebellar hypodensity along with right frontal hypodensity adjacent to a heterogeneously dense lesion. Furthermore, magnetic resonance imaging (MRI) demonstrated 3 right cerebellar (largest of 2.3 cm) and a single 2.5 cm right frontal, contrast-enhancing lesions with a significant amount of surrounding edema (Figure 5.1).

ANALYSIS OF CASE AND SURGICAL PLAN

The patient has multiple contrast-enhancing lesions with surrounding vasogenic edema. With multiple lesions, the examiner will want to make sure that you consider the differential diagnosis, whether or not surgery is indicated, and, if surgery is indicated, what surgery to offer. The differential diagnosis for multiple contrast-enhancing lesions would include embolic infarct with hemorrhagic conversion, multiple hemorrhages related to amyloid angiopathy, metastasis—from primary melanoma or other site, abscess, multifocal primary central nervous system (CNS) tumor,

demyelinating lesion, lymphoma, and immune-related lesions secondary to OPDIVO treatment such as encephalopathy/encephalitis.

In addition, it is prudent to obtain a sense of the patient's overall systemic disease. A recent CT chest, abdomen, pelvis or positron emission tomography (PET) scan for assessment of disease burden and a discussion with the primary oncologist will help. The patient's performance status must also be considered.

RATIONALE FOR SURGERY

Metastatic disease is the most common CNS tumor; up to 40% of cancer patients will present with brain metastasis[1,2] and 50% will die from neurological disease burden rather than systemic causes.[2] Management of multiple brain metastasis is still a subject of debate.

There is class 1 evidence to suggest that surgical resection followed by radiotherapy (RT) provides better control rates and overall survival for solitary lesions[3] and for oligometastatic disease.[3,4] It should be noted, though, that only the level 1 recommendation provided by the CNS Guidelines includes surgery followed by whole brain radiation for single brain metastasis.[3] The role of surgery for multiple lesions is controversial, and we lack literature for guidance[3,5]; however, multiple studies have demonstrated increased survival with aggressive treatment of metastatic lesions,[5–8] including the need for multiple craniotomies.[9,10] It has been demonstrated that multiple craniotomies during the same setting can be performed without an increase in morbidity.[9,10] The biggest, historical argument against multiple craniotomies was based on the poor prognosis of patients with brain metastasis,[10] which has changed significantly with the advances of immunotherapy, especially for diseases such as melanoma.

The caveat, for surgical resection, is that the patient must have good performance status and stable/controlled systemic

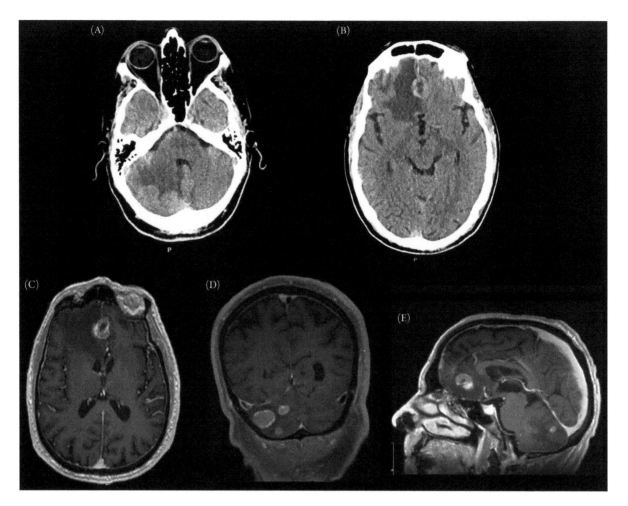

Figure 5.1 Initial CT head in the axial plane revealing the cerebellar (A) and frontal (B) lesions. Preoperative T1-weighted MRI with contrast revealing the frontal lesion in the axial view (C), cerebellar lesions in the coronal view (D) and sagittal view (E).

disease.[5] A patient with good performance status is classified as one who functions independently (Karnofsky Performance Score [KPS] >70) and spends <50% of time in bed.[5] Additionally, factors that affect prognosis include age, primary histology, and extent of extracranial disease.[2] Furthermore, number, size, and location of brain metastasis must be considered when contemplating treatment strategy.[2] It is reasonable to offer surgical resection of 1 or multiple lesions if they can be removed through the same craniotomy, are larger than 3 cm, cause significant mass effect or midline shift, are symptomatic,[5] or the patient can't be weaned off steroids.[10]

With the advent of newer technologies such as stereotactic radiosurgery (SRS), novel chemotherapeutic and immunotherapy techniques, it is a good idea to think about timing of surgery, the role of surgery, and the use of a multimodal treatment strategy.[3]

In this particular case, the patient has a good functional performance status and his systemic disease is well controlled. Given his symptomatic lesions in the right cerebellar hemisphere, it is reasonable to offer surgical resection of these lesions, with the goal of removing all 3 lesions thorough the same craniotomy. In regard to the right frontal lesion, it is 2.5 cm in size with a significant amount of edema. Concern for increased edema related to RT treatment is of concern, and therefore it is reasonable to offer up front resection of this lesion as well. The patient does suffer from significant headache, and it is possible to be a contributory factor. Alternatively, based on discussion with the patient, it is also reasonable to observe this lesion for growth, increased edema, or increased mass effect after treatment with RT and offer resection at the time of occurrence.

SURGICAL RESECTION

Resection will require coordination with frameless stereotactic navigation and the surgical team, especially if both craniotomies are to be done in the same sitting. The 3 cerebellar lesions may be resected through the same suboccipital craniotomy with the patient either in the prone or lateral position. Use of the intraoperative ultrasound may be helpful to identify resection of the deeper lesions. Intraoperative serum glucose levels should be monitored closely to minimize morbidity.

Simultaneous resection of the frontal lesion will require repositioning of the patient into the supine position or may be attempted via the lateral position if this was utilized for the suboccipital lesions. Rather than perform a large incision and frontal craniotomy, it is possible to provide a keyhole resection via an eyebrow craniotomy. This patient, however, had a wide frontal sinus. Instead, a keyhole frontal craniotomy via a wrinkle line in the forehead was offered and the lesion was resected via tubular brain retractor.

Metastatic lesions displace, rather than invade tissue. Microsurgical technique should allow for en bloc resection of the lesion, when possible, to minimize leptomeningeal dissemination. Most metastatic lesions have a capsule that will allow for shrinkage and dissection from the surrounding brain. Supratotal resection of the lesion to include 5 mm of surrounding brain, when possible, may reduce the rate of local recurrence.[11]

After surgery, radiosurgery is ultimately required to treat the resection bed. Ideally, radiosurgery may commence around 2 to 3 weeks after resection and incisional healing has occurred. At this point, the postsurgical resection cavity is at its smallest volume,[12] and morbidity is low for postsurgical complications. In addition, multidisciplinary treatment will require participation of the patient's primary oncologist for discussion of chemotherapy or immunotherapy treatment.

COMPLICATIONS

Postoperatively, the patient should be maintained in a normoglycemic range. His diabetes increases his risk of wound dehiscence and infection. Seizure prophylaxis should be maintained, per physician discretion, if the frontal lesion is resected. Postoperative imaging (Figure 5.2) is obtained to evaluate for complications, such as hemorrhage and stroke, and to assess the tumor resection. Due to the symptomatic nature, physical therapy is utilized, as the patient is likely to need some balance and gait training long term to maximize recovery.

Long-term complications include recurrence and progression of disease. Along with systemic staging, an MRI brain should be re-evaluated every few months.

PEARLS

- Currently there is only class 1 evidence for surgical resection of solitary metastatic lesions.

- Multiple studies have demonstrated aggressive treatment, including resection, of oligometastatic disease can lead to increased survival in appropriate patients.

- Surgical indications for resection include KPS >70, controlled systemic disease, lesions >3 cm, symptomatic lesions, significant cerebral edema, and lesions causing mass effect and midline shift.

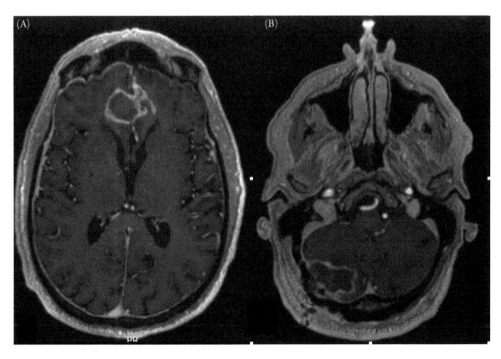

Figure 5.2 Postoperative axial MRI brain, T1-weighted image with contrast revealing the right frontal (A) and cerebellar (B) resection cavities.

- Microsurgical techniques should be used to remove lesions en bloc when possible.

- Adjuvant RT to the resection is warranted to decrease recurrence rates.

CASE 2

HISTORY AND PHYSICAL EXAMINATION

A 35-year-old, African American woman presented to her gynecologist for evaluation of amenorrhea. She was initially treated with progesterone; however, this was only temporarily successful. An endocrine panel revealed a prolactin level of 86 (normal 2–29). On review of systems, the patient acknowledged that she has been running into objects, mainly on the left-hand side, and last year was involved in a car accident where she hit someone located in her "blind spot." Given the symptoms, her gynecologist ordered an MRI, revealing a pituitary mass.

IMAGING STUDIES

Further evaluation revealed significant vision loss on visual field testing. An initial MRI revealed a large 2.8 × 2.1 × 2.1cm sellar/suprasellar lesion with upward displacement of the optic chiasm. There is no cavernous sinus extension (Figure 5.3).

CASE ANALYSIS AND SURGICAL PLAN

A patient with a pituitary lesion requires a thorough neurosurgical, endocrine, and ophthalmologic evaluation, ideally with subspecialty examination. Neurosurgical evaluation consists of identifying symptoms related to mass effect, such as optic chiasm impingement and cavernous sinus extension. An endocrine workup should include full laboratory testing that includes hormone levels for thyroid-stimulating hormone, free T4 levels, prolactin, cortisol, adrenocorticotropic hormone, insulin-like growth factor hormone, growth hormone, and sex-specific hormones of luteinizing

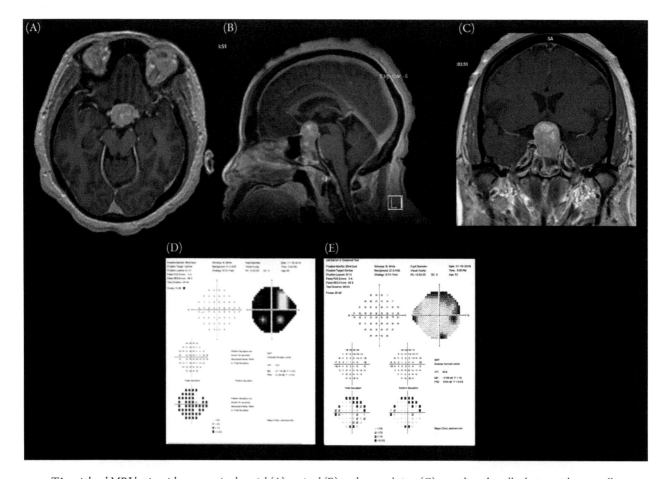

Figure 5.3 T1-weighted MRI brain with contrast in the axial (A), sagittal (B), and coronal view (C), revealing the sellar lesion with suprasellar extension. Humphrey visual field testing (D&E) revealed significant vision loss in the left eye (D) and mild visual deficits in the right eye (E).

hormone and follicle-stimulating hormone for females and testosterone for males. Estradiol may be tested for men, children, and postmenopausal women. In this case, an elevated level of prolactin (which was the same after dilutional studies) of 86 is not high enough to be considered a prolactinoma. An ophthalmologist should evaluate the patient to document presurgical visual fields and optic nerve damage. If an endoscopic approach is to be utilized, an otolaryngologist (ENT) should evaluate the patient for nasal anatomy to identify challenges in obtaining appropriate access and/or nasal septal flaps for reconstruction.

The differential diagnosis for sellar/suprasellar lesions is broad. These include, but are not limited to, sarcoid, sinonasal sarcoma/carcinoma, pituitary adenoma, aneurysm, teratoma, craniopharyngioma, hamartoma, meningioma, metastasis, and optic glioma. Intracranial lipoma can also be seen in this location.

Surgical approaches to the sella and suprasellar region include either an open craniotomy or an endonasal corridor. Cranial approaches may utilize a pterional, orbitozygomatic, or subfrontal approach. For this case, given the moderate sellar/suprasellar component as well as a pituitary tumor being at the top of the differential diagnosis, an endonasal approach is appropriate to optimize resection and be minimally invasive.[13] For extremely large macroadenomas with extensive subfrontal extension, resection may include both an endonasal and transcranial route either simultaneously or in a staged fashion. Use of lumbar drain is at the physician discretion and is based on the risk of cerebrospinal fluid (CSF) leak. We used an endonasal, endoscopic approach, harvesting a nasal septal flap. Resection of the lesion was uncomplicated and without CSF leak; therefore, no lumbar drain was used. The arachnoid web was bolstered with gelfoam, and the floor of the sella was reconstructed given the wide opening. This included replacement with a dura substitute followed by fibrin glue and a small piece of vomer to span the bony opening. The nasal septal flap then covered the sella face, and nasal packing was applied.

Make sure to spend time studying the preoperative MRI in T1 and T2 to look at the blood vessels and make sure the carotids are separated; in some cases, tortuosity of the carotids can lead to abnormal courses that may lead to inadvertently injuring this blood vessel.

COMPLICATIONS

Intraoperative complications

Given the extent of the lesion, multiple intraoperative complications can occur. These include injury to the carotid artery, optic nerve injury, and pituitary dysfunction—particularly diabetes insipidus (DI), and CSF leak.

Carotid artery injury is the most lethal complication, reportedly about 1% risk.[14] Particular anatomical anomalies such as a narrow intercavernous diameter, bulging of the internal carotid artery or dehiscence of the bony floor can place the vessel at even higher risk for injury. If this occurs, it needs to be addressed immediately. Preventative techniques include avoiding tumor traction, careful removal of the transsphenoidal septations, and avoidance of cutting burrs. If injury is suspected, one must alert the anesthesiologist and start resuscitation measures. Maintaining normotension to slight hypertension will help promote perfusion. To help with visualization, one can use multiple, large suckers; place the endoscope in the contralateral nare and apply pressure to the site of injury with cottonoids. It has been suggested that contacting the injured vessel with a crushed muscle patch or fat can aid with hemostasis. Maneuvers intraoperatively may include manual compression of the extracranial carotid at the neck to decrease blood flow in some instances. The bleeding must be controlled, and the nasal cavity packed, but care is taken not to compress and occlude the vessel. The procedure should be aborted and the vasculature should be evaluated by angiography for treatment options including vessel sacrifice, stenting, or surgical bypass.[15,16]

Optic nerve injury is rare, but devastating. Anatomical variations such as extent of sinus pneumatization, optic nerve course, and optic nerve dehiscence can increase the risk of injury[16,17] along with larger tumors, dumbbell-shaped tumors, previous surgery, and/or radiation therapy.[16,18] Nerve injury may be elicited by direct manipulation, devascularization, fracture of the orbit, postoperative hematoma, cerebral vasospasm, prolapse of the optic chiasm into an empty sella, or excessive packing during CSF leak repair.[16,18] Management is limited to treating the underlying etiology, such as decompressing an orbital fracture, angiogram with intra-arterial spasmolysis, blood pressure augmentation, or evacuation of associated hematoma.

With large tumors and long surgeries, DI may occur intraoperatively. Strict count of intake/output should be observed and controlled. If urine output acutely increases, serum sodium and osmolality should be evaluated. Make sure to review the criteria for DI diagnosis. If DI is suspected, desmopressin (DDAVP) may be given intraoperatively.

Cerebrospinal fluid leak is possible with large lesions that penetrate the diaphragma especially for lesions extending into the third ventricle. When this occurs, reconstruction of the floor with coverage by a healthy, vascularized, nasoseptal flap is imperative. Predominantly, lumbar drains are most commonly used for high flow leaks when a cistern or ventricle has been entered.[16,19] Duration of lumbar drainage is debatable and at the surgeon's discretion. Most surgeons would do 24–72 hours.

Postoperative Complications

Endocrine dysfunction can occur postoperatively, with DI the most common hormonal derangement experienced. Patient's urine output and sodium values should be followed closely. Be aware of the diagnostic criteria: urine output >250cc/hr × 3 hours, increasing sodium levels (>145 mmol/L), and urine specific gravity <1.005. Treatment for DI includes allowing the patient to drink to thirst and may involve supplementation with vasopressin. Diabetes insipidus can be a component of the triphasic response, and therefore reflex hyponatremia must be monitored. While DI is usually transient, about 0.3% of patients will experience permanent dyfunction.[14,16]

Cavernous sinus inflammation can occur if involved with tumor resection. Patients usually present in a delayed fashion with symptoms of cavernous sinus syndrome including oculomotor palsy. A CT scan can be obtained to rule out a hemorrhage and orbital fracture. If negative, an MRI should be ordered to evaluate for residual tumor, compression from sella packing, and abscess development. A lumbar puncture should be performed to rule out infection as well. If the workup is negative, a short course of steroids is prescribed, and the symptoms should resolve.[20]

Cerebrospinal fluid leaks may also present in a delayed fashion, ranging from 0% to 35% for endonasal resection of tumors.[21] Presentation may include rhinorrhea or may be more subtle such as a cough, postnasal drip, or headache. CT evaluation may reveal pneumocephalus. Bedside endoscopic inspection may help identify a nasal fluid collection. If unsure whether rhinorrhea is CSF related, a B2 transferrin level may be ordered on collected fluid. If unable to identify the presence of a CSF leak, aggressive evaluation includes high-resolution CT cisternogram with injection of intrathecal contrast dye, injection of intrathecal fluorescein with endoscopic evaluation or return to the operating room for direct invasive evaluation. Conservative treatment measures include rest and acetazolamide. When this fails, lumbar drainage with or without surgical exploration and repair follows. Ultimately, if leakage continues, surgical skull base reconstruction is undertaken followed by CSF shunting if all measures fail.

Herniation of the optic chiasm into a large, empty sella is possible, leading to visual impairment. Chiasmapexy and packing of the sella to prevent or treat herniation is offered.[22]

Nasal complications such as persistent sinusitis and empty nose syndrome may occur. Sphenoid sinusitis may present with headaches, facial pain, or nasal drainage. Endonasal is however the preferred approach. ENT evaluation and debridement may help, along with antibiotic treatment. At times, a sphenoidotomy is required. Empty nose syndrome can occur after extensive resection of intranasal contents. This includes symptoms of chronic dryness, paradoxical obstruction, neuropathic pain, and the lack of ability to feel as if one is breathing. Nasal spray and surgical remedy to narrow the nasal corridor are treatment options.[23]

In extraordinarily large tumors with attachments to the hypothalamus, the tumor capsule may descend. As this occurs, the hypothalamus may sustain injury, leading to severe hypothalamic distress. In some cases, there may be vasospasm of the surrounding microvasculature, additionally adding risk to the hypothalamus and suprasellar structure.

PEARLS

- Patients with pituitary lesions should undergo thorough neurosurgical, endocrine, rhinology, and ophthalmologic evaluation.

- Surgical indications include growth of a lesion, compression of optic apparatus, endocrine dysfunction, visual impairment, or other symptoms related to mass effect.

- Prolactinomas may be treated medically. Postoperative complications still apply due to treatment effect in large lesions.

- Surgical approach may be endonasal, transcranial, or a combination.

- Intraoperative complications include carotid injury, optic nerve injury, CSF leak, and DI.

- Postoperative complications include CSF leak, endocrine dysfunction, hypothalamic injury, vasospasm, visual impairment, cavernous sinus inflammation, sinusitis, and empty nose syndrome

- Residual lesion should be followed on serial imaging, endocrine labs, and visual evaluation.

CASE 3

HISTORY AND PRESENTING ILLNESS

A 74-year-old male presented to the local emergency room with a chief complaint of altered mental status. A few weeks prior, the family noted the patient was demonstrating some spatial issues on his left side, such as walking into objects. In addition, they noticed some weakness of his left hand to the point where he has been dropping objects. Most recently, he has demonstrated progressive confusion and disorientation.

IMAGING

An MRI of the brain was obtained and revealed a large right-sided, expansile, temporal-parietal-occipital lesion with heterogeneous contrast enhancement and significant edema (Figure 5.4).

CASE ANALYSIS AND SURGICAL PLAN

The differential diagnoses of this lesion include high-grade glioma, cerebral metastasis, CNS lymphoma, abscess, tumefactive multiple sclerosis, and subacute cerebral infarct. Given the rapid (but not sudden) progression of symptoms, age of the patient, and MRI characteristics, he is likely suffering from a high-grade glioma. General treatment options include observation, biopsy, resection, radiation therapy, or medical management. Standard treatment for high-grade glioma calls for maximal, safe cytoreduction, and combination chemotherapy/radiation.

The role of surgery in glioma patients is imperative to long-term prognosis. Patient age, KPS, location of lesion, and extent of resection (EOR) capability are all factors that should be assessed when deciding if surgery is appropriate. Extent of resection is one of the most important factors associated with long-term survival; it has been shown to be independently associated with survival[24–29] and recurrence.[29] Gross total resection, defined as resection of all

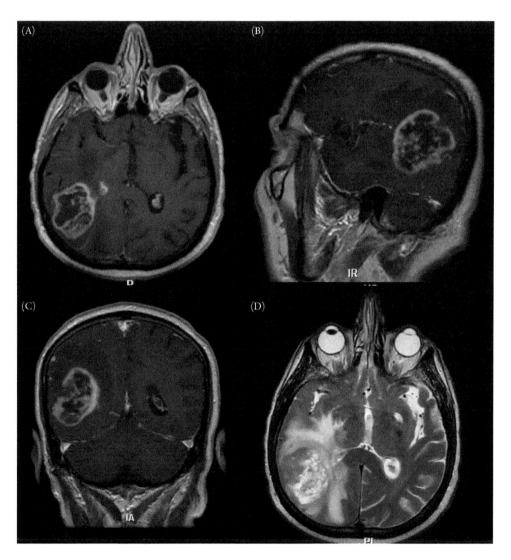

Figure 5.4 Preoperative MRI brain with contrast demonstrating a right temporoparietal/ occipital lesion with heterogeneous contrast enhancement in the axial (A), sagittal (B), and coronal (C) planes. (D) Axial image revealing significant surrounding edema.

contrast-enhancing lesion, should be attempted when possible; however, given eloquent location, this is not always feasible. The relationship between EOR and survival, in the literature, is confusing because gross total resection (GTR), near total resection, and subtotal resection are classified differently per study. To account for this, a study published in 2014 attempted to understand the minimal threshold of resection needed to improve patient survival in newly diagnosed glioblastoma (GBM) patients, regardless of location.[29] They demonstrated that the minimum amount of resection needed to statistically improve survival is 70%; survival for patients with >70% resection was 14.4 months versus 10.5 months for those who had <70% EOR.[29] Furthermore, for each 5% increase in resection, the risk of death decreased by 5.2%. Similarly, >70% EOR was associated with prolonged progression-free survival (PFS) and with every 5% increase in resection, risk of recurrence decreased by 3.2%. The median PFS was 9 months versus 7.1 months. Residual volume of 5 cm³ or less is associated with prolonged survival (14.4 months vs. 10.5 months).[29]

Gross total resection, though, still has a very important role and should be achieved outside of leaving the patient with permanent deficits. To illustrate this, patients who were deemed GTR-eligible were evaluated.[30] Unfortunately, only 29% of patients were deemed radiographically and surgically capable of having a GTR. For these patients, residual volume <2 cm³ has the biggest effect on survival (16.3 months vs. 12.1 months). In multivariate analysis, EOR >95% is needed to provide the greatest risk reduction of death. The medial survival of patients who received >95% resection was 16.3 months compared to 11.6 months.[30]

The presented patient has a lesion located in an area that is amenable to GTR; therefore, he underwent maximal, safe resection (Figure 5.5). His pathology indeed was diagnostic for GBM, including pseudopalisading necrosis, microvascular proliferation, nuclear atypia, and high mitotic index.

Postoperatively, he was treated with Stupp protocol.[31] Be familiar with this protocol, as follows: 6 weeks of fractionated radiation (60 Gy in 30 fractions) and concomitant temozolomide (75 mg/m²) daily during radiation treatment, followed by 6 cycles of adjuvant temozolomide administered at 150 to 200 mg/m² for 5 days every 28-day cycle. This regimen has been shown to statistically improve survival benefit of GBM patients.[31] Whether or not to continue temozolomide after 6 cycles or continue observation alone is controversial.[32,33]

Outside of extent of resection, a better prognosis is afforded for patients younger than 40 years old, KPS >70, cystic tumor component, healthy, and tumor genetics.

PROGRESSION OF DISEASE

The patient completed Stupp protocol, and 3 months after completion of his (6-month) adjuvant temozolomide, he radiographically demonstrated concerns for recurrence, with increased enhancement on surveillance MRI (Figure 5.6). The differential diagnosis includes progression of disease, radiation necrosis (pseudoprogression), abscess, and inflammation.

Further evaluation included laboratory testing (for infection) and MRI perfusion, which revealed increased blood volume to the region of contrast enhancement.

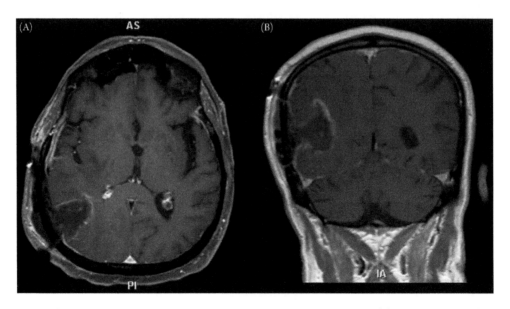

Figure 5.5 Postoperative MRI brain with contrast demonstrating gross total tumor resection in the axial (A) and coronal plane (B).

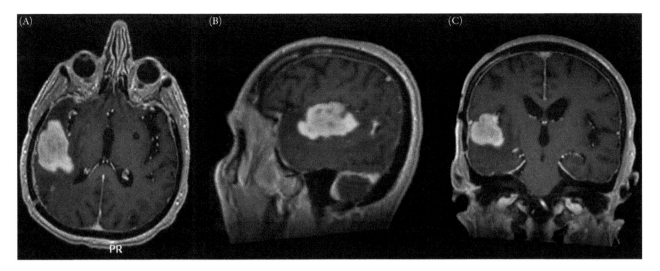

Figure 5.6 Repeat MRI brain with contrast showing recurrence of tumor in the temporal lobe, anterior to the prior resection cavity, in axial (A), sagittal (B), and coronal (C) planes.

When assessing blood volume (cerebral blood volume), a level greater than 2.6 mL blood/gram of tissue is indicative of tumor while a value less than 0.6 mL blood/gram tissue is more consistent with radiation necrosis.

Given the concern for recurrence (increased contrast enhancement, edema, and blood volume), he underwent a re-resection; pathology confirmed GBM. He was restarted on temozolomide. Unfortunately, his first posttreatment MRI revealed increased enhancement and symptomatic FLAIR signal with mass effect. He was then started on Avastin (bevacizumab) 10 mg/kg every 2 weeks and oral steroids. Subsequent MRI revealed decreased edema and mass effect with a reduction in enhancement; he was able to wean off his steroids.

Other modalities to help identify progression versus pseudoprogression include PET and magnetic resonance (MR) spectroscopy. PET scans help identify increased metabolic activity in tumors compared to hypometabolism in radiation necrosis.[34] MR spectroscopy can help pinpoint recurrence versus necrosis via metabolic analysis (Table 5.1) Assessment of recurrence versus radiation necrosis can also be evaluated by serial imaging at short intervals

to evaluate for changes in the contrast-enhancing portion and surrounding edema. Worsening of the characteristics is typically more characteristic of disease progression.

Recurrent tumors are less responsive to treatment and lack treatment options. Currently, there is no standard of care in treatment of recurrent/progressive GBM.[35] It is estimated that only 20% to 30% of recurrent GBM will be amenable to re-resection[35] due to invasion of functional areas or patient functional status. Adding to this conundrum is the overwhelming evidence that demonstrates different molecular profiles in recurrent lesions compared to the initial diagnosis,[35] in part related to differences in microenvironment, gene expression, extent of immune cell invasion,[36] mutations due to previous therapies, and further evasion of the immune system.[37]

Be familiar with the US Food and Drug Administration (FDA)-approved therapies for recurrent GBM, including Avastin (bevacizumab), Optune, and Carmustine wafers. Avastin is a recombinant monoclonal immunoglobulin G_1 antibody that arrests angiogenesis.[38] The standard dose is 10 mg/kg every other week. Be aware of the complication of hemorrhage and wound infection/dehiscence.[39] A novel antimitotic activity treatment, tumor treatment fields (OPTUNE™) was FDA-approved in 2011 for salvage monotherapy for GBM treatment and, more recently, in 2015 was approved for concomitant use with maintenance, adjuvant temozolomide in newly diagnosed patients. By providing low-intensity, intermediate frequency alternating electric fields, the device mechanism interferes with dividing cells and induces apoptosis. Compliance is key for successful outcome, which varies due to the need of 18 consecutive hours of use and requirement to shave one's head.[40]

Table 5.1. MAGNETIC RESONANCE SPECTROSCOPY METABOLITE RESULTS DIFFERENTIATING THE PRESENCE OF TUMOR VERSUS RADIATION NECROSIS

	GLIOMA	RADIATION NECROSIS
N-acetyl aspartate	↑	↓
Creatine	↓	↔
Choline	↑	↓

Carmustine wafers (Gliadel®) have been found to significantly increase overall survival in patients with both newly diagnosed and recurrent GBM.[41] Complications of this include wound dehiscence and signficant vasogenic edema.

Advanced genetic testing has become commonplace for tumor analysis. Genomic profiling helps classify primary versus secondary GBM. For example, epidermal growth factor receptor (EGFR) amplification distinguishes primary GBM versus isocitrate dehydrogenase 1/2 (isocitrate dehydrogenase [IDH] 1/2) and tumor protein 53 (TP53) mutations as secondary GBM.[42] Genomic profiling has identified primary and secondary GBM as derived from separate pathways. Primary GBM typically harbors 3 alterations: EGFR mutation/amplification (36%–60%), phosphatase and tensin homolog deletion, and homozygous deletion of CDKN2A-p16^{INK4a}.[42,43] Tumor protein 53 is the most common mutated gene in GBM.[44]

Genetic alterations which have significant clinical impact include EGFR amplification, IDH1/IDH2 mutation, and hypermethylation of O (6)-methylguanine-DNA methyltransferase (MGMT) promoter gene. For primary GBM, EGFR overexpression is the most frequent gene mutation; however, its relationship to prognosis remains controversial.[7]

IDH mutations are detected in only 5% of primary GBM and 70% to 75% of secondary GBM. In younger patients and in association with TP53 mutations, outcomes in IDH-mutated patients tend to be improved. Thus far, IDH1/IDH2 only hold prognostic information; no targeted therapy exists.[42]

MGMT promoter hypermethylation is arguably the most important prognostic indicator in GBM patients as it predicts improved response to treatment with alkylating agents, such as temozolomide.[42] The mean survival of such patients, receiving temozolomide and RT, has demonstrated 54% survival at 2 years as compared to 31% for non-MGMT methylated patients.[45]

GBM SUBTYPES

Glioblastoma can be subdivided into 4 groups: classic, mesenchymal, neural, and proneural. Proneural subtypes tend to be associated with less aggressive tumors and younger patients.[42,44] Classical subtypes tend to have EGFR amplification (97%), lack TP53 mutation, and demonstrate high expression of Notch and Sonic hedgehog signaling pathways.[44] Mesenchymal subtypes tend to have low

neurofibromatosis 1 expression and most commonly occur in conjunction with phosphatase and tensin homolog deletion. This subgroup has a higher expression of factors related to the tumor necrosis pathway and higher activity of mesenchymal markers, which has been linked to dedifferentiated tumors.[44] Focal amplification and overexpression of platelet-derived growth factor receptor A is a signature finding proneural tumors.[44] Neural tumors are identified by expression of neuron markers.[44]

COMPLICATIONS

Standard risks apply for all craniotomy patients (bleeding, seizures, infection, motor/sensory deficits, to mention a few). High-grade glioma patients commonly have multiple surgical interventions and therefore have higher potential at developing wound healing difficulties and infections. Patients who have remained on extended length steroids or have taken bevacizumab treatment are even at higher risk. In addition, patients who require steroids long term may develop adrenal insufficiency, obesity, hyperglycemia, avascular necrosis, osteoporosis, gastric ulcers, and myopathy.[46] Temozolomide can cause hematotoxicity; therefore, laboratory values must be monitored. Bevacizumab can increase the risk of intracranial and systemic bleeding with treatment.

PEARLS

- Standard postoperative treatment includes concomitant RT and temozolomide followed by 6 cycles of temozolomide.

- Bevacizumab is first line agent for symptomatic pseudoprogression and second line therapy for tumor progression.

- Reoperation is indicated for tumor progression for lesions that are accessible and are dependent on the patients' functional status.

- MRI spectroscopy, MRI perfusion and/or PET scan can help differentiate tumor progression and radiation necrosis.

- First line antiepileptic medications include levetiracetam followed by phenytoin and valproic acid. Levetiracetam has demonstrated better efficacy and fewer side-effects[47] Patients with poorly controlled seizures before surgeries should be evaluated to potentially increase their medications or add a second agent before surgery to minimize likelihood of seizures following surgery.

HISTORY AND PRESENTING ILLNESS

A 32-year-old male presented to his primary care physician secondary to new right-sided headache development. An MRI was obtained, which revealed an intracranial mass. He subsequently presented to the neurosurgical clinic for evaluation and discussion of treatment options.

IMAGING

The MRI demonstrates a homogenous FLAIR hyperintense, noncontrast-enhancing lesion in the right insular region (Figure 5.7).

CASE ANALYSIS AND SURGICAL PLAN

The differential diagnosis for this lesion includes glioma—low grade versus high grade—lymphoma, demyelinating lesion, and infectious or inflammatory pathology. This young patient likely has a low-grade glioma (LGG) in the right insular lobe. Like any new diagnosis, there are 3 potential routes of treatment; continued observation for growth, radiation treatment, or biopsy versus surgical resection.

Low-grade gliomas include both oligodendrogliomas and astrocytomas. In 2016, the World Health Organization changed the definition of LGG to include IDH mutation and 1p/19q codeletion, thereby eliminating the prior entity named mixed oligoastrocytoma.[48] In the past, the observation route was considered safe, and early resection was controversial given the diffuse infiltrative nature; however,

multiple studies have demonstrated prolonged overall survival with early safe maximal resection.[49,50]

Per the National Comprehensive Cancer Network practice guidelines, surgery is first line treatment for LGG, with the aim to obtain a GTR.[51] Surgery provides the added benefit of tissue diagnosis, improves mass effect, and is superior to biopsy in decreasing tumor progression and prolonging overall survival.[48] That being said, if the lesion is deep or the estimated resection, based on preoperative imaging, is <50%, then a biopsy alone is warranted instead.

Given the location of the lesion, and symptomatic nature, the patient was offered operative resection.

APPROACH SELECTION

Surgical intervention for this tumor requires intraoperative navigation and direct electrical stimulation was selected to allow for a safe, maximal resection. In addition, if accessible, using an intraoperative MRI can also facilitate identification of resection margins. Because of the functional/eloquent location, performing the surgery in an awake manner adds the benefit of continuous monitoring. Therefore, the patient underwent a right-sided, awake craniotomy for tumor resection with cortical and subcortical direct electrical stimulation and mapping, particularly for somatic sensorimotor responses. Of note, had the lesion presented on the dominant, left side, mapping of language function would have been performed as well.

For stimulation, a monopolar may be used; however, most prefer a bipolar handheld tool, such as the Ojemann Cortical Stimulator (Integra) or the Osiris Cortical Stimulator (Inomed), to deliver localized and specific low-frequency,

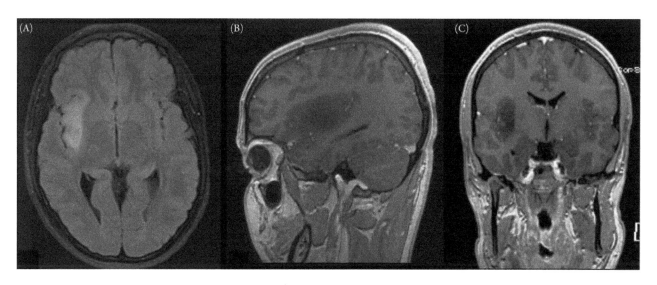

Figure 5.7 FLAIR axial (A) image identifying the right insular lesion. Sagittal (B) and coronal (C) T1-weighted image without contrast, again identifies an expansile mass within the right insula.

biphasic pulse waves to the brain. The interelectrode difference should be 5 to10 mm, as anything greater than this provides inaccuracy. Because stimulation can induce seizures, low frequency, such as 50 to 60 Hz, is used,[52] in addition to slowly increasing the power of current delivered. For awake patients, current from 2 to 8 mA is typically considered safe. That being said, after discharges should be monitored, and their appearance is indicative of potential seizure response.

Alternatives to mapping function in an awake manner include asleep direct stimulation and transcranial motor mapping, utilizing motor evoked potentials as the main response. The disadvantage of this is the limitation to only monitor motor function, and therefore for insular lesions it is not ideal given the multifunctional area as this area also is associated with working memory. Especially when located on the dominant side, awake mapping is imperative for speech identification and preservation. For asleep patients, higher electrical current delivery is needed, oftentimes reaching as high as 13 mA.

Approaches to the insula include transsylvian and transcortical routes. Yasargil was the first to describe the transsylvian approach to the insula for glioma resection and reported minimal morbidity.[46,53] Through trials of perfecting the technique, recommendations for minimizing morbidity during this approach include (i) splitting the sylvian fissure widely, (ii) awake procedure for cortical and subcortical mapping of motor and language (most prominent in left-sided insular lesions), and (iii) avoidance of coagulation to the M2 perforating vessels and lenticulostriate arteries.[53–55]

Transcortical route utilizes the overlying frontal, temporal, and/or parietal operculum as windows into the insula. Here, it is important to recognize the medial border of the insula via identification of the lenticulostriate arteries.[53,56,57]

Patient selection is key for success as well. It has been shown that favorable outcomes are likely for younger patients (<40 years), World Health Organization grade I, II, and III gliomas, high KPS, and lesions that extend into the frontal operculum. Overall survival and PFS is impacted by EOR with a cutoff of 90% resection to reach significant impact.[53,58]

MAPPING INSULAR TUMORS

Insular function is poorly understood; however, it is most likely involved in the multimodal integration and association of sensory and limbic networks. In addition, both the uncinate fasciculus and inferior fronto-occipital fasciculus run through the insula; hence, subcortical language mapping is essential when the dominant insula is involved.[53] Language tasks should include picture naming, text reading, 4-syllable repetition, auditory naming, and syntax production.[53,59] Mapping of motor, sensory, and cognitive function is essential when a transcortical route is approached. Additionally, subcortical mapping is used to identify the corticospinal tract, especially because the posterior limb of the internal capsule closely approximates the medial border of the insula.[53]

ADJUVANT THERAPY

Postoperatively, an MRI was obtained (Figure 5.8). Adjuvant treatment of RT and chemotherapy are likely to be needed; however, timing of treatment remains controversial. Four phase 3 randomized trials provide class 1 evidence that early RT increases PFS but not overall survival and that low-dose RT is equally effective as high-dose RT.[60–63]

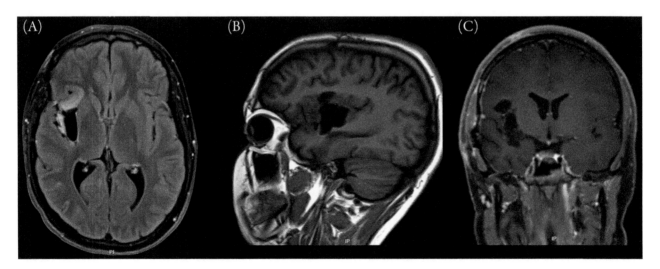

Figure 5.8 Postoperative MRI. FLAIR axial (A), sagittal (B), and coronal (C) T1-weighted noncontrast images revealing subtotal resection of the right insular lesion.

In the setting of a GTR and low-risk features, such as age <40, IDH mutant, and 1p19q codeletion, and then continued observation with regular follow-up is an appropriate choice for patients. Like IDH mutation, 1p19q codeletion is a favorable prognosis and identifies a positive predictive response to alkylating chemotherapy and RT.[53]

For patients >40 years old or who have other high-risk features including subtotal resection, large tumor size, neurological deficits, and IDH wild-type, or have other unfavorable characteristics/molecular markers, immediate adjuvant treatment is reasonable and should be considered.[51] For high-risk patients, or patients who have lesions that are in highly eloquent and potentially unresectable, treatment modalities include clinical trials, RT and procarbazine, PCV chemotherapy (procarbazine, lomustine [CCNU], and vincristine), or RT and temozolomide chemotherapy. When treatment is needed, the RTOG[64] and EOTC[65] trials have demonstrated that lesions with 1p19q codeletion are more likely to benefit from the addition of PCV to RT.

Utilization of a neuro-oncologist and radiation oncologist is integral in helping decide the best form of treatment. Whether observation or treatment is taken, MRI images should be obtained every 3 to 6 months for the first 5 years and, if stable, can be spaced to every 6 to 12 months.[51]

COMPLICATIONS

Intraoperative complications can occur with awake craniotomy. A multidisciplinary, comprehensive team approach is crucial for success. Ideally, continuous intravenous anesthetics are titrated cautiously to keep the patient comfortable, but also allowing the patient to quickly awaken when performance tasks are needed. Too much sedation, large habitus patients, little lung reserve, and sleep apnea place the patient at risk for needing airway support and intubation intraprocedurally. Overall failure to maintain an awake nature occurs 2.3% to 6.4% of cases. [66]

Direct electrical stimulation provides added electricity to the brain, thus lowering the seizure threshold. While uncommon, intraoperative seizures are estimated to occur within 3% to 54%, based on reported literature, these seem to be associated with tumor pathology. Patients at higher risk for intraoperative seizure includes those with LGG, preoperative seizures, dominant location, functional regions including motor cortex, stimulation parameters, and surgical/anesthetic team experience.[67] To prevent this, patients should receive an intravenous antiepileptic agent, such as levetiracetam, prior to the initiation of surgery, and some data indicate that a second agent should be considered

during surgery to minimize risks of seizures.[68] In addition, use of cold saline irrigation onto the cerebral cortex can help abort a seizure. If this does not work, loading the patient with a second antiepileptic agent such as phenytoin (15–18 mg/kg loading dose given at 50 mg/min) or providing a propofol bolus is an option; protection of the airway must remain a concern.

Vascular injury is a potential intraoperative complication, particularly with an insular lesion. The insula is fed by many perforating arteries from the middle cerebral artery and en passage vessels, traveling to the corona radiata, must be identified and preserved. Vascular injury in this region can be devastating.

Standard postoperative risks apply including infection, wound dehiscence, seizures, and hematoma. Depending on the location of the lesion, patients will often times develop transient neurological deficits, which resolve over the following weeks with the aid of steroids.

In general, immediate complication rates range from 20% to 26% while long-term complication rates are reported to be 3% to 9%.[53,69–71] Likewise, immediate postoperative language and motor deficits have been reported in up to 16% and 9%, respectively, but long-term affect is about 0.8% and 1.8%, respectively, of total patients.[53,69,70]

PEARLS

- The goal of glioma surgery is to maximize EOR and minimize the risk of neurological deficit in order to maintain both quality of life and survival.

- For lesions in functional areas, direct electrical stimulation provides a tool to assess and map for functional areas. This can be done awake or asleep.

- Operative approaches include transsylvian and transcortical. The transcortical window allows preservation of sylvian draining veins and potentially reduces the risk of spasm of the more proximal middle cerebral artery vessels.

- Awake craniotomy with cortical and subcortical mapping is the preferred approach

- Immediate, temporary postoperative neurological deficits occur at relatively high rates, but typically resolve over 3 months.

- Adjuvant therapy should be considered in high risk LGG patients with subtotal resection and for all LGG patients at the time of progression or transformation.

HISTORY AND PHYSICAL

A 59-year-old woman presents to the emergency department after having a tonic–clonic seizure that lasted 5 minutes and self-resolved. She reports having had a stiff neck and mild headache for the last 2 days. On examination, she is confused and agitated, but otherwise neurologically intact. Her family reports a long-standing and progressive history of personality change, disinhibition, and problems concentrating.

IMAGING

The imaging studies demonstrate a large extra-axial enhancing mass arising from the planum sphenoidale. There are significant mass effect and vasogenic edema in the bifrontal lobes (Figure 5.9).

ANALYSIS OF CASE AND SURGICAL PLAN

The patient is transferred to the intensive care unit for monitoring. The differential diagnosis of this extra-axial lesion includes meningioma, hemangiopericytoma, pituitary adenoma, dural-based metastasis, and craniopharyngioma. Initial management includes obtaining a basic metabolic panel, complete blood cell blood count, coagulation studies, and a preoperative medical evaluation for

surgery. The patient received 10 mg of intravenous dexamethasone followed by 4 mg given intravenously every 6 hours and was started on levetiracetam 1000 mg every 12 hours.

This patient should also be assessed for symptoms of Foster–Kennedy syndrome, which include anosmia, contralateral papilledema, and unilateral optic atrophy. A MR angiogram or conventional angiography can be used to assess the arterial feeders of the lesion.

Olfactory groove meningiomas differ from tuberculum sella meningiomas based on their skull base location, which affects location of the optic chiasm. In the olfactory groove meningioma, the chiasm is inferolateral to the tumor, whereas in a tuberculum sellae meningioma, the chiasm is superolateral to the tumor.

Given the symptomatic nature of the lesion, surgery is the chosen treatment option. Three potential surgical approaches can be used to resect this lesion: subfrontal, pterional, and endonasal. A subfrontal approach with or without orbital osteotomies allows for early access to vascular feeds along the skull base. A bicoronal incision provides a vascularized pericranial flap that can be used to prevent CSF leak during skull base reconstruction as well as cover the frontal sinuses. Orbital osteotomies can also be performed to help reduce the amount of brain retraction that is needed.[51] Potential complications for this approach include opening the frontal sinus, which creates a risk for CSF leak or a mucocele. A preoperative CT scan allows for evaluation of the extension of the frontal sinus in these patients. In

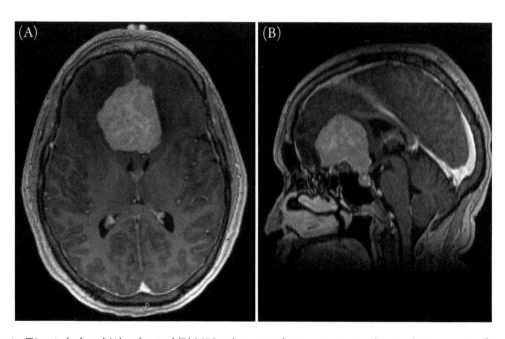

Figure 5.9 Preoperative T1-weigthed axial (A) and sagittal (B) MRI with contrast showing a contrast-enhancing lesion emerging from the planum sphenoidale, which is most consistent with a meningioma.

addition, the anterior section of the superior sagittal sinus must be sacrificed with this approach.

The pterional approach provides early exposure of the optic nerve and carotid artery, but may create a longer working distance to the contralateral side of the tumor. The access to the basal cisterns can help early drainage of CSF for brain relaxation. The disadvantages of the pterional approach include a narrow working space that may not provide adequate access to the superior portion of the tumor. Also, accessing skull base arteries or repairing skull base defects can be difficult with this approach.[72]

Endoscopic, endonasal resection is an option as well, albeit for a large lesion as long as lesions do not extend lateral to the lamina paprycea, which makes access difficult. This approach provides direct access to the tumor and early devascularization and avoids brain retraction. When performed with a highly skilled, multidisciplinary team, safe removal is possible. One should think about, and preplan for, multilayer dural closure and skull base reconstruction as CSF leak is significantly higher for this approach, reported up to 30% in the literature.[73]

For this patient, a bicoronal subfrontal approach with bilateral orbital osteotomies was used. To perform the orbital osteotomies, the facial nerve in the temporal fat pad must be protected while elevating the skin flaps. The subfrontal approach provides wide access to the anterior skull base without the need for frontal lobe retraction and allows for early devascularization of the anterior and posterior ethmoidal arteries, which are usually the vascular supply for these meningiomas. Early disconnection of the tumor arterial feeders will decrease the bleeding from the tumor, preventing obscuration of the surgical field and limiting the blood loss. The tumor can be centrally debulked using an ultrasonic aspirator. Caution must be taken along the posterior aspect of the tumor to separate it from the anterior cerebral arteries (ACAs), optic nerves, and chiasm. Frozen pathology shows a meningioma.

Aggressive resection of the tumor and dural attachments is required to reduce the chances of recurrence. This includes drilling any hyperostotic bone and removing tumor-invaded dura. Late recurrence has been shown to happen in 30% of patients with these types of tumors at 5 years and in 41% at 10 years.[33] The Simpson classification system predicts meningioma tumor recurrence after surgical resection. The extent of surgical resection and recurrence rate in this system includes 5 grades (Table 5.2).

Postoperatively, radiation can be used for recurrent tumors or meningiomas with malignant pathologies. Radiosurgery has been shown to reduce or stop tumor

Table 5.2. **SIMPSON GRADING SCALE FOR MENINGIOMA AND THE RATE OF RECURRENCE IN RELATIONSHIP TO TUMOR RESECTION**

GRADE	RESECTION	RECURRENCE RATE (%)
1	Complete tumor removal with dura and bone	10
2	Complete tumor resection with coagulation of dural attachment	15
3	Complete tumor resection without coagulation of dural attachment	30
4	Incomplete resection	85
5	Biopsy	100

growth rates in 84% to 100% of cases. Complications of radiosurgery often result from worsening edema and can result in permanent morbidity in 5.7% of cases. These morbidities can present as seizure, cranial nerve deficits, hemiparesis, mental status changes, and headaches.[74]

COMPLICATIONS

Intraoperative Complications

One potential complication that can occur intraoperatively is that after making the bicoronal incision and flipping the skin flap over the eyes to expose the orbital bar, the patient becomes severely bradycardic. In these cases, the anesthesiologist reports giving no new medication or inhalational anesthetic. The patient is likely experiencing an oculocardiac reflex, in which a decrease in pulse rate is associated with the traction applied to extraocular muscles and/or compression of the eye. The reflex is mediated by the trigeminal cranial nerve through the ciliary ganglion and the vagus nerve of the parasympathetic system.[75] Relieving the pressure of the skin flap on the orbits should reverse the bradycardia.

Another potential complication is injury to the carotid or ACA. In this situation, the bleed should be isolated and controlled, and an intraoperative or postoperative angiogram is required to assess the vascular anatomy. Preoperative computed tomography angiography, MR angiography, or conventional angiography can be used to determine the location of the ACA relative to the tumor.

When the patient is slow to wake up from anesthesia, an immediate CT scan should be done to evaluate the possibility for hematoma, edema, hydrocephalus, pneumocephalus, or ACA infarction. The patient could be experiencing frontal lobe syndrome as a result of cerebral edema or ischemia. Postoperative steroids can be used after surgery for at least 2 weeks to treat the cerebral edema.[76]

Two days after surgery the patient experiences a severe headache and a tonic–clonic seizure that resolves with intravenous lorazepam (Ativan). MRI shows extensive bifrontal edema with no residual tumor (Figure 5.10). The patient is started on dual antiepileptic treatment, levetiracetam and phenytoin, and put on a high-dose dexamethasone taper. The headache dissipates over the next few days, and seizures remain well controlled.

Other postoperative complications include vision loss that can occur after a large meningioma is removed, owing to excessive traction on the optic apparatus during resection. Care must be taken intraoperatively during the resection of the posterior component of the tumor, which can often be adhered to the optic nerve, ACA, or internal carotid arteries. Steroid use may help to reduce the swelling of the nerve.

Postoperative venous congestion and venous stroke are also potential postoperative complications of this surgery. The anterior third of the superior sagittal sinus is relatively safe to sacrifice in attempting a total resection. Care must be taken to prevent ligation or thrombosis of the posterior two-thirds of the superior sagittal sinus during tumor and frontal lobe manipulation because this may cause a venous stroke. Preoperative venography can be used to study the anatomic relation between the tumor and the sinus, sinus patency, and collateral veins.

CSF leak can present as rhinorrhea postoperatively in this type of case. The use of a pericranial flap to aid in reconstruction of the skull base helps to prevent this leak from occurring.

Long-Term Complications

During bifrontal or extended bifrontal craniotomies, if the frontal sinus is exposed during the craniotomy, simple packing of the frontal sinus with bone wax or muscle can increase the chance of mucocele formation. The posterior wall of the frontal sinus must be removed, and the sinus must then be exenterated. It is important to remove the sinus mucosa from the sinus wall down to the nasofrontal duct.[76] A diamond burr can then be used to remove the tiny remnants of mucosa found on the surface of bone, which can also lead to a mucocele. Abdominal fat, a piece of temporalis muscle, hemostatic agents, or, optimally, a piece of pericranial vascularized flap can then be used to fill the corners of the cavity if small remnants remain.[77] In addition, if the orbit is not reconstructed appropriately, patients may suffer from enophthalmos.

PEARLS

- Olfactory groove meningiomas can present with Foster–Kennedy syndrome (anosmia, contralateral papilledema, and unilateral optic atrophy).

- The optic chiasm location differs for olfactory groove and tuberculum sella meningiomas (inferolateral in

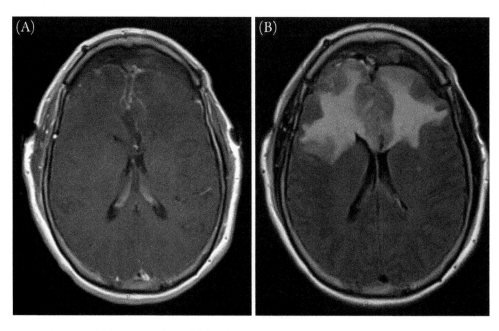

Figure 5.10 Postoperative axial T1-weigthed contrast-enhanced (A) and T2-FLAIR weighted MRIs (B) shows complete resection of the meningioma with blood products at the resection site and residual extensive frontal lobes edema as seen in the T2-FLAIR MRI.

olfactory groove meningiomas and superolateral in tuberculum sellae meningiomas).

- Subfrontal, pterional, and interhemispheric approaches, as well as endoscopic endonasal, can all be used to approach olfactory groove meningiomas.

- The Simpson classification system predicts meningioma tumor recurrence based on the extent of surgical resection and involved tissue.

- Radiosurgery can be used for recurrent meningiomas or meningiomas with higher grade (WHO grade II or III) pathologies.

- Complications include arterial injury, nerve injury, stroke, seizures, frontal lobe syndrome, vision loss, CSF leak, and mucoceles which occur following the resection of olfactory groove meningiomas.

REFERENCES

1. Gavrilovic IT, Posner JB. Brain metastases: epidemiology and pathophysiology. *J Neurooncol*. 2005;75(1):5–14. doi:10.1007/s11060-004-8093-6
2. Elaimy AL, Mackay AR, Lamoreaux WT, et al. Multimodality treatment of brain metastases: an institutional survival analysis of 275 patients. *World J Surg Oncol*. 2011;9(1):69. doi:10.1186/1477-7819-9-69
3. Nahed B V, Alvarez-Breckenridge C, Brastianos PK, et al. Congress of Neurological Surgeons Systematic Review and Evidence-Based Guidelines on the Role of Surgery in the Management of Adults With Metastatic Brain Tumors. *Neurosurgery*. 2019;84(3):E152–E155. doi:10.1093/neuros/nyy542
4. Quigley MR, Bello N, Jho D, Fuhrer R, Karlovits S, Buchinsky FJ. Estimating the additive benefit of surgical excision to stereotactic radiosurgery in the management of metastatic brain disease. *Neurosurgery*. 2015;76(6):707–713. doi:10.1227/NEU.0000000000000707
5. Kalkanis SN, Kondziolka D, Gaspar LE, et al. The role of surgical resection in the management of newly diagnosed brain metastases: a systematic review and evidence-based clinical practice guideline. *J Neurooncol*. 2010;96(1):33–43. doi:10.1007/s11060-009-0061-8
6. Al-Shamy G, Sawaya R. Management of brain metastases: the indispensable role of surgery. *J Neurooncol*. 2009;92(3):275–282. doi:10.1007/s11060-009-9839-y
7. Chi A, Komaki R, Chi A, Komaki R. Treatment of Brain Metastasis from Lung Cancer. *Cancers (Basel)*. 2010;2(4):2100–2137. doi:10.3390/cancers2042100
8. Hall W, Djalilian H, Nussbaum E, Cho K. Long-term survival with metastatic cancer to the brain. *Med Oncol*. 2000;17(4):279–286. doi:10.1007/BF02782192
9. Bindal R, Sawaya R, Leavens M. Surgical treatment of multiple brain metastases. *J. Neurosurg*. 1993;79(2):210–216.
10. Baker CM, Glenn CA, Briggs RG, et al. Simultaneous resection of multiple metastatic brain tumors with multiple keyhole craniotomies. *World Neurosurg*. 2017;106:359–367. doi:10.1016/J.WNEU.2017.06.118
11. Yoo H, Kim Y, Nam B, et al. Reduced local recurrence of a single brain metastasis through microscopic total resection. *J Neurosurg*. 2009;110(4):730–736.
12. Atalar B, Choi C, Harsh GR 4th. Cavity volume dynamics after resection of brain metastases and timing of postresection cavity stereotactic radiosurgery. *Neurosurgery*. 2013;72(2):180–185.
13. Recinos PF, Goodwin CR, Brem H, Quinones-Hinojosa A. Transcranial surgery for pituitary macroadenomas. In: Quinones-Hinojosa A, ed. Schmidek and Sweet operative neurosurgical techniques. 6th ed. Philadelphia: Elsevier; 2012:280–291.
14. Agam MS, Wedemeyer MA, Wrobel B, Weiss MH, Carmichael JD, Zada G. Complications associated with microscopic and endoscopic transsphenoidal pituitary surgery: experience of 1153 consecutive cases treated at a single tertiary care pituitary center. *J Neurosurg*. 2018. [Epub ahead of print] doi:10.3171/2017.12.JNS172318
15. AlQahtani A, Castelnuovo P, Nicolai P, Prevedello DM, Locatelli D, Carrau RL. Injury of the internal carotid artery during endoscopic skull base surgery. *Otolaryngol Clin North Am*. 2016;49(1):237–252. doi:10.1016/j.otc.2015.09.009
16. Bohnen AM, Donaldson A, Olomu N, Quinones-Hinojosa A. Endoscopic Endonasal Approach to Sellar, Para Sellar and Suprasellar lesions. In: Quinones-Hinojosa A, ed. *Schmidek & Sweet Operative Neurosurgical Techniques: Indications, Methods, and Results*. 7th ed. Philadelphia: Elsevier; 2019.
17. Cetinkaya EA, Koc K, Kucuk MF, Koc P, Muluk NB, Cingi C. Calculation of an optic nerve injury risk profile before sphenoid sinus surgery. *J Craniofac Surg*. 2017;28(1):e75–e78. doi:10.1097/SCS.0000000000003239
18. Barrow DL, Tindall GT. Loss of vision after transsphenoidal surgery. *Neurosurgery*. 1990;27(1):60–68.
19. Vemuri N V, Karanam LSP, Manchikanti V, Dandamudi S, Puvvada SK, Vemuri VK. Imaging review of cerebrospinal fluid leaks. *Indian J Radiol Imaging*. 2017;27(4):441–446. doi:10.4103/ijri.IJRI_380_16
20. Esonu C, Rincon-Torroella J, Quinones-Hinojosa A. Brain tumors. In: Levi AD, ed. *Goodman's Neurosurgery Oral Board Review*. 1st ed. New York, NY: Oxford University Press; 2017:11–24.
21. Dehdashti A, Stofko D, Okun J, Obourn C, Kennedy T. Endoscopic endonasal reconstruction of skull base: repair protocol. *J Neurol Surg Part B Skull Base*. 2015;77(03):271–278. doi:10.1055/s-0035-1568871
22. Barzaghi LR, Donofrio CA, Panni P, Losa M, Mortini P. Treatment of empty sella associated with visual impairment: a systematic review of chiasmapexy techniques. *Pituitary*. 2018;21(1):98–106. doi:10.1007/s11102-017-0842-6
23. Jiang C, Wang F, Chen K, Shi R. Assessment of surgical results in patients with empty nose syndrome using the 25-item Sino-Nasal Outcome Test Evaluation. *JAMA Otolaryngol Head Neck Surg*. May;140(5):453–458.
24. Sanai N, Polley M-Y, McDermott MW, Parsa AT, Berger MS. An extent of resection threshold for newly diagnosed glioblastomas. *J Neurosurg*. 2011;115(1):3–8. doi:10.3171/2011.7.JNS10998
25. McGirt MJ, Chaichana KL, Gathinji M, et al. Independent association of extent of resection with survival in patients with malignant brain astrocytoma. *J Neurosurg*. 2009;110(1):156–162. doi:10.3171/2008.4.17536
26. Lacroix M, Abi-Said D, Fourney DR, et al. A multivariate analysis of 416 patients with glioblastoma multiforme: prognosis, extent of resection, and survival. *J Neurosurg*. 2001;95(2):190–198. doi:10.3171/jns.2001.95.2.0190
27. Chaichana KL, Garzon-Muvdi T, Parker S, et al. Supratentorial glioblastoma multiforme: the role of surgical resection versus biopsy among older patients. *Ann Surg Oncol*. 2011;18(1):239–245. doi:10.1245/s10434-010-1242-6
28. Chaichana KL, Chaichana KK, Olivi A, et al. Surgical outcomes for older patients with glioblastoma multiforme: preoperative factors associated with decreased survival. *J Neurosurg*. 2011;114(3):587–594. doi:10.3171/2010.8.JNS1081
29. Chaichana KL, Jusue-Torres I, Navarro-Ramirez R, et al. Establishing percent resection and residual volume thresholds affecting survival

and recurrence for patients with newly diagnosed intracranial glioblastoma. *Neuro Oncol.* 2014;16(1):113–122. doi:10.1093/neuonc/not137

30. Chaichana KL, Cabrera-Aldana EE, Jusue-Torres I, et al. When gross total resection of a glioblastoma is possible, how much resection should be achieved? *World Neurosurg.* 2014;82(1-2):e257–e265. doi:10.1016/j.wneu.2014.01.019

31. Stupp R, Mason WP, van den Bent MJ, et al. Radiotherapy plus Concomitant and Adjuvant Temozolomide for Glioblastoma. *N Engl J Med.* 2005;352(10):987–996. doi:10.1056/NEJMoa043330

32. Skardelly M, Dangel E, Gohde J, et al. Prolonged temozolomide maintenance therapy in newly diagnosed glioblastoma. *Oncologist.* 2017;22(5):570–575. doi:10.1634/theoncologist.2016-0347

33. Blumenthal DT, Gorlia T, Gilbert MR, et al. Is more better? The impact of extended adjuvant temozolomide in newly diagnosed glioblastoma: a secondary analysis of EORTC and NRG Oncology/RTOG. *Neuro Oncol.* 2017;19(8):1119–1126. doi:10.1093/neuonc/nox025

34. Hou LC, Veeravagu A, Hsu AR, Tse VCK. Recurrent glioblastoma multiforme: a review of natural history and management options. *Neurosurg Focus.* 2006;20(4):E5.

35. Campos B, Olsen LR, Urup T, Poulsen HS. A comprehensive profile of recurrent glioblastoma. *Oncogene.* 2016;35(45):5819–5825. doi:10.1038/onc.2016.85

36. Pistollato F, Abbadi S, Rampazzo E, et al. Intratumoral hypoxic gradient drives stem cells distribution and MGMT expression in glioblastoma. *Stem Cells.* 2010;28(5):851–862. doi:10.1002/stem.415

37. Brennan CW, Verhaak RGW, McKenna A, et al. The somatic genomic landscape of glioblastoma. *Cell.* 2013;155(2):462–477. doi:10.1016/j.cell.2013.09.034

38. Cohen MH, Shen YL, Keegan P, Pazdur R. FDA drug approval summary: bevacizumab (Avastin) as treatment of recurrent glioblastoma multiforme. *Oncologist.* 2009;14(11):1131–1138. doi:10.1634/theoncologist.2009-0121

39. Gressett SM, Shah SR. Intricacies of bevacizumab-induced toxicities and their management. *Ann Pharmacother.* 2009;43(3):490–501. doi:10.1345/aph.1L426

40. Mittal S, Klinger N, Michelhaugh S, et al. Alternating electric tumor treating fields for treatment of glioblastoma: rationale, preclinical, and clinical studies. *J Neurosurg.* 2018;128(2):414–421.

41. Chowdhary SA, Ryken T, Newton HB. Survival outcomes and safety of carmustine wafers in the treatment of high-grade gliomas: a meta-analysis. *J Neurooncol.* 2015;122(2):367–382. doi:10.1007/s11060-015-1724-2

42. Crespo I, Vital AL, Gonzalez-Tablas M, et al. Molecular and genomic alterations in glioblastoma multiforme. *Am J Pathol.* 2015;185(7):1820–1833. doi:10.1016/j.ajpath.2015.02.023

43. Touat M, Idbaih A, Sanson M, Ligon KL. Glioblastoma targeted therapy: updated approaches from recent biological insights. *Ann Oncol Off J Eur Soc Med Oncol.* 2017;28(7):1457–1472. doi:10.1093/annonc/mdx106

44. Verhaak RGW, Hoadley KA, Purdom E, et al. Integrated genomic analysis identifies clinically relevant subtypes of glioblastoma characterized by abnormalities in PDGFRA, IDH1, EGFR, and NF1. *Cancer Cell.* 2010;17(1):98–110. doi:10.1016/j.ccr.2009.12.020

45. Weller M, Felsberg J, Hartmann C, et al. Molecular predictors of progression-free and overall survival in patients with newly diagnosed glioblastoma: a prospective translational study of the German glioma network. *J Clin Oncol.* 2009;27(34):5743–5750. doi:10.1200/JCO.2009.23.0805

46. Kostaras X, Cusano F, Kline GA, Roa W, Easaw J. Use of dexamethasone in patients with high-grade glioma: a clinical practice guideline. *Curr Oncol.* 2014;21(3):e493–e503. doi:10.3747/co.21.1769

47. Pourzitaki C, Tsaousi G, Apostolidou E, Karakoulas K, Kouvelas D, Amaniti E. Efficacy and safety of prophylactic levetiracetam in supratentorial brain tumour surgery: a systematic review and meta-analysis. *Br J Clin Pharmacol.* 2016;82(1):315–325. doi:10.1111/bcp.12926

48. Sepúlveda-Sánchez JM, Muñoz Langa J, Arráez MÁ, et al. SEOM clinical guideline of diagnosis and management of low-grade glioma (2017). *Clin Transl Oncol.* 2018;20(1):3–15. doi:10.1007/s12094-017-1790-3

49. Jakola AS, Myrmel KS, Kloster R, et al. Comparison of a strategy favoring early surgical resection vs a strategy favoring watchful waiting in low-grade gliomas. *JAMA.* 2012;308(18):1881. doi:10.1001/jama.2012.12807

50. Sanai N, Berger MS. Glioma extent of resection and its impact on patient outcome. *Neurosurgery.* 2008;62(4):753–766. doi:10.1227/01.neu.0000318159.21731.cf

51. National Comprehensive Cancer. *NCCN Clinical Practice Guidelines in Oncology: Central Nervous System Cancers, Version 2.2012.* http://www.nccn.org/professionals/physician_gls/pdf/cns.pdf.

52. Mikuni N, Miyamoto S. Surgical treatment for glioma: extent of resection applying functional neurosurgery. *Neurol Med Chir.* 2010;50:720–726.

53. Hervey-Jumper S. Insular glioma surgery: an evolution of thought and practice. *J Neurosurg.* 2019;130(1):9–16.

54. Moshel YA, Marcus JDS, Parker EC, Kelly PJ. Resection of insular gliomas: the importance of lenticulostriate artery position. *J Neurosurg.* 2008;109(5):825–834. doi:10.3171/JNS/2008/109/11/0825

55. Neuloh G, Pechstein U, Schramm J. Motor tract monitoring during insular glioma surgery. *J Neurosurg.* 2007;106:582–592.

56. Benet A, Hervey-Jumper SL, Sánchez JJ, Lawton MT, Berger MS. Surgical assessment of the insula. Part 1: surgical anatomy and morphometric analysis of the transsylvian and transcortical approaches to the insula. *J Neurosurg.* 2016;124:469–481.

57. Safaee MM, Englot DJ, Han SJ, Lawton MT, Berger MS. The transsylvian approach for resection of insular gliomas: technical nuances of splitting the sylvian fissure. *J Neurooncol.* 2016;130:283–287.

58. Simon M, Neuloh G, Lehe M von, Meyer B, Schramm J. Insular gliomas: the case for surgical management. *J Neurosurg.* 2009;110(4):685–695.

59. Duffau H, Moritz-Gasser S, Gatignol P. Functional outcome after language mapping for insular World Health Organization Grade II gliomas in the dominant hemisphere: experience with 24 patients. *Neurosurg Focus.* 2009;27(2):E7.

60. va den Bent MJ, Afra D, de Witte O, et al. Long-term efficacy of early versus delayed radiotherapy for low-grade astrocytoma and oligodendroglioma in adults: the EORTC 22845. *Lancet.* 2005;366(9490):985–990.

61. Karim AB, Maat B, Hatlevoll R, et al. A randomized trial on dose-response in radiation therapy of low-grade cerebral glioma: European Organization for Research and Treatment of Cancer (EORTC) study 22844. *Int J Radiat Oncol Biol Phys.* 1996;36(3):549–556.

62. Shaw E, Arusell R, Scheithauer B, et al. Prospective randomized trial of low- versus high-dose radiation therapy in adults with supratentorial low-grade glioma. Initial report of a North Central Cancer Treatment Group/Radiation Therapy Oncology Group/Eastern Cooperative Oncology Group Study. *J Clin Oncol.* 2002;20(9):2267–2276.

63. Karim AB, Afra D, Cornu P, et. al. Radomized trial on the efficacy of radiotherapy for cerebrallow-grade glioma in the adult: European Organization for Research and Treatment of Cancer Study 22845 with the Medical Research Council Study BRO4—an interim analysis. *Int J Radiat Oncol Biol Phys.* 2002;52(2):316–324.

64. Cairncross G, Wang M, Shaw E, et. al. Phase III trial of chemoradiotherapy for anaplastic oligodendroglioma: long-term results of RTOG9402. *J Clin Oncol.* 2013;31(3):337–343.

65. Van den Bent MJ, Erderm-Eraslan L, Idbaih A, et al. MGMT-STP27 methylation status as predictive marker for response to PCV in

anaplastic oligodendrogliomas and oligoastrocytomas: a report from EORTC study 26951. *Clin Cancer Res*. 2013;19(19):5513–5522.

66. Hervey-Jumper SL, Li J, Lau D, et al. Awake craniotomy to maximize glioma resection: methods and technical nuances over a 27-year period. *J Neurosurg*. 2015;123:325–339.

67. Szelényi A, Bello L, Duffau H, et al.; Workgroup for Intraoperative Management in Low-Grade Glioma Surgery within the European Low-Grade Glioma Network. Intraoperative electrical stimulation in awake craniotomy: methodological aspects of current practice. *Neurosurg Focus*. 2010;28:E7.

68. Eseonu C, Eguia F, Garcia O, Kaplan PW, Quiñones-Hinojosa A. Comparative analysis of monotherapy versus duotherapy antiseizure drug management for postoperative seizure control in patients undergoing an awake craniotomy. *J Neurosurg*. 2018;128(6):1661–1667.

69. Hervey-Jumper S, Li J, Osorio J, et al. Surgical assessment of the insula. Part 2: validation of the Berger-Sanai zone classification system for predicting extent of glioma resection. *J Neurosurg*. 2016;124(2):482–498.

70. Sanai N, Polley M-Y, Berger MS. Insular glioma resection: assessment of patient morbidity, survival, and tumor progression. *J Neurosurg*. 2010;112(1):1–9. doi:10.3171/2009.6.JNS0952

71. Safaee M, Englot D, Han S, Lawton MT, Berger MS. The transsylvian approach for resection of insular gliomas: technical nuances of splitting the Sylvian fissure. *J Neurooncol*. 2016;130(2):283–287.

72. Mayfrank L, Gilsbach JM. Interhemispheric approach for microsurgical removal of olfactory groove meningiomas. *Br J Neurosurg*. 1996;10(6):541–545.

73. Duffau H, Taillandier L, Gatignol P, Capelle L. The insular lobe and brain plasticity: lessons from tumor surgery. *Clin Neurol Neurosurg*. 2006;108(6):543–548. doi:10.1016/J.CLINEURO.2005.09.004

74. Kollova A, Liscak R, Novotny J Jr, Vladyka V, Simonova G, Janousková L. Gamma knife surgery for benign meningioma. *J Neurosurg*. 2007;107(2):325–336.

75. Paton JF, Boscan P, Pickering AE, Nalivaiko E. The yin and yang of cardiac autonomic control: vago-sympathetic interactions revisited. *Brain Res Brain Res Rev*. 2005;49(3):555–565.

76. Aguiar PH, Tahara A, Almeida AN, et al. Olfactory groove meningiomas: approaches and complications. *J Clin Neurosci*. 2009;16(9):1168–1173.

77. Donald P. The tenacity of the frontal sinus mucosa. *Otolaryngol Head Neck Surg*. 1979;87(5):557–566.

6.

VASCULAR NEUROSURGERY

Thomas Leipzig

Vascular neurosurgery has been a focal point of our profession. Each case requires clinical and diagnostic acumen, a solid grasp of immediate and long-term natural history risks, consideration of a variety of treatment options, and the management of potentially catastrophic complications.

Over the last 2 decades, key international studies, the development and rapid growth of endovascular neurosurgery, and computerized tomographic angiography (CTA) has led to a paradigm shift in the evaluation and management of many neurovascular disorders.

CASE 1

HISTORY AND PHYSICAL

A 35-year-old, right-handed woman is brought to the emergency department after experiencing an explosive headache during intercourse. Her husband reports that she complained of a headache 3 weeks earlier. She smokes 1 pack of cigarettes daily and has "borderline" hypertension.

Her blood pressure (BP) is 170/85 mm Hg. She has no motor deficit. Her eyes open to stimulation, and she is disoriented to year and location. She has photophobia and nuchal rigidity.

IMAGING STUDIES

Her computerized tomographic (CT) scan (Figure 6.1) demonstrates subarachnoid hemorrhage (SAH). CTA is suboptimal due to poorly timed injection of contrast. A 3-dimensional digital subtraction angiogram subsequently confirms the presence of left-sided ophthalmic artery (OA) and middle cerebral artery (MCA) aneurysms (Figure 6.2).

ANALYSIS OF CASE AND TREATMENT PLAN

General

Aneurysmal SAH (aSAH) is a classic neurosurgical emergency. The case-fatality rate is 40% to 50% with a morbidity of roughly 50% in survivors. Global cognitive impairments are present in approximately 20%. Persistent dependence is reported in 8% to 20%.

In the oral examination, acknowledge the assessment of airway, breathing, and circulation (ABCs), routine laboratory testing, and medications. Do not belabor the details. The examiners generally will apprise you of any significant issues. Her World Federation of Neurological Surgeons (WFNS) grade is 4 (Table 6.1) and her Hunt and Hess grade is 3 (Table 6.2).

SENTINEL HEMORRHAGE

A sentinel hemorrhage or "warning leak" may occur 2 to 8 weeks before an overt aSAH. It might not be an incapacitating headache. It is potentially disastrous to miss the history of an explosive, "thunderclap" onset.

Risk Factors

Aneurysmal SAH is more common in women. This patient also has risk factors including hypertension and tobacco use. Other risk factors include heavy alcohol consumption, very low body mass index, sympathomimetic drugs use, family history, and certain genetic syndromes (e.g., autosomal dominant polycystic kidney disease, Ehlers-Danlos type IV, Marfan syndrome). Aneurysmal SAH during sexual intercourse or Valsalva maneuver is not uncommon.

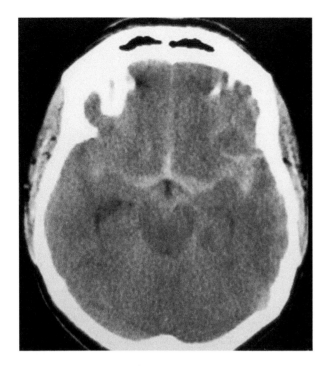

Figure 6.1 Representative cut of non-contrasted CT scan of brain demonstrates diffuse SAH, more prominent on the left side. The temporal horns are slightly prominent. Mild ventricular enlargement is seen on additional cuts.

Blood Pressure

Blood pressure is often elevated following aSAH. Keeping the systolic BP ≤ 160 mm Hg is a reasonable goal. If tolerated, systolic BP ≤ 140 mm Hg may be considered in a good grade patient (Hunt and Hess grade < 3). Use of a titratable intravenous medication such as nicardipine is preferable.

Diagnostic Studies

This patient has a modified Fisher grade 3 hemorrhage (Table 6.3) on CT scan. The sensitivity of CT scan in diagnosing aSAH within the first 3 days is nearly 100%. However, after 5 to 7 days, its diagnostic accuracy diminishes. If there is clinical suspicion for aSAH but the CT scan is negative, the patient should undergo lumbar puncture to look for red blood cells in the cerebrospinal fluid (CSF), xanthochromia, and elevated opening pressure. Obtain the minimal amount of CSF needed to decrease the risk for a rebleed created by lessening the tamponade on the aneurysmal dome. Without spectrophotometry, the utility of CSF analysis declines after 2 to 3 weeks. Certain magnetic resonance imaging (MRI) sequences (e.g., T2-weighted fluid-attenuated inversion recovery, gradient echo, susceptibility weighted imaging, diffusion-weighted imaging) may show signs of SAH when the CT scan is negative.

Although 3-dimensional digital subtraction angiography remains the "gold standard" for cerebrovascular imaging, CTA is now commonly used initially because of its ease and safety. However, aneurysms <3 mm in size may not be detected on either CTA or magnetic resonance angiography (MRA). When presented with a spontaneous SAH and a negative CTA, digital subtraction angiography (DSA) is warranted.

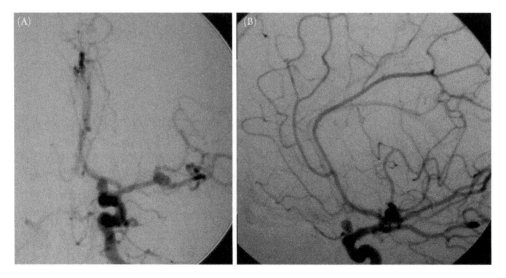

Figure 6.2 Cerebral angiogram, left side, anterior–posterior and oblique projections. ICA angiogram demonstrates an ophthalmic aneurysm and a slightly larger, lobulated MCA aneurysm.

Table 6.1. WORLD FEDERATION OF NEUROLOGICAL SURGEONS GRADING SCALE FOR ANEURYSMAL SUBARACHNOID HEMORRHAGE

WFNS SCORE	GLASGOW COMA SCALE SCORE	MOTOR DEFICIT
1	15	Absent
2	13–14	Absent
3	13–14	Present
4	7–12	Present or absent
5	3–6	Present or absent

Abbreviation: WFNS, World Federation of Neurological Surgeons.

Angiogram-negative SAH

Angiogram-negative SAH accounts for about 15% of all spontaneous SAH. Spontaneous SAH can be broken down into 4 basic radiographic patterns: CT negative with positive lumbar puncture, perimesencephalic, diffuse, and cortical.

Angiography is negative in about 95% of cases with perimesencephalic SAH (PM-SAH), which is responsible for 30% to 40% of all angiogram-negative SAH studies. The approach to PM-SAH is varied. Some question the need for any type of angiographic study in PM-SAH. We prefer DSA as our initial study in PM-SAH. If it is negative, we do not perform any additional studies. The prognosis is very favorable with negligible risk for vasospasm or recurrence.

With CT-negative or cortical SAH, we consider DSA if the initial CTA is unrevealing. There is low yield for detecting an aneurysm, but other findings such as vasculitis or a dural vascular malformation may be identified. Serial imaging is not generally performed. The prognosis is usually favorable.

On the other hand, patients with diffuse, spontaneous SAH can present with a higher Hunt and Hess grade.

Table 6.2. HUNT AND HESS GRADING SCALE FOR ANEURYSMAL SUBARACHNOID HEMORRHAGE

HUNT AND HESS GRADE	FINDINGS
0	Unruptured
1	Asymptomatic or mild headache, slight nuchal rigidity
2	Moderate-severe headache, nuchal rigidity, no neurologic deficit (other than cranial nerve palsy)
3	Drowsiness/confusion, or mild focal deficit
4	Stupor, moderate-to-severe hemiparesis
5	Deep coma, decerebrate posturing, moribund appearance

Table 6.3. MODIFIED FISHER GRADE IN THE COMPUTED TOMOGRAPHY EVALUATION OF SUBARACHNOID HEMORRHAGE

MODIFIED FISHER GRADE	FINDINGS
0	No SAH or IVH
1	Thin SAH,[a] focal or diffuse; no IVH
2	Thin SAH, focal or diffuse; with IVH
3	Thick SAH,[b] focal or diffuse; no IVH
4	Thick SAH, focal or diffuse; with IVH

Abbreviations: IVH, intraventricular hemorrhage; SAH, subarachnoid hemorrhage.

[a]Thin SAH is < 1mm in depth.

[b]Thick SAH is ≥ 1mm in depth.

If the initial CTA is negative, we perform DSA. Patients with diffuse SAH have the same risk for hydrocephalus and vasospasm as those with aSAH. If the initial studies are unrevealing, a second angiogram is obtained after 7 days, depending on the patient's clinical condition, to look for vasospasm as well as a possible underlying structural etiology.

The location of an isolated spontaneous SAH, such as in the Sylvian fissure, might also prompt an MRI scan to look for an underlying cavernous malformation if the angiogram is negative.

Hydrocephalus

The contributing role of hydrocephalus needs to be considered in a patient with a high Hunt and Hess grade (3–5) or a worsening level of consciousness. Hydrocephalus has been reported in 15% to 87% of patients following aSAH. In poor-grade patients, CSF diversion may lead to significant improvement. Again, care must be taken to avoid rapid or excessive reduction in the ventricular size with CSF drainage, which may precipitate recurrent hemorrhage. For nonobstructive hydrocephalus, a lumbar or external ventricular drain (EVD) may be used. It is convenient to place the EVD on the side contralateral to an anticipated surgical approach, unless intraoperative insertion is planned. If endovascular therapy is anticipated, the EVD may preferentially be placed on the nondominant side. Elevated intracranial pressure (ICP) is carefully lowered to 15 to 20 mm Hg.

Medications

Nimodipine should be given within 96 hours and continued for up to 21 days following aSAH. The usual dose is 60 mg every 4 hours. If significant hypotension occurs, we alter dosing to 30 mg every 2 hours. Nimodipine has been shown to improve neurological outcome despite its lack of effect on angiographic cerebral vasospasm. Statins are often utilized, but the results are mixed. A larger phase 3 trial is currently underway. Clazosentan (an endothelin-1 antagonist) and magnesium sulfate have not shown benefit.

Seizures occur in 10% to 20% of patients, often close to the time of the rupture. Use of an antiepileptic drug (AED) should be considered until the ruptured aneurysm is secured. However, extended seizure prophylaxis should be avoided since AEDs have been associated with neurological worsening, delayed fever, and poorer outcome.

Short-term (<72 hours) antifibrinolytic therapy to reduce the risk of rebleeding prior to aneurysm obliteration is at the discretion of the practitioner. The use of tranexemic or epsilon-aminocaproic acid for aSAH is "off label."

TREATMENT

Risk for recurrent hemorrhage ranges from 8% to 23% in the first 72 hours. It is associated with an even higher rate of mortality and morbidity. Once the patient is stabilized, attention should focus on securing the ruptured aneurysm as soon as possible.

Microsurgical clip ligation has been the mainstay of aneurysm treatment for decades. However, the development of Guglielmi detachable coils in 1991 opened the door for novel endovascular treatments. Unparalleled funding in research and development has led to a nearly continuous improvement in endovascular devices, capabilities, and results.

The International Subarachnoid Aneurysm Trial (ISAT), conducted primarily in the United Kingdom and Europe, assessed the treatment of ruptured intracranial aneurysms. Its results strongly favored coiling over surgery. There was a 7% absolute and a 23% relative risk reduction in death or dependency at one year. Despite the many concerns raised over ISAT, its results were embraced quickly. Key concerns included the exclusion of nearly 80% of patients with aSAH, higher recurrence and rebleed rates with coiling, and unusually poor surgical results. Also, based on ISAT data, improved outcome with coiling for patients <40 years of age cannot be assumed.

In a patient with multiple aneurysms, it is important to determine which one bled. This finding may dictate the method of treatment and approach. Usually, the pattern of hemorrhage and certain aneurysm characteristics (e.g., location, size, shape, presence of daughter blisters) indicate which aneurysm bled.

At present, the primary treatments for a recently ruptured aneurysm are Guglielmi detachable coiling or clip ligation. Acute stent-assisted coiling or flow diversion have not been utilized routinely due to the need for dual antiplatelet therapy with the current devices. There are concerns with dual antiplatelet therapy in a recently ruptured aneurysm and the potential need for intracranial procedures such as an EVD or ventriculoperitoneal shunt. Several series have reported a higher risk for radiographic and symptomatic hemorrhage in this situation.

This 35-year-old patient has left-sided OA and MCA aneurysms. In her case, it is difficult to confidently identify which aneurysm bled. The OA aneurysm appears amenable to coiling or clipping. The MCA aneurysm is handled best by surgery. Its larger size and irregularity may favor it as the source of SAH. Her young age and suspicion of MCA aneurysm rupture tips the scale toward clip ligation.

Each case must be handled individually. The progressive trend toward endovascular treatments may become a self-fulfilling prophecy as surgical volumes diminish and practitioners become less comfortable with open procedures. The examiners will scrutinize your choice. Be honest and thoughtful in your approach. Avoid appearing dogmatic. Exercise caution in recommending novel, innovative, or unproven techniques. Also, recognize that the more senior examiners may only do open surgery. They may need a very clear explanation as to why you would choose an endovascular approach.

SURGERY

Both aneurysms can be treated through a left pterional approach. Modalities such as intra-operative monitoring, navigation, indocyanine green or fluorescein videoangiography, and DSA should be mentioned only if you are familiar with them. Be ready to provide the rationale for your choices.

Proximal control is essential in any aneurysm case. For an OA aneurysm, exposure and control of the carotid vasculature in the neck is necessary. The suction decompression technique may be helpful in some OA aneurysms. Anterior clinoidectomy is accomplished extra- or intradurally. Brain relaxation through CSF drainage or osmotic diuresis is initiated with dural opening.

If an intraoperative rupture occurs, temporary occlusion or trapping will stanch bleeding to allow further controlled dissection. It may facilitate the final dissection and clipping of a difficult aneurysm. Adenosine-induced flow arrest has also been used to "soften" an aneurysm or reduce bleeding, but it has not been validated by any controlled studies.

A typical dose of 30 mg administered by rapid intravenous infusion, on average, will produce about 30 seconds of bradycardia (with 5–15 seconds of asystole) and around 60 seconds of hypotension.

The base of an MCA aneurysm will frequently incorporate one or both M2 segments. Reconstructing the base of a large or atherosclerotic aneurysm can be difficult. The clip may slide down the neck to occlude or compromise the parent or branch artery. Placing another clip in tandem above the first one and then removing the initial clip may lead to a better result.

A micro-Doppler device can check the presence of flow in the arteries and its absence in the aneurysm. Indocyanine green or fluorescein videoangiography is quick and noninvasive. However, visualization of all pertinent structures may be suboptimal in the microscopic field, especially with anterior communicating artery aneurysms.

Microsurgical clipping should routinely be considered for MCA aneurysms, those with associated intraparenchymal hematomas ≥50 ml and younger patients.

COMPLICATIONS

The development of altered consciousness in the days following aSAH should trigger an orderly cascade of assessment including:

1. *Examine the patient* yourself. Assess the degree of obtundation and look for new focal deficits (e.g., pronator drift, paresis).

2. Check *vital signs* for fever, hypertension, or hypotension.

3. Review *laboratory data* for hypoxia or metabolic derangement.

4. Review *medications* and check any appropriate blood levels.

5. Obtain a *CT scan* to look for hemorrhage, stroke, or hydrocephalus.

6. Check a *transcranial Doppler* study, especially if symptoms develop 4 to 14 days following aSAH.

7. Check an *angiographic study*.

8. Consider *electroencephalography* (EEG) to exclude the possibility of subclinical status epilepticus.

If symptomatic vasospasm is identified, the initial treatment has been "triple-H" therapy (hypertension, hypervolemia, and hemodilution). Active hemodilution has essentially been abandoned. More recently, there has been a shift away from aggressive hypervolemia to a greater reliance on induced hypertension. If there is no response, balloon angioplasty for vasospasm in proximal vessels and infusion of vasodilators for distal vessels should be considered. In a poor-grade patient, treatment of radiographic vasospasm may be performed empirically. Prophylactic angioplasty, hypervolemia, or antiplatelet therapy is not recommended.

It is best to manage a board examination case as you would in your practice and facility. Try not to anticipate what you think the examiners might do. This may take you down an unfamiliar path, which may lead to more issues. The examination is about meeting and practicing the currently accepted standard of care.

PEARLS

- *In spontaneous SAH, DSA should be performed even if CTA or MRA are negative.*

- *The best modality for treating a given aneurysm is often apparent. In ISAT, only 20% of aneurysms had true clinical equipoise.*

- *In surgery, establish "proximal control."*

- *Develop an algorithm to investigate a neurological decline.*

CASE 2

HISTORY AND PHYSICAL

A 20-year-old, right-handed, male college student experienced a grand mal seizure. He returned to normal within 30 minutes. His neurological examination in the emergency department is unremarkable. There is no papilledema. The toxicology screen and blood alcohol level are negative.

IMAGING STUDIES

CT scan shows a hyperdensity in the right frontal lobe. Subsequent MRI (Figure 6.3) demonstrates an arteriovenous malformation (AVM) without evidence of hemorrhage.

ANALYSIS OF CASE AND TREATMENT PLAN

General

In this patient, seizure precautions and an AED are initiated. A DSA is ordered. It can be performed electively (Figure 6.4).

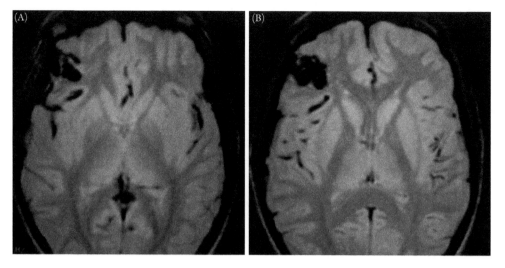

Figure 6.3 MRI scan demonstrates a compact area of flow voids in the right frontal region. No evidence of acute or prior hemorrhage detected.

MRI provides valuable information on location and size as well as evidence of prior hemorrhage. At present, standard MRA or CTA is inferior to DSA in defining the precise anatomic and circulatory details of an AVM. DSA is the best way to assess potential risk factors such as an intranidal aneurysm. Functional MRI and diffusion tensor imaging tractography may be valuable in selected patients.

The most common symptoms related to an AVM are hemorrhagic stroke (58%) and seizures (34%). The 5-year risk of developing a first seizure with an unruptured AVM is about 8%. Following an AVM-related seizure, the subsequent 5-year risk for developing epilepsy is 58%.

AVMs account for nearly 40% of spontaneous hemorrhages in patients 15 to 40 years old. The overall risk for hemorrhage from a brain AVM is about 3% per year, but

Solomon and Connolly reported a range from <1% to 33% depending on clinical and anatomic features (Table 6.4). Of patients who survive their initial hemorrhage, 45% will have severe deficits, 30% will have mild or moderate deficits, but only 25% will be free of deficit. A mortality of nearly 20% has been reported at 3 months following hemorrhage.

Management decisions are based on natural history risks balanced against the risks of treatment.

TREATMENT

Treatment options include microsurgical excision, stereotactic radiosurgery (SRS), embolization, or any combination of these. The surgical risk for resecting an AVM has been stratified by the Spetzler and Martin grading scale and

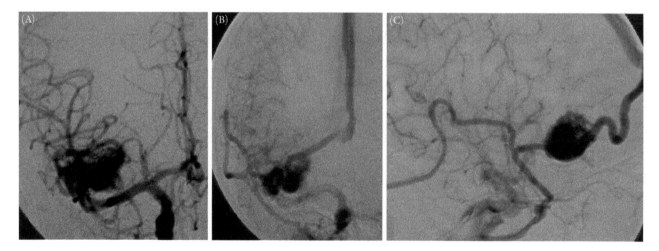

Figure 6.4 Right ICA angiogram. A: anterior–posterior projection in early arterial phase demonstrates the right frontal AVM. B: anterior–posterior projection in late arterial phase demonstrates the AVM nidus with early draining veins coursing to the sagittal, transverse, and cavernous sinuses. C: Lateral projection of the right internal carotid artery in late arterial phase again demonstrates the compact nidus located in the frontal lobe and the early draining veins.

Table 6.4. RISK FOR HEMORRHAGE WITH BRAIN ARTERIOVENOUS MALFORMATION

NUMBER OF RISK FACTORS* PRESENT	ANNUAL RISK FOR HEMORRHAGE
0	<1%
1	3–5%
2	8–15%
3	>30%

From Solomon RA, Connolly ES Jr. Arteriovenous malformations of the brain (review). N Engl J Med. 2017;376(19):1859–1866.

*Risk factors include: 1) prior bleed, 2) deep location or brainstem, 3) exclusive deep venous drainage

its variations. It is based on size, eloquent location, and deep venous drainage (Table 6.5). Microsurgical treatment for grade I and II AVMs can be performed with relatively low risk and a high expectation of cure. The risk for treatment increases substantially with each higher grade and may not result in an improvement on the natural history.

SRS obliteration rates range from 48% to 92% and generally depend on the size of the AVM. For lesions <10 cm^3 or with a diameter <3 cm, the reported cure rate is above 80%. However, it drops to less than 50% for AVMs >4 cm in diameter. The latency period to obliteration is typically 2 to 4 years. Transient symptomatic complications related to SRS are seen in 9% of patients and the risk for permanent neurologic deficit is about 3%.

Embolization is typically an adjunctive measure. It has limited benefit in grade I and II AVMs. Complication rates with embolization vary. Transient, permanent, and nonneurological problems are seen in about 7% of embolization sessions. The rate of curative embolization is traditionally low, ranging from 5% to 20%. However, a high rate of cure with a transvenous approach for selected AVMs has recently been reported by the group in Limoges, France.

Table 6.5. SPETZLER-MARTIN GRADING SYSTEM

Size of AVM	<3 cm	3–6 cm	>6 cm
Score	1	2	3
Eloquence[a]	Yes	No	
Score	0	1	
Deep venous drainage	None	Present	
Score	0	1	

Grade (I–V) is determined by adding the score from each category (size, eloquence, and deep venous drainage).

Abbreviation: AVM, arteriovenous malformation.

[a]Eloquent locations include sensorimotor, language, or visual cortices, hypothalamus, thalamus, brainstem, and cerebellar nuclei.

In 2013, the results of A Randomized Trial of Unruptured Brain AVMs (ARUBA) were released after randomization was halted. ARUBA purported that patients with an unruptured AVM do not benefit from treatment. Death or symptomatic stroke was 3 times more frequent in the interventional group compared to the medical therapy group. Criticism was strong and pointed to ARUBA's flaws including low numbers, short follow-up, and the very small percentage of patients treated with microsurgery. The Scottish Audit of Intracranial Vascular Malformation Study also supported conservative measures in the management of unruptured brain AVMs.

In 2014, Morgan and colleagues analyzed their results in 377 patients with an unruptured brain AVM and concluded that surgical intervention for grade I and II patients was quickly superior to the natural history.

This young man has a Spetzler and Martin grade 1 AVM (size = 1, location = 0, deep venous drainage = 0). His chance for a surgical cure without complication is extremely high in a large volume center. We feel that surgical treatment should be offered.

There are several principles in microsurgical resection of an AVM. Exposure should be generous to allow adequate visualization of the superficial feeding arteries and draining veins. Initially, the feeding arteries should be eliminated. Dissection proceeds circumferentially around the nidus. Major draining veins are preserved until the nidus has been devascularized. Smaller draining veins may need to be sacrificed earlier to continue with mobilization of the nidus. Intraoperative fluorescein or indocyanine green videoangiography may provide valuable information on distinguishing arterial feeders from draining veins during surgery. Complete resection should be verified with DSA.

COMPLICATIONS

Intracerebral hemorrhage (ICH) may result from residual nidus, although this risk is lessened by intraoperative DSA. A feared complication of AVM surgery is arterial–capillary–venous hypertension, which also has been called normal perfusion pressure breakthrough. It occurs in about 3% of operated cases and is usually associated with resection of a larger nidus (>4 cm in diameter). It is felt to result from occlusive hyperemia or autoregulatory failure in the surrounding ischemic bed. Eighty-three percent of new postoperative deficits are seen on emergence from anesthesia while 17% develop over the first week. One-fifth of complications are not directly related to the AVM resection (e.g., infection, pulmonary issues).

- *Only complete obliteration offers protection from hemorrhage.*

- *Microsurgical excision should be considered for a young patient with a Spetzler and Martin grade I and II AVM.*

- *Embolization should be used sparingly for low grade AVMs. Curative embolization is not currently commonplace.*

- *SRS is an alternative for a patient with a grade I or II AVM who declines surgery or is not a surgical candidate. The rate of cure is lower and there is 2- to 4-week latency period.*

- *In surgery, the major draining veins should be preserved until the nidus has been devascularized.*

- *The decision to treat patients with unruptured Spetzler and Martin grade III AVMs needs to be made carefully on a case-by-case basis. Patients with unruptured grade IV or V lesions appear to fare better with medical management.*

CASE 3

HISTORY AND PHYSICAL

A 53-year-old woman was found unconscious. Her medications are amlodipine besylate/benazepril HCl and warfarin.

The patient is intubated. Her blood pressure is 208/102 mm Hg. Her left pupil is large and sluggishly reactive. She is purposeful on her left and barely withdraws on the right. She has a right Babinski response. Her Glasgow Coma Scale score is 7T (E1,V1T, M5). Her international normalized ratio (INR) is 3.4.

IMAGING STUDIES

Her CT scan demonstrates a large left occipitotemporal ICH with intraventricular hemorrhage (IVH) and midline shift (Figure 6.5). CTA does not demonstrate any underlying vascular abnormality (Figure 6.6).

ANALYSIS OF CASE AND TREATMENT PLAN

General

Severe hypertension (systolic BP >220 mm Hg), vomiting, rapid progression of symptoms, and decreased level of consciousness or coma point toward an ICH. Most spontaneous hemorrhagic strokes, other than a hypertensive basal ganglionic hemorrhage, deserve investigation for an underlying etiology. Even though she is on an anticoagulant, CTA should be entertained.

Early deterioration following an ICH is common. ICH expansion on follow-up imaging is noted in about one-third of patients. The presence of a "spot" sign on a CTA

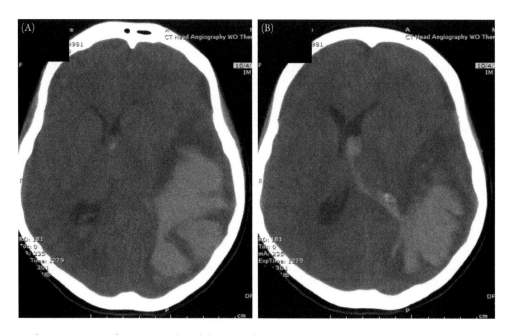

Figure 6.5 Noncontrasted CT scan images demonstrate a large left ICH with intraventricular extension and midline shift.

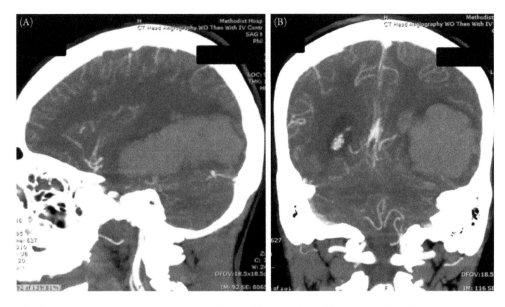

Figure 6.6 CTA (lateral and anterior–posterior reconstructions). No underlying vascular malformation is identified.

or a CT scan with contrast is a potential harbinger for clot expansion. Recombinant Factor VII can prevent hematoma growth but has not been shown to improve outcome. It is not recommended.

Blood Pressure

The 2015 American Heart Association/American Stroke Association guidelines recommended a systolic BP <140 mm Hg following ICH. However, results from more recent trials (ATACH-2 and FAST-MAG) bring this into question. It now appears that rapid or aggressive BP reduction may actually be deleterious. At present, there is no specific BP target. A systolic BP goal <160 mm Hg appears reasonable.

Medication

Up to 20% of patients with an ICH are taking an oral anticoagulant. This patient is taking warfarin and has an elevated INR. She receives intravenous vitamin K (5–10 mg) and prothrombin complex concentrate. Prothrombin complex concentrates can normalize the INR (<1.3) within 30 minutes and have essentially replaced fresh frozen plasma for rapid reversal. Reversal strategies for commonly encountered blood-thinning medications are listed in Table 6.6. Consultation may be helpful. Newer reversal agents may not be available in the formulary. Platelet transfusion is not recommended in the management of a nonoperative ICH in a patient on antiplatelet therapy.

Corticosteroids for ICH should be avoided because of increased complications without demonstrated benefit. Also, prophylactic AEDs are not recommended for ICH.

Table 6.6. **EMERGENCY REVERSAL STRATEGY FOR ANTIPLATELET AND ANTICOAGULANT AGENTS**

Antiplatelet agents (Reversal: platelet transfusion)
  aspirin/extended-release dipyridamole (Aggrenox®)
  prasugrel (Effient®)
  aspirin
  clopidogrel (Plavix®)
  ticagrelor (Brilinta®)
  cilostazol (Pletal®)
Heparins (Reversal: protamine)
  Heparin (unfractionated)
  Low molecular weight heparins[a] (LMWH)
    enoxaparin (Lovenox®)
    dalteparin (Fragmin®)
    tinzaparin (Innohep®)
Warfarin (Reversal: vitamin K, PCC, FFP)
FactorXa inhibitors (Reversal: andexanet alfa [Andexxa®])
  apixaban (Eliquis®)
  rivaroxaban (Xarelto®)
Direct thrombin inhibitors (Reversal: idarucizumab (Praxbind®))
  dabigatran (Pradaxa®)

Abbreviations: FFP, fresh frozen plasma; PCC, prothrombin complex concentrates.

[a]Protamine not as effective.

TREATMENT

Evacuation of a life-threatening ICH always needs to be considered but may be deemed inappropriate depending on the individual circumstances of the case. The role for decompressive craniectomy is not defined. The ICH score for this patient is 3 (see Table 6.7). The ICH score was first reported in 2001. It has shown that 30-day mortality steadily increases with higher scores. It has been used to stratify mortality risk. However, there are concerns that the ICH score becomes a self-fulfilling prophecy when aggressive management is withheld in those with moderate scores. It is imperative that the anticipated neurologic outcome is discussed. Her family understood and requested that she undergo craniotomy for clot evacuation.

On the other hand, the benefit of surgery for a nonlife threatening supratentorial ICH is uncertain. The Surgical Treatment for Intracerebral Hemorrhage (STICH) studies did not demonstrate any significant benefit on mortality or neurological outcome with early surgery. Recently, 2 trials focused on minimally invasive approaches to treating ICH and IVH. The Minimally Invasive Surgery plus Alteplase for Intracerebral Hemorrhage Evacuation (MISTIE III) trial investigated catheter evacuation of ICH followed by thrombolysis and the Clot Lysis Evaluation of Accelerated Resolution (CLEAR III) trial evaluated thrombolytic removal of IVH associated with a small ICH. Although safe, neither demonstrated any significant improvement in functional outcome.

Currently, the Early Minimally Invasive Removal of ICH (ENRICH) study is investigating the potential benefit of minimally invasive parafascicular surgery to evacuate subcortical ICH. Another multicenter prospective study (MIND: Artemis in the Removal of Intracerebral Hemorrhage) is investigating a minimally invasive evacuation device.

Cerebellar infarct or hemorrhage classically presents with headache, nausea, vomiting, vertigo, dizziness, dysarthria, and profound truncal ataxia. A large cerebellar stroke (>3 cm) often produces a progressively worsening level of consciousness with signs of brainstem compression (cranial nerve and gaze problems) and hydrocephalus. Patients with brainstem compression or hydrocephalus from a cerebellar stroke should undergo surgical decompression. Attempted management of obstructive hydrocephalus by EVD alone is not recommended.

PEARLS

- *There is no defined target for BP control. For most ICH, systolic BP can be lowered to 160 mm Hg. Do not use corticosteroids. Prophylactic AEDs are not recommended.*

- *Surgery is indicated for appropriate patients with life-threatening ICH or a large cerebellar ICH. Surgical intervention for a non-life threatening hematoma has not proven superior to medical management.*

- *Platelet transfusion may lead to worse results in a non-operative patient on antiplatelet therapy with an ICH.*

CASE 4

HISTORY AND PHYSICAL

A healthy, 72-year-old man presented to his family physician with progressive ambulatory difficulty, lower extremity paresthesia, and dull low back pain radiating into his legs. Symptoms worsened with walking and improved with rest.

X-rays demonstrated a mild L3–4 spondylolisthesis. He did not respond to nonnarcotic analgesics and physical therapy. An epidural steroid injection provided questionable benefit. He was placed on tamsulosin because of

Table 6.7. **INTRACEREBRAL HEMORRHAGE SCORE**

COMPONENT	ICH SCORE POINTS
Glasgow Coma Score[a]	
3–4	2
5–12	1
13–15	0
Age	
≥80 years	1
<80 years	0
Infratentorial origin of ICH	
Yes	1
No	0
ICH volume[b]	
≥30 cc	1
<30 cc	0
IVH	
Yes	1
No	0

ICH score was calculated by the sum of the ICH score points.

Abbreviations: ICH, intracerebral hemorrhage; IVH, intraventricular hemorrhage.

[a]Glasgow Coma Score score indicates the score on initial presentation (or after resuscitation).

[b]ICH volume on initial computed tomography scan calculated using ABC/2 method.

urinary difficulty. He is referred for decompression of spinal stenosis reported on MRI scan of the lumbar spine.

His examination reveals 4/5 power in the distal lower extremities. He is using a cane. He has patchy, diminished pinprick perception in both legs. Reflexes are 1⁺ in the upper extremities, 3⁺ at the knees, and 2⁺ at the ankles. There is no Babinski response but several beats of clonus are noted at the right ankle. Lower extremity tone is mildly increased.

MRI of the thoracic spine is ordered.

IMAGING STUDIES

Flexion/extension X-rays do not show abnormal motion. The lumbar MRI scan demonstrates negligible spinal stenosis, which does not account for his progressive lower extremity problems (Figure 6.7). A thoracic MRI scan is obtained and reveals signal abnormality in the lower cord and conus medullaris on sagittal T2-weighted images. Dilatation of the perimedullary veins is noted (Figure 6.8).

Spinal angiography (Figure 6.9) reveals a dural arterio-venous fistula (dAVF) at the L3 level on the right side.

ANALYSIS OF CASE AND TREATMENT PLAN

Type I spinal dAVFs are the most common vascular malformation of the spine. Initial misdiagnosis is frequent since early symptomatology is nonspecific and may mimic other conditions. Keep the diagnosis of spinal dAVF in the back

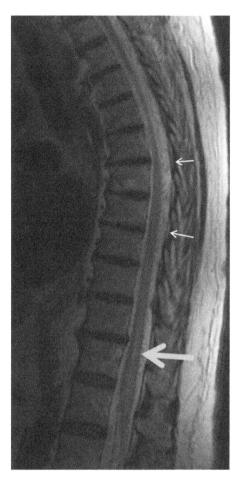

Figure 6.8 T2-weighted sagittal MRI of thoracic spine. The gold arrow points to signal alteration in the lower thoracic spinal cord and conus medullaris. The white arrows point to engorged peri-medullary veins on the dorsal spinal surface.

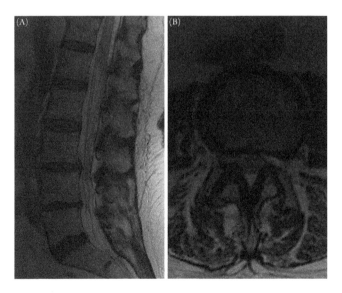

Figure 6.7 T2-weighted MRI images of the lumbar spine. A: Sagittal image shows minimal spondylolisthesis at L3–L4. B: Axial image does not demonstrate any significant foraminal, lateral recess, or canal stenosis.

of your mind when the history, physical examination, and images do not add up. This patient's lumbar MRI scan is underwhelming. His disproportionate symptomatology and mild myelopathic findings should detour any thought of a decompressive surgery.

The abnormal T2 signal in the spinal cord could also potentially represent demyelination, inflammation, or tumor. The presence of enlarged perimedullary veins on sagittal imaging points to a possible spinal dAVF. MRA or CTA can image the perimedullary venous drainage noninvasively and may assist in localizing the dAVF segmentally. Spinal angiography allows precise localization of the fistula located on the dural root sleeve. They are predominantly located on the left side, usually from T8 to L2.

Type I spinal dAVFs lead to an inexorable progression of symptoms from venous congestion, which produces hypertension in the spinal cord. Hemorrhage is exceedingly rare. Two to three percent of patients may have multiple lesions.

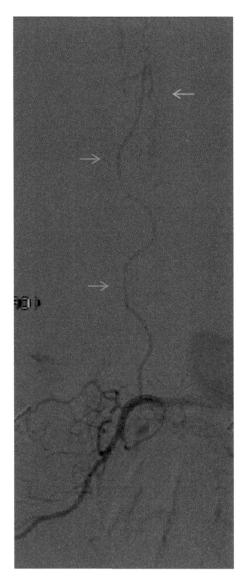

is easily identified and traced to the root sleeve (Figure 6.10A). Classically, the fistulous connection at the dura is occluded by a clip (Figure 16.10B). However, the clip may complicate dural closure. An alternative strategy is to coagulate and divide the fistulous venous segment, which allows removal of the clip to facilitate dural closure (Figure 6.10C). Angiographic confirmation of obliteration should be completed.

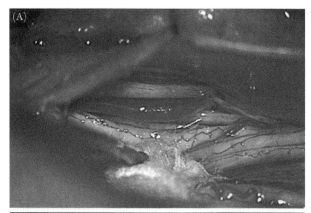

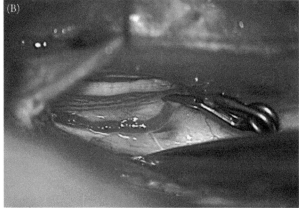

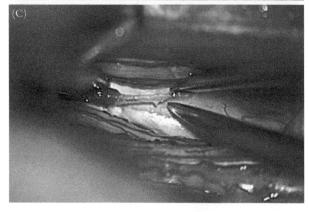

Figure 6.9 Spinal angiogram, right L3 segmental artery, right anterior oblique projection. The enlarged medullary vein is identified as it flows in retrograde manner to the dilated coronal venous plexus.

TREATMENT

Treatment options include endovascular therapy and microsurgical obliteration. Embolization has a higher rate of recurrence. Navigating tortuous radicular arteries in older patients, increased radiation exposure, and difficulty depositing embolic material proximally into the fistulous vein are some of the problematic challenges. The presence of a spinal medullary artery arising from the segmental artery supplying the dAVF is a contraindication to embolization.

On the other hand, surgical obliteration via a limited laminectomy has very low morbidity and an extremely high rate of durable occlusion. Precise intraoperative localization is necessary. Following durotomy, the arterialized vein

Figure 6.10 Intraoperative images following a partial L2–L3 laminectomy. A: The enlarged, arterialized vein is identified as it arises from the fistula (green arrow) located at the dural root sleeve. B: A clip is placed across the medullary vein at the fistula. Change in caliber is already noted. C: The fistulous vein is coagulated and divided to allow removal of the clip. This may facilitate dural closure. Note the darkened color of the residual medullary venous segment.

The vast majority of patients experience stabilization or improvement following treatment. Motor symptoms tend to improve more readily than sensory or sphincter disturbances. Timely diagnosis and treatment is critical to the recovery of function.

COMPLICATIONS

There is risk for CSF leakage. Water-tight dural closure should be attempted. It may be supplemented with collagen sponge and/or tissue glue. Use of a wound drain with a suction device is a personal preference.

This patient's initial postoperative examination is unremarkable. However, after his period of flat bedrest, he perceives increased weakness in his legs with ambulation and a greater sense of numbness in his feet. Proprioception and pinprick perception are preserved. Early postoperative worsening is unusual, and a MRI scan is warranted. It reveals a postoperative hematoma (Figure 6.11). He returns to the operating room for evacuation. If the postoperative MRI scan is unremarkable, follow-up angiography should be obtained.

Neurological worsening months or years after obliteration (especially by embolization) merits repeat imaging, first with MRI scan to look for cord signal change and then, if necessary, MRA or CTA followed by spinal angiography.

PEARLS

- *Misdiagnosis or delay in diagnosis is not uncommon. If history, examination, and imaging studies do not add up, consider the possibility of a Type I spinal dAVF.*

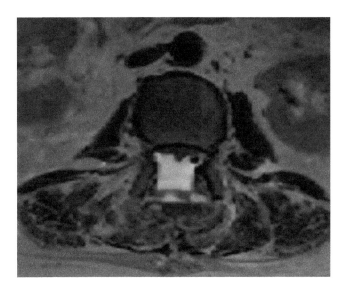

Figure 6.11 Axial T2-weighted image at L3 level. A hyperintense epidural hematoma is compressing the thecal sac.

- *Symptoms will progress if not treated. Motor symptoms tend to be most responsive to treatment.*

- *Although many Type I spinal dAVF can be treated endovascularly, surgery is simple, safe, and more durable.*

CASE 5

HISTORY AND PHYSICAL

A 70-year-old right-handed man experienced a 15-minute episode of nausea, dizziness, visual disturbance, and right arm weakness. He continued to have mild expressive dysphasia for another 2 hours. He has a history of hypertension and smokes 1 pack of cigarette per day.

His blood pressure is 157/90 mm Hg, and there is a left carotid bruit. His neurological examination is now normal.

IMAGING STUDIES

The CT scan is normal, and the CTA of the neck reveals significant carotid stenosis on the left (Figures 6.12 and 6.13). CTA of the brain demonstrates a patent circle of Willis. MRI study is unremarkable.

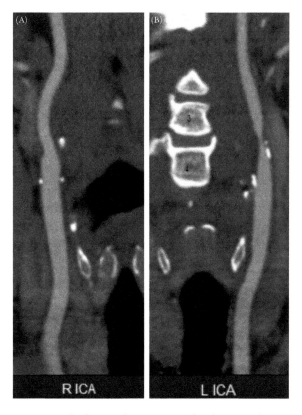

Figure 6.12 Coronal reformatted CTA images of neck. Minimal stenosis is identified on the right (A), and there is significant stenosis of the left carotid artery (B). Calcification in the plaque is also detected.

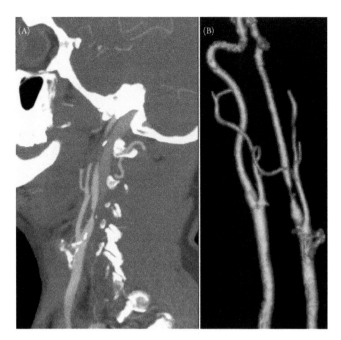

Figure 6.13 CTA of left cervical carotid artery. A: Sagittally reformatted image shows significant ICA stenosis with calcification. B: Three-dimensional reconstruction demonstrates severe left carotid stenosis with an ulceration in the mid-portion of the plaque.

ANALYSIS OF CASE AND TREATMENT PLAN

General

This patient presents with a classical transient ischemic attack (TIA). Hemodynamic TIAs tend to resolve within minutes, whereas embolic TIAs usually last for several hours. About one-third of patients who experience a TIA eventually suffer a stroke. The risk for stroke is 5% in the first month and 12% during the first year following a TIA. Extracranial atherosclerotic disease of the carotid arteries and aortic arch account for more than 50% of all strokes, with 20% to 30% related to problems at the carotid bifurcation. Complex ulceration in the carotid plaque increases the risk of stroke.

Risk factors for stroke include hypertension, hypercholesterolemia, tobacco use, diabetes, sedentary life style, and excess body weight. This patient has a cervical bruit, which is the most common physical sign of extracranial vascular disease. However, bruit has a very broad differential diagnosis. Up to 50% of patients with significant stenosis may not have a bruit. A thorough cardiac evaluation is also needed.

He is started on low dose acetylsalicylic acid (ASA; 81–325mg) and a "statin." Hepatic hydroxymethyl glutaryl coenzyme A reductase inhibitors have been shown to lower the risk of stroke in patients with carotid atherosclerosis by 19% to 32%.

His CTA shows significant carotid stenosis. We also perform an intracranial CTA to assess the circle of Willis and look for tandem lesions. MRA tends to overestimate the degree of narrowing and may give a false impression of occlusion. Duplex ultrasound may be more accurate than angiography in demonstrating ulceration, but it tends to underestimate the degree of stenosis.

TREATMENT

There is compelling evidence to recommend carotid endarterectomy (CEA) for this patient. With carotid stenosis > 69%, the North American Symptomatic Carotid Endarterectomy Trial (NASCET) found there was a 65% relative risk reduction for stroke with CEA compared to medical management after 2 years. The absolute risk reduction from CEA was 16% at 5 years. For symptomatic stenosis of 50% to 69%, the benefit is smaller (absolute risk reduction of 4.6% at 5 years). Pooled data from 3 additional large studies on CEA showed benefit in men. The benefits for women are less certain.

We recommend expeditious treatment. Following the last symptomatic event (TIA or nondisabling stroke), treatment within 2 weeks is associated with better results. The Carotid Revascularization Endarterectomy vs. Stenting Trial (CREST) did not find any significant difference in outcomes for stroke, myocardial infarction (MI), or death between CEA and carotid angioplasty with stenting (CAS). The periprocedural risk for stroke was higher with CAS and the risk for MI was greater with CEA. Younger patients (<70 years) had slightly better outcomes with CAS and older patients (>69 years) had better outcomes with CEA. Most randomized studies have shown that CAS is durable with regard to the long-term reduction in ipsilateral stroke.

Given the patient's age and lack of surgical risk factors, the decision is made to perform a CEA. CEA can be performed under local or general anesthesia. Following exposure, dissection is carried from the common carotid artery (CCA) to beyond the end of the plaque in the internal carotid artery (ICA). The common facial vein may need to be ligated and divided near the bifurcation. The ansa cervicalis is kept medially. It is important to place the medial blades of the self-retaining retractor superficial to the trachea to avoid injury to the trachea and its nerve supply.

Before cross clamping, a fixed dose (5,000 U) or a weight-based dose of heparin is administered intravenously. The ICA, CCA, and ECA (and superior thyroid artery) are cross-clamped or occluded in sequential order

(I–C–E). Various strategies to detect significant ischemia during vessel occlusion include monitoring stump pressure, EEG, transcranial Doppler, or neurological assessment during surgery under local anesthesia. If ischemia is detected, induce moderate hypertension to increase collateral flow. If this fails to rectify the situation, a shunt is needed. The use of a shunt can create some technical difficulties with the CEA as well as be a source for emboli or intimal injury. The shunt should first be inserted into the ICA and then the CCA. Alternatively, some surgeons employ EEG burst suppression or the routine use of a shunt during the period of cross clamping. You should have your personal algorithm prepared for the examination.

Following removal of the plaque, the proximal and distal ends of the endarterectomy are inspected for any residual filaments of plaque or intimal flaps. Closure is initiated. Debris and air bubbles are expelled by back bleeding each vessel. Removal of the clip on the superior thyroid artery allows continuous back bleeding during placement of the final few sutures. The ECA is then reopened and the CCA is temporarily reopened to flush debris into the ECA system. The ICA is then temporally reopened to flush debris into the ECA. The clamps are then permanently removed from the CCA and then the ICA (reverse I–C–E order).

Generally, the heparin is not reversed. Bleeding from the suture line is controlled by the application of a hemostatic sponge. Low-dose ASA (81–325 mg) is recommended before and for at least 3 months after surgery. Blood pressure is tightly controlled during the postoperative period.

The best management for asymptomatic, severe carotid stenosis is being evaluated. The rate of ipsilateral stroke in a medically treated patient with any degree of stenosis may presently be as low as 0.5% to 1% annually. CREST-2 is utilizing 2 parallel arms to assess the management of asymptomatic patients with severe carotid stenosis. Each arm will evaluate the effectiveness of medical management, one compared to CEA and the other to CAS. All 3 modalities may yield comparable results.

COMPLICATION

Following CAS and CEA, cerebral hyperperfusion can develop in 1% and 2% of patients, respectively. It develops more quickly following CAS. It is characterized by unilateral headache, face and eye pain, seizures, and focal neurological symptoms. There may be cerebral edema. ICH occurs in less than 1%. The development of ICH following endarterectomy is avoided by tight blood pressure control. SAH is more common following CAS, but it is not correlated to blood pressure management.

If an intimal flap or dissection occurs with CEA, it should be tacked down with a 7-0 monofilament double-ended suture, placed from the intimal side.

Risk for perioperative MI is 2% to 3%. Wound hematoma is seen in about 5% of cases. If airway obstruction develops, the hematoma must be evacuated. Awake fiber-optic intubation can be performed if ventilation is adequate. If fiber-optic intubation is unsuccessful, or if the patient is unstable, direct laryngoscopy should be performed before or after anesthetic induction. Reopening the surgical incision to facilitate direct laryngoscopy or emergency tracheostomy may be required.

A variety of nerve injuries can be seen with CEA. Most of these are stretch injuries and resolve within 3 to 6 months. Injury to the mandibular branch of the facial nerve at the inferior margin of the parotid gland can affect the lip depressor. Recurrent laryngeal nerve injury has been reported in 6%. This risk is lessened by proper placement of the medial blade of the retractor. Superior laryngeal nerve injury can occur during high dissection medial to the ICA and ECA. It is disabling due to difficulty sensing and swallowing food. Injury to the spinal accessory nerve as it courses under the sternocleidomastoid muscle paralyzes both the trapezius and sternocleidomastoid muscles ipsilaterally. Hypoglossal nerve injury occurs in about 5% of cases.

PEARLS

- *CEA is very effective for high grade (>69%) stenosis. It should be performed within 2 weeks following a TIA or minor stroke.*

- *Low dose ASA should be used preoperatively and for a minimum of 3 months after CEA.*

- *In CEA, apply cross clamps using the I–C–E mnemonic. Remove in reverse sequence.*

- *CAS has been shown to be noninferior to CEA. It is currently reimbursed for treatment of symptomatic carotid stenosis and in asymptomatic patients with difficult surgical anatomy.*

- *Risk for MI is higher with CEA compared to CAS.*

- *CAS has a higher risk for stroke in the perioperative period. Stroke has a greater adverse effect on quality of life than MI.*

- *Older patients (age ≥70 years) have fewer events with CEA compared to CAS.*

- *Younger patients have slightly fewer events with CAS than CEA.*

HISTORY AND PHYSICAL

A 45-year-old female did not show up for work. Her co-workers became concerned when she again failed to show the following morning and notified the police. She was found in her apartment. She had been incontinent, was dehydrated and dysphasic, and had right hemiplegia. No prescription medications were found.

She is admitted to the intensive care unit. Her vital signs are stable and rehydration is initiated. She has early signs of skin breakdown. She has a left-sided Horner's syndrome.

IMAGING STUDIES

CT scan of the brain demonstrates ischemic changes in the left MCA distribution (Figure 6.14). CTA reveals a left carotid occlusion from dissection.

ANALYSIS OF CASE AND TREATMENT PLAN

General

A partial Horner's syndrome can be seen with carotid dissection. Typically, it is painful. There will be miosis and ptosis. Anhidrosis is not seen since the sympathetic fibers supplying the facial sweat glands are carried on the ECA. Patients may also experience pulsatile tinnitus from stenosis related to the carotid dissection.

"Malignant" MCA infarction is typically characterized by a higher initial National Institute of Health Stroke Scale score, larger infarct volume (involvement of >50% of the MCA territory or additional territories), and the development of transtentorial herniation. Malignant MCA infarction has a mortality rate of 50% to 80% despite aggressive medical management. These large infarcts traditionally represent 10% to 15% of all strokes.

Three European studies (Decompressive Surgery for the Treatment of Malignant Infarction of the Cerebral Artery [DESTINY], Decompressive Craniectomy in Malignant Middle Cerebral Artery Infarction [DECIMAL], and Hemicraniectomy after Malignant Cerebral Artery Infarction with Life-Threatening Edema Trial [HAMLET]) evaluated the potential benefit of hemidecompression (HD) surgery for massive stroke in patients <60 years-old. A pooled analysis demonstrated a reduction in mortality from 71% to 22% (49% absolute risk reduction) with HD.

This pooled analysis also looked at functional outcomes using the modified Rankin Scale (mRS). Surgery did not produce an increase in the rate of survival with severe disability (mRS =5: bedridden, incontinent, requiring constant nursing care and attention). However, it did result in an increased rate of moderately severe disability (mRS =4) from 2% to 31%. These patients are unable to walk or attend to their own bodily needs without assistance. The number of surgical survivors with lesser disabilities also increased to some degree.

In another review of survivors, favorable results (mRS ≤3) were seen in 41%, poor outcomes (mRS =5) in 11%, and 47% were moderately severely disabled (mRS =4).

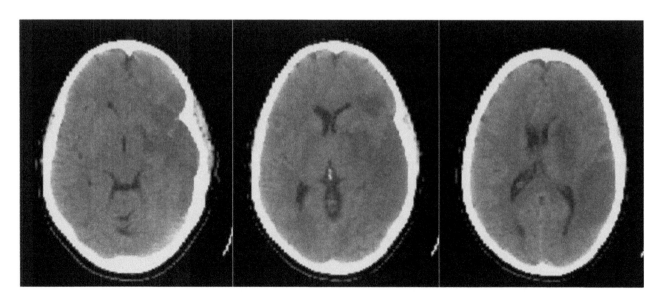

Figure 6.14 CT images of early changes of left MCA infarction.

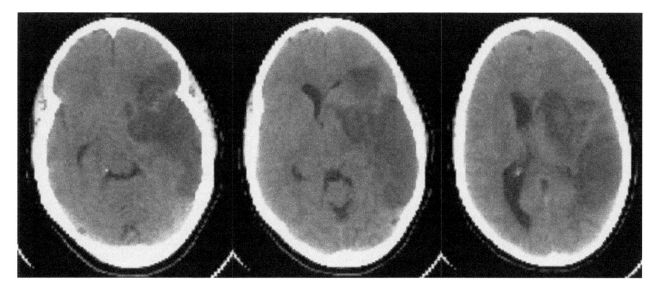

Figure 6.15 CT scan demonstrates evolution of the malignant MCA infarct with increasing mass effect.

DESTINY II looked at HD in older patients (>60 years old). Surgery again resulted in a higher rate of survival, but with a worsened profile of outcomes. More survivors were left with a mRS of 4 to 5.

Earlier surgery (<48 hours) is associated with the best outcomes and survival. Patients under 60 years of age are better candidates. The side of a malignant infarct should not play a significant role in the decision process; hemineglect is considered as detrimental as aphasia from a rehabilitation perspective. Also, aphasia improves over time in the majority of patients.

As soon as possible, the situation is discussed at length with her family. It is important to do this early, before the decision on surgery becomes critical. Most patients will be left with notable permanent disabilities and may be dependent on the assistance and care of others to manage their daily activities of living. The family needs an opportunity to consider the implications of their decision on outcome as well as survival. They need to consider her goals and what matters most to her.

She begins to deteriorate over the day with increasing somnolence. A repeat CT confirms worsening mass effect (Figure 6.15). The family wishes to proceed with HD.

Surgery

The hemicraniectomy should be >12 cm in diameter. It is centered over the area of the stroke. It may be advisable to extend bony removal to the floor of the middle cranial fossa. HD alone will reduce ICP by 15%. If duroplasty is also performed, ICP will be reduced by 55%.

COMPLICATIONS

Common complications include bone flap infection, bone flap resorption, and seizures. The syndrome of the trephined may occur. It responds well to replacement of the bone flap or cranioplasty. Replacement of the bone flap within 10 weeks is associated with a higher risk for infection (13.5%) and lower rate of epidural hematoma (2.7%) compared to bone flap replacement after 10 weeks (8.1% and 5.4%, respectively).

PEARLS

- *The mortality associated with a large territory MCA infarct is extremely high.*

- *HD has a dramatically positive impact on survival. Functional outcomes are better in survivors <60 years old.*

- *Results are better when HD is performed early (<48 hours). However, even patients with early signs of transtentorial herniation may benefit.*

- *HD should be at least 12 cm in diameter.*

- *The side of the stroke is not a major rehabilitation consideration.*

REFERENCES

1. Adamczyk P, Amar AP, Mack WJ, Larsen DW. Recurrence of "cured" dural arteriovenous fistulas after Onyx embolization. *Neurosurg Focus.* 2012;32(5):E12.
2. Al-Shahi Salman R, White PM, Counsell CE, et al; Scottish Audit of Intracranial Vascular Malformations Collaborators. Outcome

after conservative management or intervention for unruptured brain arteriovenous malformations. *JAMA*. 2014;311(16):1661–1669.

3. Anderson CS, Heeley E, Huang Y, et al; INTERACT 2 Investigators. Rapid blood-pressure lowering in patients with acute intracerebral hemorrhage. *N Engl J Med*. 2013;368:2355–2365.

4. Baharoglu M Irem, Cordonnier C, Al-Shahi Salman R, et al; PATCH Investigators. Platelet transfusion versus standard care after acute stroke due to spontaneous cerebral hemorrhage associated with antiplatelet therapy (PATCH): a randomized, open-label, phase 3 trial. *Lancet*. 2016;387:2605–2613.

5. Bervini D, Morgan MK, Ritson EA, Heller G. Surgery for unruptured arteriovenous malformations of the brain is better than conservative management for selected cases: a prospective cohort study. *J Neurosurg*. 2014;121(4):878–890.

6. Brott TG, Hobson RW 2nd, Howard G, et al; CREST Investigators. Stenting versus endarterectomy for treatment of carotid-artery stenosis. *N Engl J Med*. 2010;363(1):11–23.

7. Brott TG, Howard G, Roubin GS, et al; CREST Investigators. Long-term results of stenting versus endarterectomy for carotid-artery stenosis. *N Engl J Med*. 2016;374(11):1021–1031.

8. Campi A, Ramzi N, Molyneux AJ, et al. Retreatment of ruptured cerebral aneurysms in patients randomized by coiling or clipping in the International Subarachnoid Aneurysm Trial (ISAT). *Stroke*. 2007;38(5):1538–1544.

9. Chaturvedi S, Bruno A, Feasby T, et al. Carotid endarterectomy—an evidence-based review: Report of the Therapeutics and Technology Assessment Subcommittee of the American Academy of Neurology. *Neurology*. 2005;65(6):794–801.

10. Chung P-W, Kim J-T, Sanossian N, et al; FAST-MAG Investigators and Coordinators. Association between hyperacute stage blood pressure variability and outcome in patients with spontaneous intracerebral hemorrhage. *Stroke*. 2018;49(2):348–345.

11. Colby GP, Coon AL, Sciubba DM, Bydon A, Gailloud P, Tamargo RJ. Intraoperative indocyanine green angiography for obliteration of a spinal dural arteriovenous fistula. *J Neurosurg Spine*. 2009;11(6):705–709.

12. Connolly ES Jr, Rabinstein AA, Carhuapoma JR, et al. Guidelines for the management of aneurysmal subarachnoid hemorrhage: a guideline for healthcare professionals from the American Heart Association/American Stroke Association. *Stroke*. 2012;43(6):1711–1737.

13. Derdeyn CP, Zipfel GJ, Albuquerque FC, et al; American Association Stroke Council. Management of brain arteriovenous malformations. A scientific statement for healthcare professionals from the American Heart Association/American Stroke Association. *Stroke*. 2017;48:e200–e224.

14. Gross BA, Du R. Natural history of cerebral arteriovenous malformations: a meta-analysis. *J Neurosurg*. 2013;118(2):437–443.

15. Gurm HS, Yadav J, Fayad P et al; SAPPHIRE Investigators. Long-term results of carotid stenting versus endarterectomy in high-risk patients. *N Engl J Med*. 2008;358(15):1572–1579.

16. Hanley DF, Lane K, McBee N, et al; CLEAR III Investigators. Thrombolytic removal of intraventricular hemorrhage in treatment of severe stroke: results of the randomized, multicenter, multiregion, placebo-controlled CLEAR III trial. *Lancet*. 2017;389(10069):603–611.

17. Hanley DF, Thompson RE, Rosenblum M, et al; MISTIE III Investigators. Efficacy and safety of minimally invasive surgery with thrombolysis in intracerebral haemorrhage evacuation (MISTIE III): a randomized, controlled, open-label, blinded endpoint phase 3 trial. *Lancet*. 2019;393(10175):1021–1032.

18. Hemphill JC 3rd, Bonovich DC, Besmertis L, Manley GT, Johnston SC. The ICH score: A simple, reliable grading scale for intracerebral hemorrhage. *Stroke*. 2001;32(4):891–897.

19. Hemphill JC 3rd, Greenberg SM, Anderson CS, et al. Guidelines for the management of spontaneous intracerebral hemorrhage: a guideline for healthcare professionals from the American Heart Association/American Stroke Association. *Stroke*. 2015;46(7):2032–2060.

20. Hofmeijer J, Jaap Kappelle L, Algra A, et al; HAMLET investigators. Surgical decompression for space-occupying cerebral infarction (the Hemicraniectomy After Middle Cerebral Artery infarction with Life-threatening Edema Trial [HAMLET]). *Lancet Neurol*. 2009;8(4):326–333.

21. Hudson JS, Nagahama Y, Nakagawa D, et al. Hemorrhage associated with ventriculoperitoneal shunt placement in aneurysmal subarachnoid hemorrhage patients on a regimen of dual antiplatelet therapy: a retrospective analysis. *J Neurosurg*. 2018;129:916–921.

22. Hudson JS, Prout BS, Nagahama Y, et al. External ventricular drain and hemorrhage in aneurysmal subarachnoid hemorrhage patients on dual antiplatelet therapy: a retrospective cohort study. *Neurosurgery*. 2019;84(2):479–484.

23. Johnston SC, Dowd CF, Higashida RT, et al. Predictors of rehemorrhage after treatment of ruptured intracranial aneurysms: the Cerebral Aneurysm Rerupture After Treatment (CARAT) study. *Stroke*. 2008;39(1):120–125.

24. Juttler E, Schwab S, Schmiedek P, et al; DESTINY Study Group. Decompressive surgery for the treatment of malignant infarction of the middle cerebral artery (DESTINY): a randomized, controlled trial. *Stroke*. 2007;38:2518–2525.

25. Juttler E, Unterberg A, Woitzik J, et al; DESTINY Investigators. Hemicraniectomy in older patients with extensive middle-cerebral-artery stroke. *N Engl J Med*. 2014;370:1091–1100.

26. Kano H, Lunsford LD, Flickinger JC, et al. Stereotactic radiosurgery for arteriovenous malformations. Part 1: Management of Spetzler-Martin grade I and II arteriovenous malformations. *J Neurosurg*. 2012;116(1):11–20.

27. Kung DK, Policeni BA, Capuano AW, et al. Risk of ventriculostomy-related hemorrhage in patients with acutely ruptured aneurysms treated using stent-assisted coiling. *J Neurosurg*. 2011;114:1021–1027.

28. Marulanda-Londono E, Chaturvedi S. Carotid stenosis in women: time for a reappraisal. *Stroke Vasc Neurol*. 2016;1:192–196.

29. Mayberg MR, Wilson SE, Yatsu F, et al; Veterans Affairs Cooperative Studies Program 309 Trialist Group. Carotid endarterectomy and prevention of cerebral ischemia in symptomatic carotid stenosis. *JAMA*. 1991;266(23):3289–3294.

30. McCracken DJ, Lovasik BP, McCracken CE, et al. The intracerebral hemorrhage score: a self-fulfilling prophecy? *Neurosurgery*. 2019;84(3):741–748.

31. McDougall CG, Spetzler RF, Zabramski JM, et al. The Barrow Ruptured Aneurysm Trial. *J Neurosurg*. 2012;116(1):135–144.

32. Mendelow AD, Gregson BA, Fernandes HM, et al. Early surgery versus initial conservative treatment in patients with spontaneous supratentorial intracerebral haematomas in the International Surgical Trial in Intracerebral Haemorrhage (STICH): a randomised trial. *Lancet*. 2005;365(9457):387–397.

33. Mendelow AD, Gregson BA, Rowan EN, et al. Early surgery versus initial conservative treatment in patients with spontaneous supratentorial lobar intracerebral haematomas (STICH II): a randomised trial. *Lancet*. 2013;382(9890):397–408.

34. Mendes GAC, Kalani MYS, Iosif C, et al. Transvenous curative embolization of cerebral arteriovenous malformations: a prospective cohort study. *Neurosurgery*. 2018;83(5):957–964.

35. Mitchell P, Kerr R, Mendelow AD, Molyneux A. Could late rebleeding overturn the superiority of cranial aneurysm coil embolization over clip ligation seen in the International Subarachnoid Aneurysm Trial? *J Neurosurg*. 2008;108(3):437–442.

36. Mohr JP, Parides MK, Stapf C, et al. Medical management with or without interventional therapy for unruptured brain arteriovenous malformations (ARUBA): a multicentre, non-blinded, randomised trial. *Lancet*. 2014;383(9917):614–621.

37. Molyneux A, Kerr R, Stratton I, et al. International Subarachnoid Aneurysm Trial (ISAT) of neurosurgical clipping versus endovascular coiling in 2143 patients with ruptured intracranial aneurysms: a randomised trial. *Lancet*. 2002;360(9342):1267–1274.

38. Molyneux AJ, Kerr RS, Birks J, et al. Risk of recurrent subarachnoid haemorrhage, death, or dependence and standardised mortality ratios after clipping or coiling of an intracranial aneurysm in the International Subarachnoid Aneurysm Trial (ISAT): long-term follow-up. *Lancet Neurol.* 2009;8(5):427–433.

39. Ogasawara K, Sakai N, Kuroiwa T, et al. Intracranial hemorrhage associated with cerebral hyperperfusion syndrome following carotid endarterectomy and carotid artery stenting: retrospective review of 4494 patients. *J Neurosurg.* 2007;107(6):1130–1136.

40. Ogilvy CS, Stieg PE, Awad I, et al. AHA Scientific Statement: Recommendations for the management of intracranial arteriovenous malformations: a statement for healthcare professionals from a special writing group of the Stroke Council, American Stroke Association. *Stroke.* 2001;32(6):1458–1471.

41. Oldfield EH, Doppman JL. Spinal arteriovenous malformations. In Little JR, ed. *Clinical Neurosurgery.* Vol 24. Baltimore, MD: Williams & Wilkins; 1986:161–183.

42. Ondra SL, Troupp H, George ED, Schwab K. The natural history of symptomatic arteriovenous malformations of the brain: a 24-year follow-up assessment. *J Neurosurg.* 1990;73(3):387–391.

43. Quershi AI, Palesch YY, Barsan WG, et al; ATACH-2 Trial Investigators and the Neurological Emergency Treatment Trials Network. Intensive blood-pressure lowering in patients with acute cerebral hemorrhage. *N Engl J Med.* 2016;375(11):1033–1043.

44. Rabinstein AA. Optimal blood pressure after intracerebral hemorrhage still a moving target (editorial). *Stroke.* 2018;49:275–276.

45. European Carotid Surgery Trialists' Collaborative Group. Randomised trial of endarterectomy for recently symptomatic carotid stenosis: final results of the MRC European Carotid Surgery Trial (ECST). *Lancet.* 1998;351(9113):1379–1387.

46. Rosenfield K, Matsumura JS, Chaturvedi S, et al; ACT I Investigators. Randomized trial of stent versus surgery for asymptomatic carotid stenosis. *N Engl J Med.* 2016;374(11):1011–1020.

47. Rosengart AJ, Huo JD, Tolentino J, et al. Outcome in patients with subarachnoid hemorrhage treated with antiepileptic drugs. *J Neurosurg.* 2007;107(2):253–260.

48. Rothwell PM, Eliasziw M, Gutnikov SA, et al; Carotid Endarterectomy Trialists Collaboration. Endarterectomy for symptomatic carotid stenosis in relation to clinical subgroups and timing of surgery. *Lancet.* 2004;363(9413):915–924.

49. Saladino A, Atkinson JL, Rabinstein AA, et al. Surgical treatment of spinal dural arteriovenous fistulae: a consecutive series of 154 patients. *Neurosurgery.* 2010;67(5):1350–1357; discussion 1357–1358.

50. Solomon RA, Connolly ES Jr. Arteriovenous malformations of the brain (review). *N Engl J Med.* 2017;376(19):1859–1866.

51. Spence JD, Naylor AR. Endarterectomy, stenting, or neither for asymptomatic carotid-artery stenosis (editorial). *N Engl J Med.* 2016;374:1087–1088.

52. Spetzler RF, Martin NA. A proposed grading system for arteriovenous malformations. *J Neurosurg.* 1986;65(4):476–483.

53. Spetzler RF, McDougall CG, Albuquerque FC, et al. The Barrow Ruptured Aneurysm Trial: 3-year results. *J Neurosurg.* 2013;119(1):146–157.

54. Spetzler RF, McDougall CG, Zabramski JM, et al. The Barrow Ruptured Aneurysm Trial: 6-year results. *J Neurosurg.* 2015;123(3):609–617.

55. Vahedi K, Hofmeijer J, Juettler E, et al; DECIMAL, DESTINY, and HAMLET investigators. Early decompressive surgery in malignant infarction of the middle cerebral artery: a pooled analysis of three randomized controlled trials. *Lancet Neurol.* 2007;6(3):215–222.

56. Vahedi K, Vicaut E, Mateo J, et al; DECIMAL Investigators. Sequential-design, multicenter, randomized, controlled trial of early decompressive craniectomy in malignant middle cerebral artery infarction (DECIMAL Trial). *Stroke.* 2007;38(9):2506–2517.

7.

ENDOVASCULAR NEUROSURGERY

Ahmad Sweid and Pascal Jabbour

Endovascular neurosurgery has evolved dramatically since the first description of aneurysm coiling in 1991, and it is now employed as a primary treatment strategy for managing a multitude of cerebrovascular pathologies, including aneurysms, arteriovenous malformations (AVMs), and management of acute ischemic stroke.

Endovascular treatment of cerebral aneurysms has frequently replaced craniotomy for clipping in a large proportion of aneurysms since the publication of the International Subarachnoid Aneurysm Trial (ISAT), which demonstrated better outcomes for endovascular coil occlusion of ruptured aneurysms compared with surgical clipping in selected cases. The endovascular approach offers an attractive, minimally invasive alternative for aneurysm treatment with low procedure-related morbidity and mortality. The durability and long-term efficacy of endovascular interventions is continuously evolving, especially with the introduction of newer coils, stents, and flow-diversion techniques.

With the development of catheter and guidewire technology and novel embolic materials, endovascular management of AVMs has gained significant popularity and has become common practice. Endovascular management of AVMs can be used for presurgical embolization, preradiosurgical intervention, or palliative embolization or as a primary treatment for curative embolization, depending on the characteristics of the lesion.

Over the past few decades, the management of stroke has progressed exponentially, beginning with US Food and Drug Administration (FDA) approval of intravenous recombinant tissue plasminogen activator (r-tPA). Advances in endovascular management of acute stroke have further increased the therapeutic window of r-tPA administration using the intraarterial route, which led to the introduction of new devices for clot removal and vessel recanalization.

CASE 1

HISTORY AND PHYSICAL EXAMINATION

A 58-year-old woman with a history of migraines presented to the emergency department with the worst headache of her life, accompanied by nausea, vomiting, and dizziness. On physical examination, the patient was lethargic but oriented ×3. She had corneal, gag, and cough reflexes. Pupils were equal and reactive to light. Extraocular muscles were intact. Face was symmetrical. All other cranial nerves were intact. She was moving all extremities with 5/5 strength.

IMAGING STUDIES

Brain computed tomography (CT) demonstrates extensive subarachnoid hemorrhage (SAH) bilaterally, mainly in the region of the anterior aspect of the corpus callosum/ cingulate gyrus (Figure 7.1). No hydrocephalus or evidence of large territorial infarction is noted. An angiogram is performed and shows a 2 × 1.5-mm anterior communicating artery aneurysm (Figure 7.2).

ANALYSIS OF CASE AND SURGICAL PLAN

In patients with suspected SAH, a noncontrast-enhanced head CT should be obtained. If CT is nondiagnostic but suspicion is high, a lumbar puncture can be performed. Digital subtraction angiography (DSA) with three-dimensional rotational angiography is indicated to confirm the presence of an aneurysm and to devise a treatment plan. A multidisciplinary team is required to determine the best treatment strategy depending on patient and aneurysm characteristics. For ruptured aneurysms amenable to both microsurgical clipping and endovascular coiling, careful consideration of each treatment option should be given.

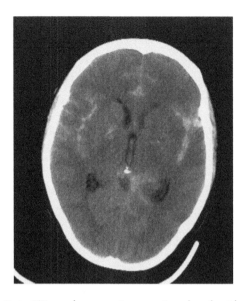

Figure 7.1 Brain CT scan demonstrating extensive subarachnoid hemorrhage bilaterally, mainly in the region of the anterior aspect of the corpus callosum/ cingulate gyrus. No hydrocephalus or evidence of large territorial infarction are seen.

Endovascular management of the ruptured aneurysm should be performed early, within 24 to 72 hours, aiming at complete obliteration of the aneurysm to reduce the rate of rebleeding after aneurysmal SAH. Aneurysm rebleeding is associated with very high mortality and poor prognosis for functional recovery. The risk for rebleeding is maximum in the first 2 to 12 hours, occurring at a rate of 3% to 4% within the first 24 hours.

The ISAT showed a reduction in death and disability from 31% in patients treated with microsurgery to 24% in the endovascular group (relative risk reduction, 24%). The risk for epilepsy and significant cognitive decline was also decreased in the endovascular treatment arm. However, the rate of late rebleeding (2.9% after endovascular repair vs. 0.9% after open surgery) was higher with endovascular treatment, and the rate of complete aneurysm obliteration was lower in coiled aneurysms (58% vs. 81% of clipped aneurysms). In patients with ruptured intracranial aneurysms, endovascular coiling may be favored in older patients (>65 years of age), patients with poor-grade SAH, patients with concomitant vasospasm, and those with posterior circulation aneurysms (e.g., basilar apex aneurysms). Patients with ruptured middle cerebral artery (MCA) aneurysms, wide-necked aneurysms, aneurysms with one or more branches incorporated into the neck or dome of the aneurysm, and large intraparenchymal hematomas should be considered for microsurgical clipping instead of coiling.

Arterial access for endovascular treatment is usually obtained by inserting a sheath through the common femoral artery connected to a heparinized flush, although radial artery access is becoming more commonplace. A guiding catheter is advanced over a guidewire into the aortic arch. Multiple runs in multiple views are obtained to identify the aneurysm, and then a microcatheter is advanced over a micro-guidewire into the aneurysm. Coils are available in many lengths, diameters, and shapes, and some coils have bioactive coatings or volume expanding gels. Coils are designed to be stretch resistant during manipulation or retrieval. The platinum coil wire is delivered through the microcatheter. When coils are inserted into the lumen of

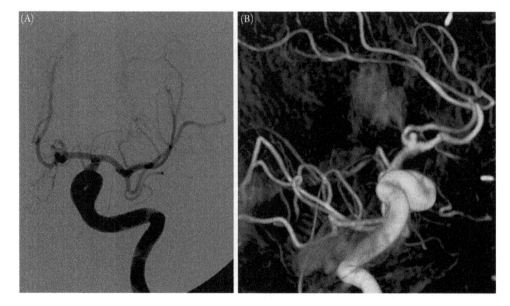

Figure 7.2 A: Cerebral angiogram showing a 2 × 1.5 mm anterior communicating artery aneurysm. B: Three-dimensional reconstruction showing the aneurysm.

the aneurysm, a local thrombus forms that leads to obliteration of the aneurysmal sac. Endovascular coiling is usually performed under general anesthesia for appropriate hemodynamic management and to obtain high-quality images. Neurophysiologic monitoring, including somatosensory evoked potential, electroencephalography, and brainstem auditory evoked potential monitoring, is often used. Patients with high-grade SAH should have intracranial pressure monitoring with a ventriculostomy and hemodynamic monitoring with a Swan-Ganz catheter and radial arterial line.

Between the time of SAH onset and aneurysm obliteration, blood pressure should be controlled with a titratable agent (decrease in systolic blood pressure to <160 mm Hg) to control the risk for stroke, rebleeding, and maintenance of cerebral perfusion pressure. Patients are managed in the intensive care unit after aneurysm therapy with continuous hemodynamic and neurological monitoring. Imaging follow-up should be performed at 6 months and 1 year and at later time intervals depending on the occlusion status of the aneurysm. If magnetic resonance angiography (MRA) or computed tomographic angiography (CTA) shows evidence of recurrence, an angiogram should be performed. Long-term aneurysm recurrence after coiling occurs in about one-fifth of all coiled cerebral aneurysms, and 10% of coiled aneurysms require another intervention.

Cerebral vasospasm affects approximately 60% to 70% of patients after SAH, resulting in symptomatic ischemia in approximately half of these patients. Vasospasm occurs most frequently 7 to 10 days after aneurysm rupture. Transcranial Doppler can be used to monitor for the development of arterial vasospasm. Oral nimodipine should be administered to all patients with aneurysmal SAH. Initial management of vasospasm consists of hyperdynamic therapy including hypervolemia, hemodilution, and induced hypertension. In patients who are refractory to medical therapy, cerebral angioplasty or intraarterial vasodilator therapy in the affected territory may be beneficial in improving angiographic and clinical outcome, if performed in a timely manner. Patients who develop acute hydrocephalus are usually managed by external ventricular drainage or lumbar drainage.

The patient had placement of a ventriculostomy catheter and was emergently taken to the interventional neuroradiology suite for an angiogram, which showed an anterior communicating artery aneurysm. The decision was made to coil the aneurysm. With a Seldinger technique, the right-sided femoral artery was catheterized with a 7-French sheath hooked to continuous heparinized flush. A guidewire and a catheter were introduced into the descending aorta up to

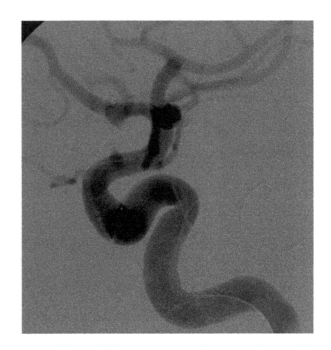

Figure 7.3 A 16-month follow-up angiogram showing complete occlusion of the aneurysm.

the arch. Selectively, the left internal carotid artery (ICA) was catheterized. Super selectively, the aneurysm was catheterized, then embolization with coils was performed. A 16-month follow-up angiogram in this case shows complete occlusion of the aneurysm (Figure 7.3).

COMPLICATIONS

Complications related to endovascular treatment of intracranial aneurysms can arise during different phases of treatment. Complication rates depend on patient characteristics (e.g., vascular tortuosity, atherosclerotic disease, and resistance to antiplatelet therapy), on aneurysm-related factors (e.g., size, shape, and location), and on operator experience. The main complications related to endovascular treatment include thromboembolic complications, intraprocedural aneurysm rupture, and access-related complications.

Thromboembolic complications with resultant ischemic symptoms occur at a rate of about 5% and depend highly on the use of antiplatelet treatment before intervention and on the concurrent use of balloon- or stent-assisted techniques. If thromboembolic complications are detected during the procedure, adequate heparinization should be confirmed by activated clotting time measurements. If the patient is adequately heparinized and a branch occlusion is seen, pharmacologic thrombolysis using tPA or intraarterial antiplatelet agents (glycoprotein IIb/IIIa receptor antagonists) can be used, or mechanical thrombolysis can be performed in the case of significant branch occlusions.

The aneurysm should be well coiled before thrombolytic treatment to avoid aneurysm rerupture.

Intraprocedural aneurysm rupture has been reported to occur in 1% to 5% of coil embolization procedures. Risk factors for intraprocedural rupture include ruptured aneurysm status, lower initial Hunt and Hess Stroke Scale grade, small aneurysm size, and low operator experience. Intraprocedural aneurysm rupture is associated with a significant risk for permanent neurological disability and death (38% for ruptured aneurysms and 29% for unruptured aneurysms). It may be accompanied by a sudden and massive rise in blood pressure with or without bradycardia attributable to an elevation in intracranial pressure. When intraoperative aneurysm rupture is encountered, protamine should be given if the patient is heparinized. For perforations at the aneurysm dome, rapid packing with coils can be performed, and a balloon can be inflated for temporary parent artery occlusion. For aneurysms perforated at the neck or parent vessel, parent vessel occlusion or a salvage technique using a balloon and liquid embolic agents can be considered. Intracranial pressure should be aggressively controlled after securing the aneurysm with ventricular drainage and medical management (e.g., hyperventilation and osmotic diuresis). A CT scan should be performed to rule out a large intraparenchymal hemorrhage that may require evacuation. Finally, if antiplatelet agents were administered, the patient should receive platelet transfusions when indicated.

Aneurysm rerupture and rehemorrhage following endovascular coiling is strongly related to the degree of aneurysm occlusion. Long-term follow-up is necessary to monitor for that risk.

CASE 2

HISTORY AND PHYSICAL EXAMINATION

A 68-year-old woman presented to the clinic with persistent headaches of several months' duration and 2 recent episodes of diplopia. The patient has a family history of aneurysmal SAH. On physical examination, the patient was neurologically intact.

IMAGING STUDIES

A head CT does not show any evidence of acute intracranial hemorrhage (Figure 7.4). CT angiography shows the presence of a 10-mm, wide-necked aneurysm arising from the right cavernous ICA and projecting anteromedially (Figure 7.5). It is lobulated in appearance. An angiogram

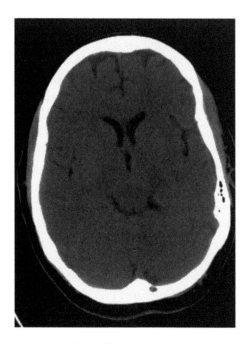

Figure 7.4 Noncontrast-enhanced brain CT showing no acute intracranial hemorrhage and no abnormal extra-axial fluid collection.

is performed and shows the right cavernous ICA aneurysm (Figure 7.6).

ANALYSIS OF CASE AND SURGICAL PLAN

Unruptured intracranial aneurysms (UIAs) are found in about 3.2% of the adult population. They are being found with an increasing frequency because of the wide-spread use of magnetic resonance imaging (MRI). UIAs may also be discovered when patients present with cranial nerve deficits (most commonly a third nerve palsy), seizures, mass effect, or motor and sensory deficits. Initial imaging should provide a complete evaluation of the anatomy of the aneurysm with accurate measurement of the neck size, neck-to-dome ratio, and relationship to the surrounding vessels. The techniques of aneurysm imaging have expanded greatly, with MRA, CTA, and DSA being performed with high sensitivity and specificity. CTA is frequently added to the non–contrast-enhanced head CT to assist diagnosis. DSA remains the "gold standard" of aneurysm diagnosis.

Overall, the annual rupture rate of UIAs is about 1%. Risk factors for rupture include patient characteristics that consist of increasing patient age, female sex, cigarette smoking, hypertension, prior personal history of SAH from a different aneurysm, and family history of SAH. Risk factors related to aneurysm features include larger aneurysm size; aneurysm morphology (increased rupture risk with aneurysms that have daughter sacs); documented

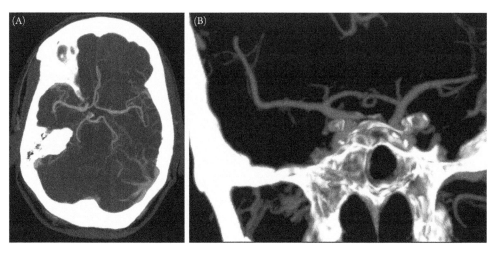

Figure 7.5 CTA showing the presence of (A) a 10-mm wide-necked aneurysm arising from the right cavernous internal carotid artery and (B) projecting anteromedially. It is lobulated in appearance.

aneurysmal growth during follow-up; aneurysm location in the posterior circulation, posterior communicating artery, or anterior communicating artery; and symptomatic status of the UIA. All these factors should be considered in selecting the optimal management of UIAs. The treatment strategies for UIA include conservative management, endovascular intervention, and surgical treatment. Given that the patient in our case had a positive family history of SAH, a symptomatic aneurysm, and an aneurysm at least 10 mm in size, she was strongly considered to undergo aneurysm treatment. For patients with small aneurysms (<5 mm) without a family or personal history of SAH, with small asymptomatic UIAs, and with low hemorrhage risk by location, size, and morphology, observation with

periodic follow-up imaging can be performed. If changes in aneurysm size or morphology are documented, treatment should be strongly considered. Although surgical clipping is an effective treatment for UIAs, treatment strategies of UIAs have shifted dramatically toward endovascular therapy. Patients with UIAs who are considered for treatment should be fully informed about the risks and benefits of both strategies. Patient age, presence of medical comorbidities, and aneurysm characteristics should be carefully taken into consideration because these are strong predictors of perioperative morbidity and rupture risk. In older patients (in this case, a 68-year-old patient), the benefit of endovascular treatment compared with surgery appears to be greater, especially because the rate of surgical

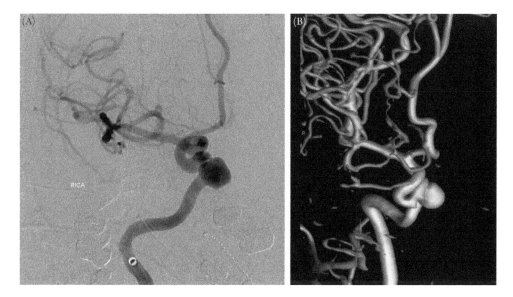

Figure 7.6 A: Cerebral angiogram, right internal carotid artery injection showing a 10-mm right cavernous carotid artery aneurysm. B: Three-dimensional reconstruction showing the 10-mm aneurysm.

complications is higher in this age group. Endovascular management is associated with a reduction in procedural morbidity, length of hospital stay, and mortality compared with surgical clipping in selected cases; however, endovascular treatment has an overall higher risk for recurrence than microsurgical treatment, and the latter confers more durable protection against aneurysm regrowth.

Coiling represents the most commonly employed endovascular strategy. However, large, giant, and wide-necked aneurysms tend to have higher recurrence and retreatment rates after coiling. Several technologies are available to target these lesions, including stent placement, stent-assisted coiling, and flow diversion. Recanalization and retreatment rates are lower with these techniques. The Pipeline Embolization Device (PED) was used in this case because of the size and wide neck of the aneurysm. The PED is FDA approved for the treatment of large and giant wide-neck aneurysms in the ICA, from the petrous to the superior hypophyseal segments. The PED belongs to a family of devices known as flow diverters, which work by acting as a scaffold for endothelial overgrowth of the aneurysm neck and cause parent vessel remodeling. The main structural differences from previous stents are the higher metal surface area coverage and the low porosity, which allows more flow reduction into the aneurysm neck. The PED has gained popularity because it provides a more physiologic and durable treatment strategy compared with other endovascular interventions, and studies have confirmed its high success rate in achieving aneurysm occlusion and low aneurysm recurrence and retreatment rates.

For endovascularly treated aneurysms, follow-up imaging with DSA or noninvasive methods is usually performed 6 months to 1 year after treatment. Later follow-up imaging can be obtained depending on the occlusion status of the aneurysm because residual aneurysms can still present with late hemorrhages and aneurysm recurrences.

This patient's UIA was treated using the PED. She was started on 75 mg/day of clopidogrel and 81 mg/ day of aspirin 10 days before the intervention. Preoperative P2Y12 reaction unit values were checked to assess platelet inhibition in response to clopidogrel, with a target therapeutic range between 60 and 240. During the procedure, the patient received a bolus of intravenous heparin to maintain an activated clotting time that was 2 to 3 times her baseline. Treatment was performed under general anesthesia. Her motor evoked potentials, somatosensory evoked potentials, and brainstem evoked potentials were monitored, and they were stable throughout the procedure. An angiographic evaluation was obtained to assess the dimensions of the aneurysms. An 8-French femoral sheath was used for access. A 6- French shuttle sheath was placed in the carotid bulb, and a catheter was placed at the level of the petrocavernous carotid junction. A microcatheter was then introduced distally to the M1-M2 junction. The PED was sized according to the width of the inflow vessel to avoid any endoleak. The PED was introduced through the microcatheter. After embolization was accomplished, a control angiogram was obtained. Heparin was stopped at the end of the procedure. After conclusion of the procedure, the catheters and sheaths were removed, and manual compression was applied for 20 minutes to achieve hemostasis. The site was checked for further bleeding, and the leg was immobilized. After discharge, the patient was scheduled for clinical follow-up and a follow-up angiogram. A follow-up angiogram performed at 6 months in this case showed complete obliteration of the aneurysm (Figure 7.7).

COMPLICATIONS

Risks common to all procedures with endovascular access include vascular injury, vessel dissection, and perforation or aneurysm rupture. Patients with access-related complications (groin complications), including groin hematomas, retroperitoneal hematomas, fistulas, and pseudoaneurysms, may present with severe pain at the puncture site with or without hemodynamic instability. Management consists of manual compression, abdominal and pelvic CT to check for hemorrhage, volume expansion with intravenous fluids, transfusion if needed, and reversal of antithrombotic treatment if necessary.

The main complications related to treatment with the PED and other stents can be grouped into thromboembolic and hemorrhagic complications. Because the PED consists of a bare metal stent that aids in neointimal tissue formation, platelet activation can result in local thrombosis with cerebral infarction or distal embolization. For this reason, patients who are scheduled to undergo stent placement require a preoperative administration of a dual antiplatelet therapy including clopidogrel and aspirin for about 10 days before the intervention to prevent stent thrombosis. This, however, may facilitate the occurrence of hemorrhagic complications, mainly intraparenchymal hemorrhage.

CASE 3

HISTORY AND PHYSICAL EXAMINATION

A 61-year-old man with a family history of brain aneurysms developed a stroke where workup revealed an incidental 6-mm anterior communicating artery aneurysm (ACoA) on

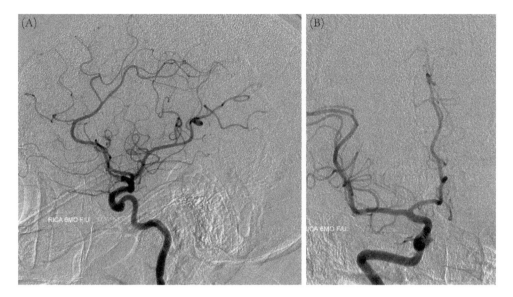

Lateral (A) and anterior (B) views on a 6-month follow-up angiogram with right internal carotid artery injection showing complete occlusion of the aneurysm with no in-stent stenosis.

MRA. The patient denies a history of smoking and sudden severe headaches.

IMAGING STUDIES

MRA showed a 6-mm saccular aneurysm originating from the right side of the anterior communicating artery (Figure 7.8). Cerebral angiography was performed for a better evaluation of the aneurysm morphology, size, neck, and branching vessels pattern. Angiogram showed a wide-necked ACoA aneurysm measuring 6.8 × 5.7 mm (Figure 7.9).

ANALYSIS OF CASE AND SURGICAL PLAN

In the early era of endovascular aneurysms treatment, wide-necked aneurysms were challenging to treat. The procedures were associated with high risk of coil herniation, migration, parent artery occlusion, and poor obliteration rates with high recurrence. The cornerstone for treating wide-necked aneurysms was surgical clipping. Different types of coils have been developed and refined to achieve better results. Balloon-assisted coiling and stent-assisted coiling have been introduced to provide protection and support to the coil

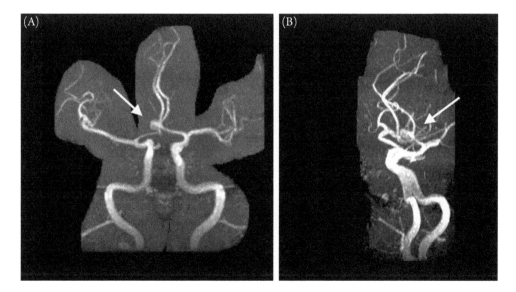

Figure 7.8 (A) antero-posterior and (B) lateral MRA 3D reconstruction showing a 6-mm saccular aneurysm originating from the right side of the anterior communicating artery (white arrow).

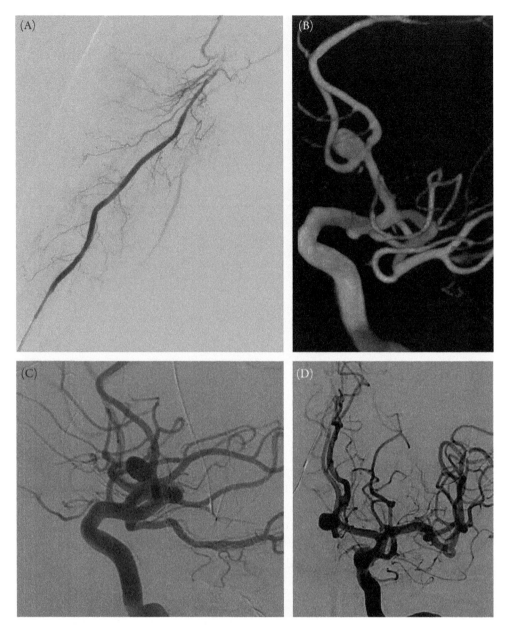

Figure 7.9 A transradial diagnostic angiogram showing a 6.8 × 5.7 mm ACoA. (A) Digital subtraction angiogram of a transradial run. (B) 3D reconstruction, (C) lateral, and (D) antero-posterior DSA showing a wide-necked ACoA.

mass. An intracranial stent can also provide a scaffold for neoendothelization in addition to the reduction of the flow into the aneurysm.

The first report of intracranial stent was reported by Higashida et al. in 1997. They used a balloon-expendable cardiac stent in combination with Guglielmi coils. The first FDA-approved intracranial open cell design stent was the Neuroform™ (Boston Scientific Corporation, USA). The device was approved for "humanitarian device exemption" in 2002. A succeeding stent was introduced in Europe, which was a closed cell design, Leo™ (Balt, Montmorency, France), followed by Enterprise™ (Cordis Neurovascular, Miami,

USA). The modification introduced to the Enterprise, which is a closed cell design, was that it was resheathable after partial deployment in contrast to Neuroform. Lastly, the most recent innovation is the Atlas stent™ (Stryker Neurovascular, Fremont, USA), which is an open cell design laser cut open cell stent with a diameter of 3.0 mm to 4.5 mm that is delivered through a 0.017-inch microcatheter.

Stent-assisted coiling is indicated for wide-necked aneurysms (neck larger than 4 mm, where dome-to-neck ratio is <2, or ASPECT ratio is >1.6) or unfavorable anatomy. Careful assessment of candidates for this treatment option as it warrants proper adherence to dual antiplatelet therapy.

Any reason for suspected noncommitment could be a relative contraindication. In addition, caution should be taken in the setting of ruptured aneurysm where the patient would require dual antiplatelet therapy, as those patients may require surgical procedures such as ventriculostomy, ventriculoperitoneal shunt, or decompressive surgery. In such cases, a staged approach may be performed where the aneurysm dome is protected and then complement the procedure with stent-assisted coiling.

Wide-necked aneurysms located at bifurcations are more complex to treat, as they require double stent placement in either an X or Y fashion, which carries increased risk of complications. Three devices have been developed for such bifurcating aneurysms: the Woven EndoBridge (WEB; Sequent Medical, Aliso Viejo, California), the pCONus (phenox, Bochum, Germany), and the PulseRider device (Pulsar Vascular, San Jose, California). The Web device is similar in concept to flow diverting stents, such as Silk, PED, and Surpass; however, it is an intrasaccular braided-wire flow disruptor that does not need dual antiplatelet therapy. In this case, a PulseRider assisted coiling was performed because of the wide neck nature of the aneurysm.

The PulseRider has a frame configuration that opens to conform to the vessel walls. It is designed to maintain luminal patency and hemodynamic flow through the parent vessel bifurcation by protecting both bifurcating vessels with wings, while securely retaining coils within the aneurysm sac. It is a self-expanding retrievable implant. It comes in either a T or a Y configuration to fit in the geometry of the daughter vessels with 8- or 10-mm diameters. The device can be delivered via a standard microcatheter and can electrolytically detached from the delivery wire.

The patient was started on 75 mg/day of clopidogrel and 81 mg/ day of aspirin 10 days before the intervention. Preoperative P2Y12 reaction unit values were checked to assess platelet inhibition in response to clopidogrel, with a target therapeutic range between 60 and 240. During the procedure, the patient received a bolus of intravenous heparin to maintain an activated clotting time that was 2 to 3 times her baseline. The procedure was performed under moderate sedation using a trans radial approach. The right wrist is prepped and draped. Radial artery catheterization is achieved using ultrasound guidance via the double wall puncture technique with a 6 Fr Slender sheath (Terumo). Then, a mix of 2000 units of heparin, 5 mg of nicardipine, and 200 mcg of nitroglycerin are administered intra-arterially through the sheath. Then the sheath is exchanged to a sheathless Neuron Max 90 cm (Penumbra Inc., Alameda, California) or a 6-French Shuttle sheath 90 cm (Cook Medical Inc., Bloomington, Indiana). Once the sheath is in place, we check the blood pressure to ensure it is within the desired target goal. Sometimes the cocktail given intra-arterially can cause systemic hypotension, requiring the administration of intravenous fluids or vasopressors. Then, a Simmons 2 Penumbra catheter is inserted into the access sheath through the radial artery all the way to the brachial artery, which is followed by sliding the access sheath on top of the Simmons 2 catheter the internal carotid artery is catheterized. Super selectively, the aneurysm was catheterized with a Prowler Select Plus® (Codman, Raynham, Massachusetts) and then deployment of a pulse Ryder device was performed covering the neck of the aneurysm with the 2 wings (Figure 7.10 A and B). Following that, the aneurysm was supraselectively catheterized with an Echelon™ 10 (Medtronic, Irvine, California) and coils were deployed (Figure 7.10 C). Control angiogram showed 100% occlusion of the aneurysm (Figure 7.10 D). After completion of the procedure, the radial sheath is removed, and a radial artery compression (Terumo TR Radial compression device) is placed on the wrist and inflated with air for 1 hour. It is gradually deflated after 1 hour and temporarily reinflated if hemostasis is not achieved according to protocol. A follow-up angiogram performed at 6 months in this case showed complete obliteration of the aneurysm (Figure 7.11).

COMPLICATIONS

Preoperative planning should be carefully performed for proper selection of candidate patients for such a procedure to avoid failure. Potential complications include but are not limited to aneurysm perforation or rupture, incomplete aneurysm occlusion and/or recanalization, device misplacement or migration, intracranial or intracerebral hemorrhage, stenosis or occlusion of treated vessel segment or device, and vascular sequelae including vasospasm, thrombosis, dissection, and perforation.

CASE 4

HISTORY AND PHYSICAL EXAMINATION

A 66-year old man had an incidental finding of a left-sided 6-mm ICA bifurcation aneurysm.

IMAGING STUDIES

Angiogram showed a left-sided ICA bifurcation aneurysm 6.5 × 4.4 mm and a smaller 1 × 1.6 mm bifurcation MCA aneurysm (Figure 7.12).

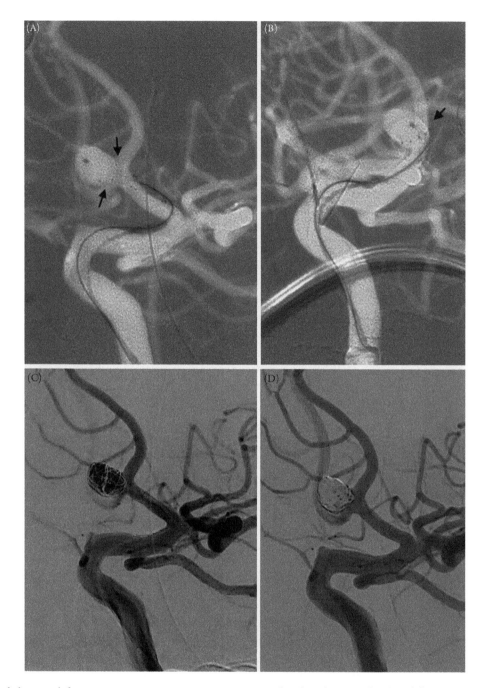

Figure 7.10 A transradial approach for treating an anterior communicating artery with PulseRider assisted coiling. (A) Lateral and (B) antero-posterior DSA showing the deployment of the PulseRider. The arrows points toward the wings of the PulseRider. (C) Lateral DSA showing coils deployed in the aneurysm sac. (D) Final run lateral DSA showing complete aneurysm occlusion.

ANALYSIS OF CASE AND SURGICAL PLAN

This is also a wide-necked bifurcating aneurysm that warrants treatment mainly due to the risk of rupture because of its size. The presence of multiple aneurysms is another variable to take into consideration. Treatment options include open surgical treatment or endovascular treatment using stent assisted coiling placed in a Y configuration, PulseRider stent-assisted coiling, or Web device. Flow-diverting stents are not an option in bifurcating aneurysms. Both stent-assisted coiling and the PulseRider requires dual antiplatelet therapy for at least 6 months.

The WEB Aneurysm Embolization System (Sequent Medical Inc., Aliso Viejo, California) was introduced in 2011 and recently received FDA approval. It is approved for bifurcating aneurysms originating from the internal carotid artery terminus, middle cerebral artery bifurcation, anterior communicating, and basilar apex wide-neck aneurysms.

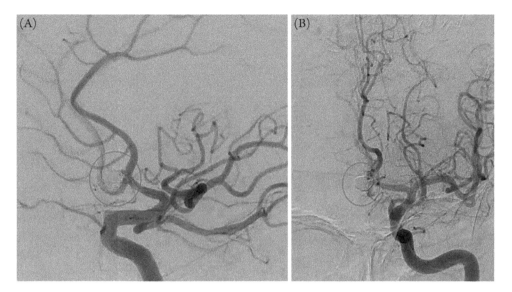

Figure 7.11 Follow-up angiogram showing complete aneurysm occlusion. (A) lateral and (B) antero-posterior DSA showing complete aneurysm occlusion.

It is an intrasaccular device consisting of a dense nitinol mesh that provides immediate flow disruption through the aneurysm ostium, resulting in subsequent thrombosis of the aneurysm sac. It is placed entirely within the aneurysm without affecting the parent vessel, hence not requiring antithrombotic medications. Due to these properties, the WEB is suitable for a broad range of aneurysms, including wide-necked, bifurcation, and ruptured aneurysms.

The devices available range in diameter from 4 mm to 11 mm and are deployed using 0.021 to 0.033-inch microcatheters (VIA 21, 27, 33). Aneurysms larger than 11 mm are not suitable for the device. An important benefit of the WEB device is the ability to perform an angiographic run after deployment but prior to detachment where the neurointerventionalist can safely evaluate placement prior to

detachment and retrieve the device if the desired positioning is not achieved.

The right wrist is prepped and draped. Radial artery catheterization is achieved using ultrasound guidance via the double wall puncture technique with a 6 Fr Slender sheath (Terumo). Then, a mix of 2000 units of heparin, 5 mg of nicardipine, and 200 mcg of nitroglycerin are administered intra-arterially through the sheath. Then the sheath is exchanged to a sheathless Neuron Max 90 cm (Penumbra Inc., Alameda, California) or a 6-French Shuttle sheath 90 cm (Cook Medical Inc., Bloomington, Indiana). Once the sheath is in place, we check the blood pressure to ensure it is within the desired target goal. Sometimes the cocktail given intra-arterially can cause systemic hypotension, requiring the administration of intravenous fluids

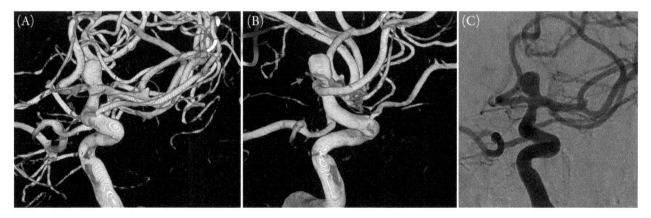

Figure 7.12 A transradial diagnostic angiogram showing a left sided ICA bifurcation aneurysm 6.5 × 4.4 mm and a smaller 1 × 1.6 mm bifurcation MCA aneurysm. (A) anteroposterior and (B) lateral 3D reconstruction, and (C) anteroposterior DSA showing ICA bifurcation aneurysm (red arrow) and smaller MCA aneurysm (red circle).

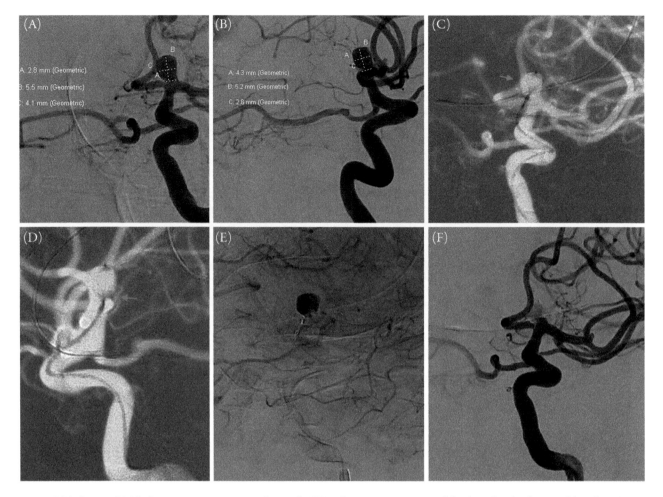

Figure 7.13 DSA showing ICA bifurcation aneurysms treated using the WEB device. Measurements of the dome height, dome width and aneurysm neck are performed on (A) antero-posterior and (B) lateral DSA. (C) Antero-posterior roadmap view showing the microcatheter and initial deployment of the WEB device (red arrow). (D) Lateral roadmap view showing final deployment of the WEB device (red arrows). (E) Showing contrast stasis following device deployment. (F) Anteroposterior control DSA showing aneurysm occlusion (red arrow).

or vasopressors. Then, a Simmons 2 Penumbra catheter is inserted into the access sheath through the radial artery all the way to the brachial artery, which is followed by sliding the guide catheter on top of the Simmons 2 catheter. A 6 envoy was brought all the way up to the internal carotid artery. Superselectively with a Via 21, the aneurysm was catheterized then embolization with WEB SL 6 × 3 was performed. Final run showed adequate placement of the WEB (Figure 7.13).

CASE 5

HISTORY AND PHYSICAL EXAMINATION

A 21-year-old man presented after having a new-onset secondary generalized tonic-clonic seizure accompanied by 30 minutes of postictal confusion. On presentation, the patient was awake, alert, and oriented ×3. He was neurologically intact on physical examination.

IMAGING STUDIES

A head CT shows a focal hyperdensity in the left temporal lobe which has a tubular configuration and may represent an arteriovenous malformation (Figure 7.14). An angiogram is performed and shows a left temporal lobe arteriovenous malformation, 2.4 × 2 × 2.3 cm with superficial venous drainage (Figure 7.15).

ANALYSIS OF CASE AND SURGICAL PLAN

Patients with brain AVM most commonly present with hemorrhage, with intraparenchymal hemorrhage being the most common followed by SAH and intraventricular hemorrhage. The second most common presentation is seizures.

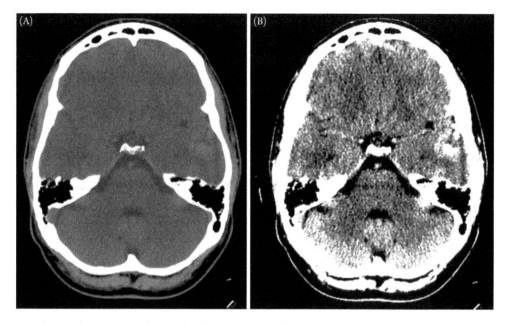

Figure 7.14 Noncontrast-enhanced brain CT scan showing focal hyperdensity in the left temporal lobe that has a tubular configuration. Both on (A) above windows and (B) below windows.

Less common presentations include headache, focal neurological deficit, and as an incidental finding.

The risks of treating unruptured brain AVMs must be weighed against the natural history of the lesion. The annual risk of first hemorrhage has been reported to be 2% to 4%.

The features most consistently associated with an increased risk for hemorrhage include deep venous drainage, a single draining vein or stenosis of the draining vein, associated aneurysms, and deep or posterior fossa locations. ARUBA (A Randomized Trial of Unruptured Brain Arteriovenous

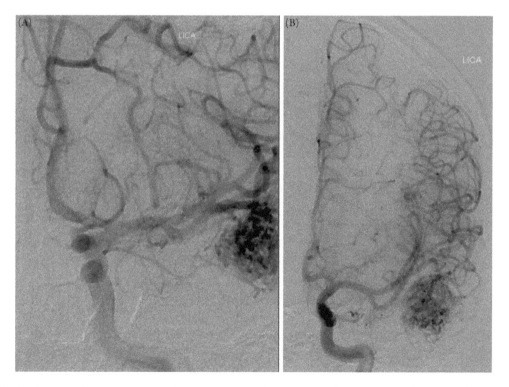

Figure 7.15 Lateral (A) and anterior (B) views on a cerebral angiogram with left internal carotid artery injection showing a 2.4 × 2 × 2.3-cm anterior pole arteriovenous malformation with superficial venous drainage and arterial feeders from the distal M3 and M4 branches.

Malformations), however, concluded that medical management alone is superior to combined medical and interventional treatment for the prevention of death or stroke in unruptured brain AVMs followed for 33 months. Longer follow-up is still required to confirm these findings.

Complete angiographic evaluation should be performed to assess the arterial supply of the AVM, the characteristics of the nidus, and identification of the venous drainage for planning the treatment strategy. AVMs demonstrate arteriovenous shunting on angiography, resulting in early opacification of the draining veins and a decrease in the arteriovenous transit time.

Definitive treatment of a brain AVM requires its complete obliteration to prevent subsequent hemorrhage. Therapeutic options include endovascular embolization, surgery, stereotactic radiosurgery, or combined therapies. Although surgical resection remains the standard for the definitive treatment of most intracranial AVMs, endovascular management can be used for presurgical embolization to improve the safety and efficacy of the procedure. Presurgical embolization can be used for large or giant cortical AVMs to reduce the blood flow within the nidus, to embolize deep and surgically inaccessible arterial feeders, or to occlude associated intranidal aneurysms. This can be achieved with low morbidity and mortality. Preoperative embolization of AVMs can reduce operative time and intraoperative blood loss, makes surgical resection easier, results in fewer postoperative neurological deficits and less postoperative epilepsy compared with surgical treatment alone, and does not present with significantly more complications than surgery alone. Presurgical embolization can also convert inoperable Spetzler-Martin high-grade lesions to lower grade AVMs that can be amenable to surgical treatment.

Endovascular management can be used for embolization of AVMs before radiosurgical treatment to reduce the nidus size. Smaller lesions (<3 cm in diameter) have a higher cure rate and a lower morbidity rate after radiosurgery. Preradiosurgical embolization may also be used to occlude arterial feeder or intranidal aneurysms to reduce the risk for hemorrhage and to target large high-flow AVMs, which are less sensitive to radiosurgery. Endovascular embolization can also be used to treat residual lesions that persist after radiosurgery.

Endovascular treatment can be employed for palliative embolization in patients with progressive or refractory neurological deficits secondary to high flow or venous hypertension and seizures. However, palliative embolization does not eliminate the risk for bleeding. Partial AVM embolization is not recommended as the only strategy for AVM management; however, it can be used as part of a treatment plan aimed at staged AVM obliteration.

Endovascular embolization can be used as the primary treatment for some AVMs for curative embolization. Several factors determine the efficacy of embolization for curative purposes. Smaller AVMs and AVMs with a low number of arterial feeders are more likely to achieve complete cure following endovascular embolization. Superficial AVMs, lesions in noneloquent locations, and those with an overall lower Spetzler-Martin grade are more likely to be cured as well.

Embolic agents used in brain AVM management consist of solid agents (e.g., coils, silk threads, balloons, and particulates such as polyvinyl alcohol) and liquids agents (e.g., cyanoacrylates, Onyx, and ethanol). The most commonly used agents are the liquid agents n-butyl cyanoacrylate (NBCA) and Onyx, which is a premixed, liquid embolic agent that consists of ethylene-vinyl alcohol copolymer and tantalum powder for radiopacity, dissolved in dimethyl sulfoxide. Onyx was preferred in this case for multiple reasons: it has a lower thrombogenicity and causes less inflammation than NBCA; it has a nonadhesive nature that decreases the risk for adherence of the catheter to the vessel wall; it allows for longer, slower, and more controlled injections with better penetration into the AVM; it offers better handling during later surgical intervention; and recent studies have demonstrated that embolization using Onyx results in complete occlusion in 50% of appropriately selected cases.

Patients are observed in the neurointensive care unit following AVM embolization. Mild hypotension may be induced for 24 hours after embolization of a large, high-flow AVM. In patients for whom the treatment plan includes other sessions, additional embolization procedures are staged every 3 to 4 weeks. Follow-up imaging is crucial for any incompletely obliterated lesion.

In the present case, initial endovascular embolization was performed for management of seizures. Because the AVM had accessible arterial feeders from the distal M3 and M4 branches, endovascular management was attempted. Two embolization sessions using Onyx resulted in angiographic cure of the AVM (Figure 7.16). For both procedures, general anesthesia was induced. The right common femoral artery was catheterized with a 7-French sheath, hooked to continuous heparinized flush. With a 6-French catheter and a guidewire, the aorta was ascended up the arch. Selectively, the left ICA was catheterized. At that point, superselectively, the M3 and M4 pedicles were microcatheterized followed by embolization using Onyx. The microcatheter was then removed. A control cerebral angiogram showed a significant decrease in the size of the AVM after the first intervention and angiographic cure

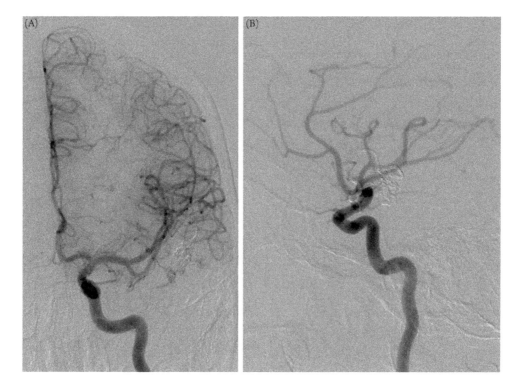

Figure 7.16 Lateral (A) and anterior (B) views on a postembolization cerebral angiogram with left internal carotid artery injection showing no evidence of an arteriovenous malformation, no clear nidus, no shunting, and no abnormal venous drainage.

after the second treatment session. Manual compression was held for 20 minutes in the right groin. The patient was neurologically intact.

COMPLICATIONS

Most complications related to AVM embolization are related to hemorrhagic and ischemic events. The combined major morbidity and mortality rates from embolization with ethylene-vinyl alcohol copolymer are quoted to be 10%. Complication rates that have been reported depend on patient selection, AVM characteristics, and agents used. Intracerebral hemorrhage can be the result of technical factors, including arterial dissection or perforation by the microwire or microcatheter, rupture of an associated aneurysm, and vascular injuries during catheter retrieval. Hemorrhage may also be the result of hemodynamic changes related to the embolization procedure, which may result in a reduction of flow through the fistulous nidus with stagnation in the draining veins. This can lead to venous outflow thrombosis and a delayed hemorrhage or a venous infarct. Embolization of large, high-flow AVMs can result in normal perfusion pressure breakthrough and hemorrhage. This is due to a sudden elevation in arterial pressure and a decrease in venous pressure, decreasing cerebral perfusion pressure in patients with impaired autoregulation.

The resulting parenchymal hyperperfusion can cause cerebral edema or hemorrhage. If a hematoma is encountered, immediate intubation, hyperventilation, osmotic diuresis, barbiturate anesthesia, and emergent surgical evacuation are indicated.

Ischemic stroke may result from arterial dissection related to microcatheter or guidewire manipulation, occlusion of normal arterial branches by the embolic agent, reflux of the embolic material into normal cerebral vasculature, and showering of glue droplets during retrieval of the microcatheter. Brain AVM embolization requires advancing a suitable microcatheter into the distal aspect of the arterial feeder to the nidus. Neurological deficits may be caused by embolization of branches arising from feeders that supply normal brain parenchyma. Provocative testing (the superselective Wada test) can be performed to determine the safety of embolization. Intraarterial injection of amobarbital through the micro-catheter placed at the site of planned embolization is performed, and appropriate neurological and neurophysiologic testing is carried out.

Pulmonary emboli are uncommon but have occurred with the use of embolic agents. Complications such as groin hematoma or dissection and other complications related to endovascular intervention such as contrast allergy, infection, and nephrotoxicity may occur as well.

HISTORY AND
PHYSICAL EXAMINATION

A 77-year-old man with a history of hypertension and hyperlipidemia presents with a right-sided hemiplegia and aphasia. The patient was last seen normal 5 hours ago. On neurologic examination, the patient has global aphasia and is not following commands. Cranial nerves are notable for left gaze preference and right facial weakness. Motor strength is notable for antigravity spontaneously in the left upper and lower extremity, 3/5 in the right upper and 2/5 in the right lower extremity. The National Institutes of Health Stroke Scale score is 22.

IMAGING STUDIES

Non–contrast-enhanced head CT shows loss of gray-white differentiation within the left insular ribbon consistent with early left MCA territory infarct, without evidence of hemorrhage (Figure 7.17). CTA shows focal tapering cutoff of the left ICA just distal to the bifurcation (Figure 7.18). The left ICA reconstitutes intracranially at the level of the left posterior communicating artery. Focal cutoff of the left MCA at the proximal M1 segment, with no significant

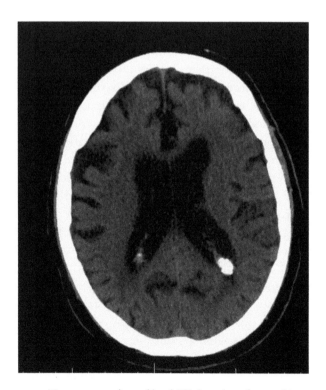

Figure 7.17 Noncontrast-enhanced head CT shows loss of gray–white differentiation within the left insular ribbon consistent and early left middle cerebral artery territory infarct, without hemorrhage.

opacification of distal MCA branches, is seen. CT perfusion shows increased mean transit time (Figure 7.19) and decreased cerebral blood flow (Figure 7.20) involving nearly the entire left MCA territory, with a smaller area of decreased cerebral blood volume (Figure 7.21).

ANALYSIS OF CASE AND
SURGICAL PLAN

Given the narrow therapeutic window for treatment of acute ischemic stroke, timely evaluation and diagnosis are vital. The initial evaluation of a potential stroke patient begins with immediate stabilization of the airway, breathing, and circulation. This is quickly followed by an assessment of neurological deficits and possible comorbidities. Emergency non–contrast-enhanced head CT is recommended before initiating any specific therapy to treat acute ischemic stroke to exclude intracerebral hemorrhage. Laboratory tests to consider in all patients include blood glucose, electrolytes with renal function studies, complete blood count with platelet count, cardiac markers, prothrombin time, international normalized ratio, and activated partial thromboplastin time. Intravenous fibrinolytic therapy with r-tPA (0.9 mg/kg, maximal dose 90 mg) is recommended in patients presenting within 4.5 hours of onset of ischemic stroke and should not be delayed while awaiting coagulation studies unless a coagulopathy is suspected.

Timely brain imaging and interpretation are critical. A noninvasive intracranial vascular study (CTA, MRA) should be performed during initial imaging if either intra-arterial fibrinolysis or mechanical thrombectomy is being considered to evaluate the size, location, and vascular distribution of the infarction and document the presence of large-vessel occlusion. CT perfusion and MRI perfusion and diffusion imaging provide measures of infarct core and penumbra size to evaluate the degree of reversibility of ischemic injury. They play an important role in the selection of patients with "salvageable" tissue for acute reperfusion therapy. A scan consistent with a mismatch between cerebral blood volume and cerebral blood flow or mean transient time is a favorable patient selection criterion. Stroke imaging should not delay intravenous r-tPA therapy.

Mechanical thrombectomy devices seek to salvage ischemic but not yet fully infarcted brain tissue by restoring perfusion through the occluded artery. It can be used as a primary reperfusion strategy or in conjunction with pharmacologic fibrinolysis. It is most effective when performed as early as possible. The initial goal of mechanical thrombectomy is to achieve recanalization, defined by a Thrombolysis in Cerebral Infarction (TICI) grade of 2b (complete filling

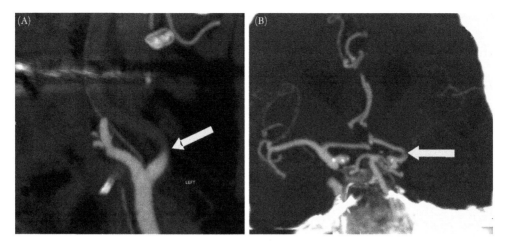

Figure 7.18 A: Computed tomographic angiogram shows focal tapering cutoff of the left ICA just distal to the bifurcation (arrow). The left ICA reconstitutes intracranially at the level of the left posterior communicating artery. B: Focal cutoff of the left MCA at the proximal M1 segment (arrow), with no significant opacification of distal MCA branches.

of all of the expected vascular territory is visualized but the filling is slower than normal) or 3 (complete perfusion).

Mechanical thrombectomy should be considered in patients with neuroimaging excluding hemorrhage, with a small infarct core (patients with large territorial infarcts on CT scan are at a higher risk for hemorrhagic conversion following treatment) and large artery occlusion in the proximal anterior circulation, as demonstrated on CTA, MRA, or DSA. Mechanical thrombectomy should not prevent the initiation of intravenous thrombolysis when indicated. If intravenous thrombolysis is contraindicated, mechanical thrombectomy should be considered as first-line treatment if the patient is eligible. Mechanical thrombectomy should be performed as soon as possible and within 8 hours of

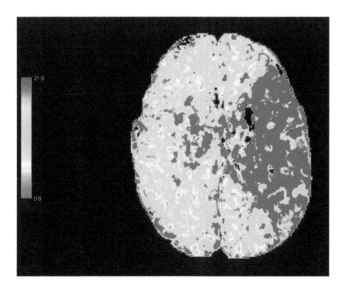

Figure 7.19 There is increased mean transit time involving nearly the entire left middle cerebral artery territory, with sparing of a small portion of the left basal ganglia.

stroke symptom onset when indicated. The decision to proceed with mechanical thrombectomy should be made by a multidisciplinary team and performed by an experienced neurointerventionalist in centers providing comprehensive stroke care.

There are currently many mechanical thrombectomy devices. The Penumbra system (Penumbra, Alameda, California) is an aspiration device that employs vacuum aspiration to remove the thrombus from the occluded vessel. The Solitaire device™ (Medtronic, Irvine, California) the Trevo® device (Stryker, Fremont, California) and the Embotrap® device (Cerenovus, Johnson and Johnson, New Jersey) are stent-retriever devices that employ a self-expanding stent deployed within the thrombus, pushing it aside and incorporating it within the stent's struts followed by extraction of the thrombus. Intraarterial treatment with mechanical thrombectomy reduces disability, improves outcomes and functional independence, and is superior to intravenous thrombolysis alone in eligible patients with proximal large artery occlusions in the anterior circulation. Second-generation stent-retriever devices seem to have the best safety and efficacy profiles. For this reason, the Solitaire flow-restoration device was used in the present case.

Acute interventions are most commonly performed under general anesthesia to improve procedural safety and efficacy. Femoral access is established in the symptomatic lower extremity, if possible. An angiogram is performed for a detailed examination of the cerebrovascular anatomy and to note any proximal stenosis or occlusion. Proximal vessel disease may require immediate treatment with balloon angioplasty or stenting, or both, to allow access to the intracranial pathology. Patients are

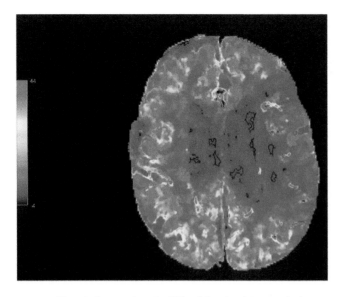

Figure 7.20 There is decreased cerebral blood flow involving nearly the entire left MCA territory, with sparing of a small portion of the left basal ganglia.

admitted to the neurointensive care or stroke unit after treatment with monitoring of hemodynamic and neurological status.

This patient was treated using the Solitaire device. Bilateral groins were prepared and draped in a sterile fashion. With a Seldinger technique, the right femoral artery was catheterized with a 6-French sheath hooked to a continuous heparinized flush. A guidewire and a catheter were introduced into the descending aorta up to the arch. Selectively, the left ICA was catheterized showing an M1 occlusion. Superselectively, the M2 was catheterized.

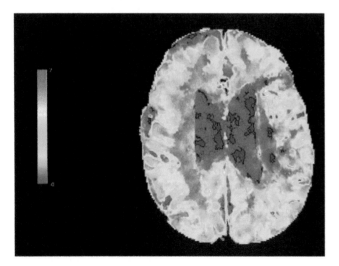

Figure 7.21 There is a much smaller area of decreased cerebral blood volume involving a portion of the left basal ganglia, left corona radiata, and insular cortex, extending into the left anterior temporal lobe. In the more peripheral left MCA territory, there is normal to increased cerebral blood volume.

Mechanical thrombectomy with Solitaire was then performed. TICI grade 3 recanalization was achieved after two passes (Figure 7.22, before mechanical thrombectomy; Figure 7.23, after thrombectomy). The patient had an excellent recovery and had a modified Rankin scale score of 2 at the 3-month follow-up.

COMPLICATIONS

Mechanical thrombectomy for acute ischemic stroke is associated with several risks. Symptomatic intracerebral hemorrhage occurs in 10% of patients with first-generation Merci and Penumbra devices but is substantially lower with stent-retriever devices (2% to 6%). A head CT can be obtained after the endovascular procedure. In patients with asymptomatic and small hemorrhages, conservative treatment is warranted (heparin reversal, fresh frozen plasma and platelet transfusion, tight blood pressure control). In patients with symptomatic and significant hemorrhage, medical measures, intubation, mannitol, ventriculostomy (in the case of

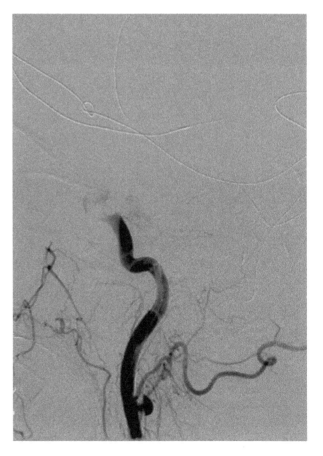

Figure 7.22 Cerebral angiogram with left ICA injection shows an M1 occlusion.

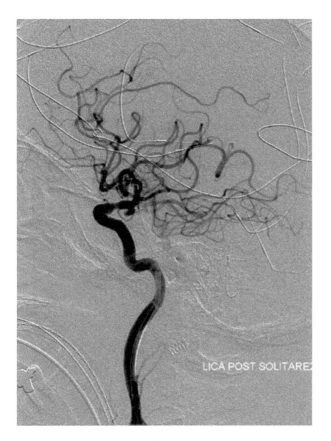

Figure 7.23 Cerebral angiogram with left ICA artery injection after mechanical thrombectomy with the Solitaire device™ shows resolution of the occlusion with a thrombolysis in cerebral infarction grade 3 recanalization.

symptomatic hydrocephalus), and craniotomy for clot evacuation should be considered.

Trauma to the vessel wall can arise from endovascular manipulation resulting in permanent vascular injury, vessel rupture, and SAH. This is especially of concern in old, friable vessels.

Fragmentation of the target thrombus during clot removal may result in embolization of dislodged clot material to the distal circulation, resulting in additional ischemic threats.

REFERENCES

1. Berkhemer OA, Fransen PS, Beumer D, et al. A randomized trial of intraarterial treatment for acute ischemic stroke. *N Engl J Med.* 2015;372(1):11–20.
2. Connolly ES Jr, Rabinstein AA, Carhuapoma JR, et al. Guidelines for the management of aneurysmal subarachnoid hemorrhage: a guideline for healthcare professionals from the American Heart Association/American Stroke Association. *Stroke.* 2012;43(6):1711–1737.
3. Gory B, Spiotta AM, Mangiafico S, et al. PulseRider stent-assisted coiling of wide-neck bifurcation aneurysms: periprocedural results in an international series. *Am J Neuroradiol.* 2016;37(1):130–135.
4. Maldonado IL, Bonafé A. Stent-assisted techniques for intracranial aneurysms. In: Murai Y, ed. *Aneurysm.* London: IntechOpen, 2012. https://www.intechopen.com/books/aneurysm/stent-assisted-techniques-for-intracranial-aneurysms. Accessed June 16, 2019.
5. Molyneux AJ, Kerr RS, Yu LM, et al. International subarachnoid aneurysm trial (ISAT) of neurosurgical clipping versus endovascular coiling in 2143 patients with ruptured intracranial aneurysms: a randomised comparison of effects on survival, dependency, seizures, rebleeding, subgroups, and aneurysm occlusion. *Lancet.* 2005;366(9488):809–817.
6. Morgan MK, Davidson AS, Koustais S, Simons M, Ritson EA. The failure of preoperative ethylene-vinyl alcohol copolymer embolization to improve outcomes in arteriovenous malformation management: case series. *J Neurosurg.* 2013;118(5):969–977.
7. UCAS Japan Investigators, Morita A, Kirino T, et al. The natural course of unruptured cerebral aneurysms in a Japanese cohort. *N Engl J Med.* 2012;366(26):2474–2482.
8. Ogilvy CS, Stieg PE, Awad I, et al. Recommendations for the management of intracranial arteriovenous malformations: a statement for healthcare professionals from a special writing group of the Stroke Council, American Stroke Association. *Circulation.* 2001;103(21):2644–2657.
9. Saver JL, Jahan R, Levy EI, et al. Solitaire flow restoration device versus the Merci Retriever in patients with acute ischaemic stroke (SWIFT): a randomised, parallel-group, non-inferiority trial. *Lancet.* 2012;380(9849):1241–1249.
10. Starke RM, Komotar RJ, Otten ML, et al. Adjuvant embolization with N-butyl cyanoacrylate in the treatment of cerebral arteriovenous malformations: outcomes, complications, and predictors of neurologic deficits. *Stroke.* 2009;40(8):2783–2790.
11. Thompson BG, Brown RD Jr, Amin-Hanjani S, et al. Guidelines for the management of patients with unruptured intracranial aneurysms: a guideline for healthcare professionals from the American Heart Association/American Stroke Association. *Stroke.* 2015;46(8):2368–2400.
12. Wiebers DO, Whisnant JP, Huston J 3rd, et al. Unruptured intracranial aneurysms: natural history, clinical outcome, and risks of surgical and endovascular treatment. *Lancet.* 2003;362(9378):103–110.

8.

CRANIAL TRAUMA AND ICU MANAGEMENT

Gary Simonds

Head injury is a commonly encountered disorder in neurosurgery and is felt by some to be relatively limited in its technical challenges. By rights, head trauma cases should therefore be straightforward opportunities to pick up steam in the general section of the examination. The more command the test-taker has over a subject, the more confidence he or she will build and store for perhaps more challenging questions. It is therefore wise to review and master the subject in preparation. I would advise paying particular attention to published head injury guidelines.[1] Remember that these are subject to modification every so many years, so check them out online rather than in a textbook. If you are taking the focused practice component of the exam in the realm of Trauma and Critical Care, there will likely be some further but perhaps more complicated (multisystem injury, comorbidities, refractory pathologies) head injury cases mixed in with considerably more general critical care issues. Know the pathophysiology and medical management of the major neurological illnesses (including stroke) and of the major comorbidities and complicating disorders such as hypertension, infection, lung dysfunction, cardiac ischemia, acid-base imbalance, shock, diabetes, heart failure, renal dysfunction, nontraumatic coma, associated injuries, and so on—basically anything you were called about as a resident when you were covering an intensive care unit (ICU). In this chapter, we will focus predominantly on the neurosurgical side of the cases but throw in some critical care questions and complications for those focusing on Trauma and Critical Care (marked by an *). When preparing for the exam, I would advise practicing answering questions aloud and describing any surgery you might do in detail, all the while contemplating the many associated complications that might occur. Articulating your answers aloud will make this rather foreign and artificial experience more familiar and less anxiety provoking when you get to the actual examination. Consider describing the surgical portion of your response as you would in an operative dictation. If this becomes too tedious for the examiners, they will "fast-forward" you to another stage of the case.

CASE 1

HISTORY AND PHYSICAL EXAMINATION

A previously healthy 18-year-old woman is involved in a motor vehicle collision in which she is thrown through a windshield at high speed and sustains multiple trauma. She arrives by helicopter intubated. She has significant facial trauma and swelling. She is in a coma. Her best motor response is reported to be decorticate. Her right pupil is dilated and unresponsive. Her left pupil is normal and responsive to light and she has a brisk corneal response.

IMAGING STUDIES

Right pneumothorax and several fractured ribs are seen on the chest x-ray.

ANALYSIS OF CASE AND SURGICAL PLAN

Stop for a moment, take a deep breath, and think! This may not be a surgical case at all. No surgical lesions have been given to you, although you are concerned about the dilated right pupil. This might be a closed head injury management question. If part of the focused practice exam, perhaps they want you to think about lung injury, hemopericardium, abdominal injury, shock, and so on. Do not run to the operating room quite yet—start with the basics. We know that airway and breathing are controlled, but what is the blood pressure? 80/40 mm Hg. Heart rate is 120 beats/minute. So first things first—this patient needs to be resuscitated, and you might mention we have not ruled out a spinal cord injury, although this does not sound like spinal shock because of the elevated heart rate.

The trauma team gives her 2 liters of lactated Ringer's solution and places a chest tube, and her vital signs respond well. Laboratory tests including a toxin and pregnancy screen are requested. The trauma team performs a survey, and you evaluate for any other neurological findings, but they are obfuscated by sedatives and paralyzing agents. Next stop then would be a computed tomography (CT) scan of the brain as part of the CT trauma survey, which will include chest, abdomen, and pelvis, as well as cervical, thoracic, and lumbar imaging. The mechanism of injury and lack of an obtainable spinal cord neurological examination warrant the latter studies. Major concomitant injury is probably unlikely due to her rapid response to simple resuscitation but keep it in mind nonetheless. Please do get the spine imaging; we were confronted with this very case this past week, and the patient had a horrific T6-T7 fracture dislocation.

CT of the brain shows scattered deep white matter punctate hemorrhages with no mass lesions or mass effect. Cisterns are "tight." The right orbit shows multiple fractures (Figures 8.1). Direct trauma to the globe or optic nerve may explain the dilated pupil rather than a cranial nerve III palsy. The CT scans of the chest, abdomen, and spine are "unremarkable."

SAMPLE QUESTIONS AND REASONABLE ANSWERS

What do you want to do next?

I would like to make sure the patient goes to an ICU and is stabilized (no hypotension or hypoxia), and I would like to place a right frontal ventriculostomy for intracranial pressure (ICP) measurement and control. The patient thus far has a Glasgow Coma Scale (GCS) of less than 8 and an abnormal CT of the head. Guidelines (IIb level evidence) suggests that employment of ICP monitoring decreases 2-week and in-hospital mortality of this type of patient.[1]

Why not a simple parenchymal ICP monitor?

Guidelines do not necessarily favor the use of ventriculostomy in patients with severe closed head injury (no Level I or II evidence) but ventriculostomies allow for cerebrospinal fluid (CSF) drainage to assist in ICP control. They also can be readily recalibrated—allowing ICP monitoring without the inherent "drift" that parenchymal systems are prone to. Prolonged use of a ventricular catheter is relatively well tolerated with low incidence of infection, particularly since the introduction of antibiotic impregnated catheters. Guidelines do favor continuous CSF drainage over intermittent, but the evidence is weak (Level III only).[1]

Why didn't you use advanced cerebral monitoring such as PtiO2 or SjvO2?

At our institution, we have not found such methods improved our outcomes. There is currently no Level I or II evidence to support their employment although it has been suggested (Level II evidence) that patients with desaturation have poorer outcomes.[1]

*What is angular acceleration with reference to head injury?

Head injury victims may be subjected to a number (and mix) of forces in a traumatic incident. If the head is

Case 1 - DAI

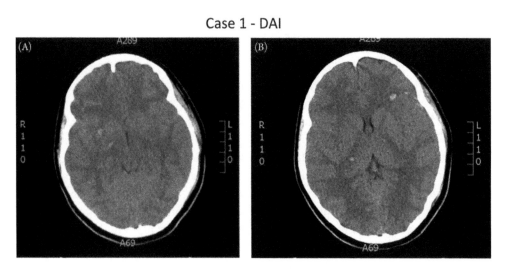

Figure 8.1 A and B. Noncontrast CT scan of the brain in an 18-year-old in coma status post motor vehicle accident.

subjected to linear acceleration-deceleration, the brain moves within the head linearly and can collide with the surrounding skull. This can result in contusions of the poles at various surfaces but unless the forces are extreme leaves the bulk of the brain without too much injury. Angular acceleration (a.k.a. rotational acceleration) means the head is rapidly turned on its axis. Because of differentials in brain density, this can result in a "wringing" motion of the cerebrum on the brainstem, stretching, damaging, and tearing millions of axons. This can result in the diffuse injury of neurons throughout the brain with terrible sequelae, and this is known as diffuse axonal injury. Someone thrown through a car windshield at high velocity is subjected to all sorts of horrific forces in combination.

The ICP is 44 mm Hg. What do you want to do?

I would like to initiate a series of maneuvers and interventions to bring the ICP to below 20 mm Hg if at all possible. These would include raising the head of the bed, assuring no constriction around the neck with the head in a neutral position, CSF drainage, sedating lightly to prevent Valsalva maneuver and coughing (fighting the endotracheal tube), administering judicious intravenous fluids with no free water or dilute solutes (use, for example, Normal Saline), and considering employment of concentrated (hypertonic) saline or mannitol. Although guidelines do not offer a specific recommendation here (no Level I, II, or III evidence) I generally use intermittent mannitol and/or 3% saline when the ICP will not respond to other measures—INTERRUPTION (this is common).

Should you hyperventilate the patient?

No, particularly in the early stages of injury (first 24 hours) this would be contraindicated (Level III evidence). If no other measures were working and we were headed toward a more aggressive intervention such as barbiturate coma or surgery, guidelines weakly support its employment as a temporizer (Level III evidence) but recommend against prolonged prophylactic use (Level IIB evidence).[1]

Why not?

Hyperventilation lowers Paco2 which results in vasoconstriction and may contribute to further local and regional injury of the traumatized brain. The head-injured patient appears to be particularly vulnerable during the first 24 hours after the trauma (Level III evidence).[1]

Should you "dry the patient out" with diuretics?

No, although diuretics may indeed lower ICP, they also create a hypovolemic state which may compromise perfusion of damaged regions of the brain as well as contribute to cardiovascular instability.

Should you give anticonvulsants?

I generally would, although this is debatable. Acute use of anticonvulsants in traumatic brain injury will lower the chances of early seizures but will not lower the rate of late or downstream seizures. Guidelines do not currently recommend this (insufficient evidence). Anticonvulsants may certainly have side effects. I generally administer 1000 mg of Keppra (Levetiracetam) twice daily in the acute phase of severe brain injury, although there is currently insufficient evidence to recommend over phenytoin.[1]

*What is the action of Keppra?

Keppra binds to a synaptic vesical protein SV2A and presumably alters neurotransmitter release, but the effect of this activity is not well understood.

*What is nonconvulsive status epilepticus (NCSE)?

A continuous epileptic condition without convulsive manifestations lasting more than 10 minutes.[2]

*What is comatose-NCSE?

Periodic or continuous epileptic/rhythmic discharges without convulsive motor movements. Minor motor manifestations may be seen. The condition may contribute to a diminished level of consciousness. It may be difficult to distinguish from typical electroencephalogram (EEG) findings in a patient with coma.

*What are typical EEG findings of a patient in coma?

Diffuse polymorphic delta activity, burst suppression, spindles and sleep-like patterns, alpha/theta coma patterns, prolonged bursts of slow-wave activity, periodic ictal and rhythmic discharges, periodic lateralized epileptiform discharges.[2]

Ictal patterns with typical spatiotemporal evolution or epileptiform discharges faster than 2.5 Hz. Rhythmic delta activity. Fluctuation. Response to antiepileptic medications. Subtle motor manifestations concomitant with EEG findings.[2]

What cerebral perfusion pressure (CPP) do you aim for in a patient with a severe CHI?

Guidelines support the use of managing CPP to lower 2-week mortality.[1] If possible, I would like to get the CPP to the 60 to 70 mm Hg range (Level IIb evidence).[1] Aggressively pushing CPP above 70 mm Hg may increase the risk of respiratory failure (Level II evidence).[1]

How much dexamethasone (Decadron) will you give?

Steroids are contraindicated in the care of patients with severe closed head injuries (Level I evidence).[1] I would not use any. The CRASH study demonstrated a significant increase in 2-week mortality, worse outcomes at 6 months, and no demonstrable benefit after a 48-hour infusion of methylprednisolone after closed head injury. [3]

COMPLICATIONS

ICPs are well controlled for a day and you are called because they suddenly have shot back up into the high 40s. What do you want to do?

I would evaluate the patient and make sure the ventriculostomy is working and is calibrated correctly. I would look for straightforward reasons for the elevation (e.g., neck kinked, low sodium/hypervolemic, hypoventilation, seizure, coughing and Valsalva, etc.). I would evaluate the neurological status for new lateralizing findings that might indicate a developing expanding intracranial lesion. I would initiate ICP lowering administrations. If I did not have a readily identifiable and reversible reason, I would take the patient to CT to rule out a new mass lesion.

CT scan shows that a good 1 cm of your ventricular catheter is in the left thalamus. What should you do?

If the catheter is working well with good CSF access and waveforms, I would leave it in.

You also see a 2-centimeter hematoma around the catheter in the right frontal lobe. What should you do?

If the ICP is well controlled, I would leave the hematoma alone and follow it. If the ICP is uncontrollable, I might consider evacuation as a component of a decompressive craniectomy.

*What is the evidence supporting your decompressive craniectomy?

Well, to be frank, it is not overwhelming. The RESCUEicp Decompressive Craniectomy Trial demonstrated that 6-month mortality was reduced, but long-term vegetative state rates were increased.[4] Guidelines recommend against bifrontal craniectomies for the sake of improving 6-month outcomes, even though it does help control ICPs and lessen days in the ICU (Level IA evidence).[1] The long and short of it is that a long discussion would be necessary with family members prior to engaging in such an intervention.

*Under what circumstances would the pneumothorax be of concern?

If a pneumothorax is large enough or is continuing to expand as a "tension pneumothorax," ventilation and oxygenation may be affected. If severe, cardiac function may be compromised and there may be a cardiovascular collapse.

*When is the diagnosis suspected in a traumatic coma patient?

Physical exam may be suggestive to include decreased breath sounds and jugular venous distention. Ventilator alarms may be triggered reference increased resistance (increased airway pressure) and the patient may demonstrate hypotension, tachycardia and hypoxia. Any of these findings should trigger immediate x-ray and/or CT evaluation.

CASE 2

HISTORY AND PHYSICAL EXAMINATION

A previously healthy 19-year-old man is involved in a motor vehicle collision in which he is thrown through a windshield at high speed and sustains multiple traumas. At your center, he undergoes a full trauma evaluation and resuscitation. He is in a coma with symmetrical flexor posturing

Case 2- DAI

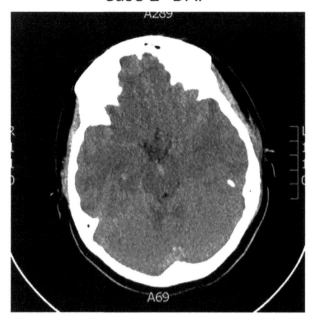

Figure 8.2 Noncontrast CT scan of the brain in a 19-year-old coma status post a motor vehicle accident.

to noxious stimuli. CT scan of the brain shows scattered deep white matter petechial hemorrhages, "tight cisterns," and no space-occupying lesions or shift (Figure 8.2). CT scans of the spine are normal. In the ICU, a ventriculostomy was placed. ICPs were in the 40 mm Hg range, and your team has struggled to lower the ICP using positioning, CSF drainage, sedation with propofol and low-dose pentobarbital, hypertonic saline, and even some limited hyperventilation to no avail. The EEG shows slowing but no seizure activity. ICP is 45 mm Hg, CPP is 60 mm Hg, serum sodium level is 152, Pco2 is 34. A repeat CT scan of the brain is performed. What do you want to do next?

IMAGING STUDIES

The CT scan of the brain is essentially unchanged from the original with only a small amount of "blossoming" (expansion) of petechial hemorrhages. A ventricular catheter sits in the appropriate position in the right frontal horn of the lateral ventricles.

ANALYSIS OF CASE AND TREATMENT PLAN

This is an example of a case for which there is no definitive single answer to the problem. There is no class I or II evidence to guide your answer. There is evidence that argues for *and* against surgical intervention (see previous case). *Do*

not play a game of guessing what the examiners are thinking! Put yourself in the situation described, and go ahead with what you would do in your institution and be prepared to defend it. Resorting to "barbiturate coma" (pentobarbital 10 mg/kg load over 30 minutes, then 5 mg/kg/hr × 3 doses, then 1 mg/kg per hour) with burst-suppression EEG (or serum levels of 3–4 mg%) would be a viable alternative to surgery. At our institution, we have had a somewhat light trigger to go to decompressive craniectomy—particularly in young patients without evidence of associated severe hypoxic injury. From here, the most appropriate type of craniectomy also is not well delineated. We tend to perform a very large hemicraniectomy (Guidelines recommend at least 12 × 15 × 15 cm by Level IIA evidence),[1] when one side has a preponderance of contusions or extra-axial hematoma and/or mass effect. If there is pretty equivalent bilateral diffuse swelling, we still might employ a large bifrontal craniectomy. No matter your choice, be prepared to describe the procedure "from skin to skin."

SAMPLE QUESTIONS AND REASONABLE ANSWERS
So what do you want to do?

I think we are failing to control ICPs with aggressive maneuvers, although we are maintaining a good CPP. With this young patient who was originally flexor on examination, I would resort to decompressive craniectomy to assist in ICP control.

Why not try "pentobarbital coma"?

Guidelines support the use of "barbiturate coma" for elevated ICPs refractory to medical and surgical therapy—but not for prophylaxis (Level IIB evidence).[1] I think barbiturate coma is an option and can be quite effective in lowering ICP, but it depresses functions throughout the body and can lead to significant systemic complications. It also might delay definitive ICP reduction through craniectomy. Furthermore, it completely obfuscates the neurologic examination,—often for a prolonged period. Craniectomy will usually lower ICP to acceptable levels immediately allowing for earlier assessment of examination.

What kind of craniectomy do you plan?

With neither side of the brain bearing the brunt of contusions and no substantial extra-axial collections, I would perform a bifrontal decompressive craniectomy with duraplasties.

I would transfer the patient to the operating room and position the patient supine with the table in reverse Trendelenberg. After an appropriate "prep and drape," I would initiate a full time-out—INTERRUPTION (Note: It is good to be very descriptive about your procedures, but be prepared for the examiner to cut you off and "fast forward" you to the components of the procedure he or she wants to hear.)

What kind of incision will you make and where will you place your burr holes?

I would make a bicoronal incision behind the coronal suture and reflect the scalp anteriorly down to the orbital rims. I usually place burr holes 2 cm behind the coronal suture on either side of midline and anteriorly above the orbital rims. I also may place a single burr hole bilaterally 2 to 3 cm below the temporalis insertion over the temporal fossa. (You will have a model to demonstrate these locations.)

Okay, then what do you do?

I will use a Penfield dissector #3 to separate the dura from the skull, particularly over the sagittal sinus. I will then raise a single craniotomy flap using a side-cutting drill with a foot plate. When the flap is raised, I will pass it off for deep freezing. I will then open the dura in a cruciate fashion, flapping one component toward the sagittal sinus. I will evaluate the brain for lesions that could be evacuated such as a discrete hematoma or obviously necrotic brain as well as obtaining meticulous hemostasis. I will then use a dural substitute to cover the exposed brain and lightly re-reflect the patient's own dura over it. Usually, I place bilateral subdural drains and bring them out of distant stab incisions posteriorly. I then close the scalp in multiple layers.

How far behind the coronal suture is the motor strip?

Approximately 5 cm.

On the head surface, where approximately is the sylvian fissure?

Along a line from the lateral canthus to a point three-fourths of the way along a line from the nasion to the inion. (Note: this type of question is not "make or break" for the exam—but could come up as a probe of your knowledge depth.)

Where is the angular gyrus?

Just above the pinna.

COMPLICATIONS

You make your craniotomy and you notice you entered the frontal sinus. What do you do?

If it is a small opening and the mucosa is intact, I would use bone wax to seal it. If it is a large opening with torn mucosa, I would have to exenterate it, pack the ostia with temporalis muscle, eventually flap a pedicle-based pericranial flap over it, and seal it with fibrin glue.

In raising your craniotomy flap, you see profound bleeding from the sagittal sinus. How do you handle this?

I would ask for greater reverse Trendelenberg positioning and apply gentle compression over the sinus with sheets of thrombin soaked Gelfoam and large Cottonoid pads. If this controlled the bleeding, I would inspect for large rents.

Anesthesiology reports a drop in the end tidal CO2 and hypoxia, what do you suspect?

A possible air embolus.

What are some other manifestations of air embolus in this setting?

Increased end tidal nitrogen and $PaCO_2$. If severe, hypotension, tachycardia, cardiac arrhythmia, and potential cardiovascular collapse.

What is heard in an esophageal stethoscope?

A "mill-wheel" murmur.

What should you do?

Lower the head of the bed, flood the field with saline, and pack the wound with saline-soaked sponges, wax bone edges.

How much embolized air is fatal?

It has been estimated to be in the 200 to 300 cc range (approximately 3–4 cc/kg).

Turn off any nitrous oxide. Give 100% oxygen. If a central line is in place, aspirate the air. Give volume. Support blood pressure. Consider jugular compression. Consider left lateral decubitus position if possible.

What if you open your dura and initially the brain appears relatively relaxed, but as you are preparing to close the brain, it suddenly starts swelling?

I would ask for increased reverse Trendelenberg positioning. I would ask the anesthesiologist if something had changed significantly on their side. Are we ventilating appropriately? Is there a kink in the endotracheal tube? What are the end tidal Po_2 and Pco_2? Is the patient fully anesthetized? I would ask for some hyperventilation and 25 g of mannitol. I would inspect the brain for evidence of regional extra-axial or intraparenchymal bleeding. We could even inspect using an ultrasound.

Actually, your patient does well, and the ICPs immediately come under good control, until the next morning when the nurse calls you and states that the ICPs are up in the 50s. What will you do?

I would evaluate the patient immediately. I would make sure the ICP monitor was functioning appropriately. Raise the head of the bed, make sure there is no kinking or compression of the neck, make sure the ventilator is working appropriately, and make sure the patient is ventilating well. Initiate ICP control measures, remove any potentially constrictive head wraps, and feel the decompression flap for fullness. If there were no obvious explanations, I would obtain a stat CT scan of the head.

*Five days post-op, the patient declines in what was an improving neurological status, is febrile, and demonstrates a CSF profile highly suspicious for meningitis/ventriculitis. What antibiotic therapy should you initiate?

Barring drug sensitivities and other contraindications, I would initiate a regimen that would include Vancomycin (15–20 mg/kg intravenous [IV] 8 to 12 hours), an antipseudomonal beta-lactam such as Ceftazidime, Cefepime, or Meropenem.[5,6]

*What type of organisms are you trying to cover?

Postoperative meningitis tends to see a much greater percentage of gram negative bacilli, Staph Aureus, and other Staphlococcal species than community-acquired meningitis.[5,6]

*How does prophylactic antibiotics affect the preponderance of organisms found in postoperative meningitis?

Without prophylactic antibiotics, the majority of species tend to be skin flora. With prophylactic antibiotics, enteric organisms become more common.[5,6]

*If Meropenem and beta-lactams are contraindicated in the patient, what additional antibiotic would you employ?

Aztreonam (2 gm IV q 6–8 hrs) or ciprofloxacin (400 mg IV Q 8–12 hrs).[5,6]

CASE 3

HISTORY AND
PHYSICAL EXAMINATION

A previously healthy 21-year-old man is in your trauma bay with a gunshot wound to the head. Preliminary trauma evaluation and resuscitation have been completed. He is intubated. There is a small round scalp wound in the right forehead and a ragged laceration in the right parietal occipital region with bone fragments and brain material in the adjacent hair. There is no active bleeding. The patient does not open his eyes or follow commands but does reach toward noxious stimulus with the right hand. He is hemiplegic on the left. The right pupil is dilated and unreactive, and the left pupillary function is normal.

IMAGING STUDIES

CT scan of the brain demonstrates a 2.5-cm diameter holo-hemispheric right subdural hematoma with mass effect and 3 cm of midline shift. There are some scattered contusion and boney fragments along a track through the high right hemisphere (Figure 8.3).

ANALYSIS OF CARE AND
TREATMENT PLAN

Management of gunshot wounds to the brain is controversial and will vary between institutions. Patients with a very low GCS and bihemispheric injuries, and/or very low projectile trajectories are often treated expectantly. However, this is a case that really leads to a surgical solution. The examiners likely want to hear your surgical management and are presenting you with a young patient who has a

Case 3- GSW with SDH

Case 3 GSW w/ SDH

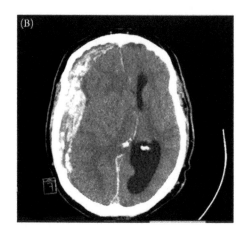

Figure 8.3 A and B. Noncontrast CT scan of the brain in a 21-year-old who sustained a gunshot wound to the head. Not shown: slices of the right brain that show scattered contusion and boney fragments along a track in the high right hemisphere, no retained bullet.

large space-occupying hematoma, and is likely herniating, yet is still localizing, and whose injury is predominately contained to the nondominant hemisphere—it is well supported to go to surgery.[7]

In gunshot wounds to the head, initial medical maneuvers are similar to those for severe closed head injury: elevate the head of bed, ventilate, use judicious amounts of higher osmolarity fluids, consider mannitol and hypertonic saline, and keep the neck unrestricted. Entry and exit wounds should be shaved and inspected. Bleeding should be controlled. In this case, the patient should be rapidly prepared for surgery. Remember, there will be no single correct way to perform the surgery—describe the surgery as you would perform it if you had to at your institution.

SAMPLE QUESTIONS AND REASONABLE ANSWERS

So what do you want to do?

I would make sure the patient is stabilized and resuscitated working with my trauma colleagues as quickly as possible and would head emergently to the operating room for surgical decompression of the hematoma and debridement of the gunshot wounds.

Where would you make your incision and craniotomy?

I would perform a large trauma flap. This would entail a large right fronto-temporal-parietal question mark shaped incision that would be flapped anteriorly with the temporalis musculature. (Remember: you will have a model of the head to demonstrate this.) The incision would either include or incorporate the posterior scalp laceration from the bullet. I would make burr holes in the "key point," in the temporal fossa just above the zygoma and far posteriorly in the parietal region. I would raise as large a fronto-temporal-parietal craniotomy flap as possible from the burr holes, approaching to within 1.5 cm of the midline.

You evacuate the hematoma and control bleeding. What do you do about the bullet track?

I would inspect the entry and exit sites in the brain. I would debride clearly macerated, pulped, devitalized tissue and any easily accessible foreign material (bone, etc.) at these sites and evacuate any sizable coalesced contusions or hematomas but would not aggressively pursue the track deep into the brain or try to debride every fleck of skull from its depths.

Why not?

Aggressive debridement of the track and small skull fragments has not been shown to lower infection rates and may damage viable tissue or precipitate bleeding in difficult to access depths. Outcomes of aggressive debridement have generally been less than optimal.[7]

What if there were a large fragment of bullet three-fourths of the way through the track?

There is some argument to remove large, readily accessible bullet fragments because of propensity to migrate.

Will you replace the bone flap?

Generally, I do not. Aggressive decompressive craniectomy was shown to be of benefit in military gunshot wounds to the head, although it may be of less benefit in lower-velocity civilian cases. Gunshot wounds are prone to postoperative swelling and increased ICP. I therefore usually perform the procedure as a decompressive craniectomy and place a ventriculostomy for postoperative ICP monitoring.

What is the difference between a high-velocity and low-velocity bullet wound to the brain?

Low-velocity bullets injure the most immediate tissue to their track through direct mechanical trauma (tearing, contusing). High-velocity rounds cause direct injury as well but also cause distant injury through shock waves and cavitation. Thus brain injury is generally far more extensive and severe.

Are there any other postoperative concerns?

Sure, there are many. Postoperative hemorrhage must be watched for. Seizures are not uncommon, and I use prophylactic phenytoin (or other anticonvulsants such as Keppra at 1000 mg twice daily) although this has not been shown to reduce late onset "downstream" seizures. Infection is a major concern to include meningitis but also deep brain abscess. I tend to use prophylactic antibiotics (cefazolin [Ancef]) for 1 week, although this regimen is not well established. There is also a risk for traumatic aneurysm formation, and I tend to obtain a vascular study about 5 days after injury, particularly if the bullet traversed near major intracranial vasculature.[7]

How do you handle a surface vessel that is "pumping" out hemorrhage?

I generally tamponade it with a Cottonoid pad. I then peel back the Cottonoid until I can see the vessel clearly without bleeding and use bipolar electrocautery to eliminate the bleeding. I usually then leave a piece of thrombin soaked Gelfoam over the site. (Examiners may want to hear your straightforward surgical techniques—these are not trick questions!)

What do you do about hematoma along the sagittal sinus or coursing into the interhemispheric fissure?

Generally, I do not "chase" hematoma all the way up to the sinus or into the interhemispheric fissure unless it is very large. This region tends to bleed a fair amount with manipulation, and there is a risk for damaging important draining cortical veins. I prefer to leave a light covering of hematoma in the region and to pack thrombin soaked Gelfoam along it before closing.

*What are the effects of Propofol and Thiopental on cerebral blood flow (CBF), CRMO2, and ICP in a coma patient with a severe head injury?

These agents reduce all three.[8]

*Are there any concerns about using Propofol in a patient with severe brain injury?

Propofol infusion syndrome can be seen with prolonged or high-dose usage, particularly in children. It also may reduce MAP, and thus CPP.[8]

*Benzodiazepines?

They reduce CRMO2, ICP, and CBF. The effects on CRMO2 and ICP are less marked than in barbiturates and they may reduce MAP and CPP. They do increase the seizure threshold, however.[8]

*What are the effects of Ketamine on CRMO2, CBF, and ICP?

This is not entirely clear. Earlier work suggests it increases all three; later larger studies suggest it decreases all three. Some authors argue that it is contraindicated in severe head injury; some argue that it is a valuable asset. It tends not to compromise MAP (or CPP). It therefore may have particular value as an induction agent in someone who is hemodynamically unstable.[8]

*Comment on the use of opioids in a patient with a severe brain injury.

They are used at times to supplement sedation and reduce pain. They, however, can increase ICP and decrease MAP and CPP. They can confound a neurological exam. They tend to accumulate and thus may take quite some time to clear. Remifentanil is rapidly broken down and tends to be well tolerated, even in the setting of severe head injury.

COMPLICATIONS

Surgery is going well, but as you are cleaning up the exit site of the brain, you notice increased bleeding from all plains, and the blood has a dilute "Kool-Aid" type appearance. What is going on?

I would be very concerned about disseminated intravascular coagulation (DIC), which can occur in massive head injuries. It is thought to be related to a large-scale release of tissue thromboplastin and other procoagulants. It results in consumption of platelets and components of the coagulation cascade. It can result in diffuse bleeding from "raw" sites, and this can be very difficult to combat mechanically (through surgical maneuvers).

How would you handle this?

I would seek to minimize any further surgical manipulation of tissue and obtain mechanical hemostasis as best as possible. I would ask for assistance from my anesthesia colleagues in the manner of transfusion of appropriate supportive materials such as platelets, fresh frozen plasma, and cryoprecipitate. I would seek to obtain hemostasis and close up as soon as possible with no further manipulations.

*The patient does well and regains consciousness and some movement on the left side. One week out, he develops a descending rigidity from his face down. He then develops diffuse spasms set off by the lightest stimuli. Any ideas?

My first thought would be meningitis, and I would obtain CSF for culture either by ventriculostomy if it is still in place or by lumbar puncture if the CT scan appeared benign. One other thought might be to question the trauma team and the emergency department about whether the patient received a tetanus toxoid shot on admission—this presentation has the markings of tetanus. (Note: This is a "way out there" question, but the examiners may have wanted to hear about tetanus toxoid administration in the initial management of the patient. If so, they will make it obvious.)

CASE 4

HISTORY AND PHYSICAL EXAMINATION

A 17-year-old male high school football player is knocked unconscious during a game. He "comes to" in less than a minute and sits on the bench for the remainder of the half. He slumps over onto a teammate and is found to be unresponsive. At your center, he is found to be hemiplegic on the right with a left dilated and unreactive pupil. He localizes with his left side but does not open his eyes or follow commands.

IMAGING STUDIES

Imaging is pending.

ANALYSIS OF CARE AND TREATMENT PLAN

This has all the markings of a classical traumatic brain injury syndrome, but you should not jump to conclusions immediately. Address the case as if you were arriving at the emergency department to find the patient unattended. The examiners may want to hear components of your initial evaluation and management. They will move you along to the "meat" of the case. Work through the case in an orderly, succinct, and efficient manner.

SAMPLE QUESTIONS AND REASONABLE ANSWERS
So what do you want to do?

I would make sure the patient was attended to, reference airway, breathing, and circulation. If he were not intubated, he would need to be so. I would ask my trauma colleagues to evaluate for other major injuries and to resuscitate the patient as needed. This would be considered a full "trauma code." I would complete my initial neurological survey and then proceed to imaging.

What images do you want?

I would want a CT scan of the head as soon as possible because I suspect an intracranial hematoma with mass effect and herniation. I would also want CT studies of the entire spine, particularly the cervical spine, because of my inability to fully evaluate the patient.

CT scan of the spine is okay. CT scan of the brain reveals a left epidural hematoma (Figure 8.4). What would make you bring the case to surgery?

Guidelines suggest that an epidural hematoma with a volume greater than 30 cm³ should be evacuated no matter what. Other criteria that lean one toward surgery would include thickness greater than 1.5 cm, associated focal neurological deficits, GCS score of less than 9, and midline shift greater than 5 mm. Anisocoria and GCS score of less than 9 suggest the need for immediate surgery.[9]

Case #4- EDH

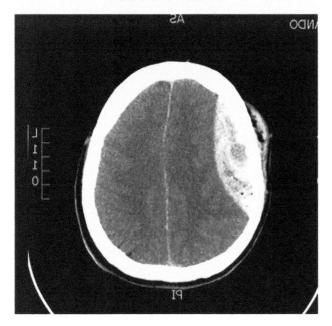

Figure 8.4 Noncontrast CT scan of the brain in a 17-year-old injured in football and now in a coma.

How do you measure epidural hematoma volume?

A decent estimate of volume is thickness by length by height divided by 2.

What is Kernohan's notch phenomenon?

This is known as a false localizing sign. With temporal lobe (uncal) herniation, the brainstem (cerebral peduncle) can be pushed against the contralateral incisura (temporal notch) causing ipsilateral rather than contralateral hemiparesis.

This patient has a 2.5 cm thick epidural hematoma on the left. What do you want to do?

This patient needs to go to surgery immediately for emergent evacuation of the hematoma.

The operating room says it will be 2 hours before the next neurosurgical room is available.

I would argue that this is not acceptable. Survival in this situation is time dependent. The longer the herniation is allowed to transpire, the higher the chances of irreversible brainstem injury. This is a bona fide emergency and a room needs to be made available preferably within minutes.

What if there were a flood in the operating room, or a mass casualty situation, or you were out in the "boonies"—where would you put your burr holes if you had to perform a life-saving procedure in the emergency department?

Evacuation of an epidural or subdural clot can be problematic because of the consistency of the hematoma. In a desperate situation, however, such a maneuver could be life-saving. The first choice for a generous burr-hole placement would be over the middle fossa to obviate uncal herniation. This burr hole would be created just above the zygomatic arch and just anterior to the ear (through temporalis muscle). Another burr hole should be located over the thickest portion of the hematoma. Classical teaching talks about creating trauma burr holes in the advent of similar clinical findings to this case but with no brain imaging available. Here, the first burr hole would be placed over the middle fossa as described previously, ipsilateral to the side of the dilated pupil. If no epidural hematoma is found, the dura should be opened. If this is negative, a second burr hole would be made over the middle fossa on the other side (in case of a falsely localizing Kernohan's notch phenomenon). If this is negative, two further burr holes can be made on the side ipsilateral to the dilated pupil over the parietal and frontal lobes.

What procedure will you perform?

I will perform a fronto-temporal craniotomy centered on and encompassing the width of the hematoma. (Be prepared to demonstrate your incision and describe your opening, hematoma evacuation, and closure.)

What will you do to prevent reaccumulation of hematoma?

I would make sure there is meticulous hemostasis of the field. I use hemostatic agents on the field such as thrombin soaked Gelfoam. I usually place a small drain and bring it out of a separate stab incision. I would use 4-0 Nurolon dural tack-up sutures circumferentially and centrally in the craniotomy field.

How do you do this?

I would make small "wire-passing" holes in the bone surrounding the craniotomy defect. I would pass the suture through the outer layer of the dura immediately adjacent to the bone edge and then through the circumferential holes and tightly tie the dura up to the bone edges. I would also place 1 or 2 tack up sutures in the center of the dural field and bring them up through holes in the craniotomy flap. These are tied taut after the craniotomy flap is secured in place.

So you replace the bone flap?

Yes, almost always.

Why almost always?

Epidural hematomas are generally not associated with significant underlying diffuse injury, so we generally do not anticipate severe brain swelling and increased ICP. If the underlying brain is full and tight, something else is going on. (Please note: you almost "stepped in it" here by throwing in an editorial comment rather than just the facts—"almost always" rather than just a simple yes.)

Do you almost always replace the bone flap in a subdural hematoma evacuation? If not, what is the difference?

The mechanism of injury is often different between the two. Generally, epidural hematomas arise from focal trauma with little diffuse brain injury. They are more often the result of torn vessel than brain pulping. On the other hand, subdural hematomas are often associated with more profound traumatic forces and more extensive brain injury. The brain may be pulped and abraded causing surface bleeding that coalesces into a subdural hematoma. Even with evacuation of the subdural hematoma, the diffusely injured brain may be too swollen to replace the bone flap.

What then are your criteria for evacuation of an acute subdural hematoma?

Many factors go into the decision to evacuate a subdural hematoma. Many subdural hematomas are small compared with the adjacent brain injury and thus will be followed unless ICPs become unmanageable. Guidelines suggest that clots thicker than 10 mm thickness with greater than 5 mm of midline shift should be evacuated. They also suggest evacuation for smaller clots when the GCS score drops by 2 points, the pupils are asymmetrical, or ICP cannot be lowered medically below 20 mm Hg.[5]

In surgery for acute subdural hematoma, do you always leave the bone flap out?

No. I prefer to replace it. I go by the swelling of the brain. If the brain looks in good shape and is relaxed with the hematoma evacuation, I replace the flap over subdural drains. If the brain is particularly pulped up and swollen, I will perform a duroplasty and leave the craniotomy flap out.

What kind of outcomes do you anticipate in the two types of hematomas?

If the epidural hematoma is caught early enough, particularly in a patient with a lucid interval history, the patient can make a spectacular recovery, although a small percentage of these patients die or are left in a coma. Neurological outcomes run a broad gamut depending on the original injury and timing.

*In the ICU, what PEEP and tidal volume do you generally use on your coma patients with severe head injuries?

Historically, tidal volumes of more than 8 ml/kg IBW and PEEPs of less than 3 cm H20, have been employed; but there is momentum in the literature for lower tidal volumes in the 6 to 7 ml/kg range and higher levels of PEEP, above 5 cm H20. Evidence seems to be suggesting that increased PEEP does not increase ICP or lower CPP and may improve cerebral oxygenation.[10]

*What criteria do you use for extubation?

This issue is open to some debate. Neurosurgeons have generally wanted to see return to vigorous consciousness. Evidence suggests that reintubation rates are reasonable below this level if the patient is stable medically and neurologically, coughs and swallows, and demonstrates visual pursuits.[10]

COMPLICATIONS

Your patient does great during surgery and is awake and alert without deficit within 2 hours. He is extubated. The following morning you are called because he is unresponsive with fixed and dilated pupils. What do you do?

I would evaluate the patient. (Note: Please *do not* order a CT scan from your breakfast table!) I would assess his airway and vitals and potentially intubate as needed. I would assess his neurological examination and his operative site and drains.

He is rigid throughout with labored breathing and clutched teeth. He then starts rhythmic jerking of the upper extremities. What now?

He is likely seizing. I would ask the nurse how long he had been this way and ask for an intubation team to head to the patient's room (it is likely this has been going on for some time and the patient is in status epileticus). I would place an oxygen mask and make sure he has appropriate IVs. I would have electrolyte and blood chemistries drawn. Thiamine and glucose are given to an unknown patient but would not be strongly indicated in this setting. I would administer 0.1 mg/kg of lorazepam initially (2–4 mg). I would repeat if no response after a minute. At the same time, I would be starting 20 mg/kg of phenytoin in the form of fosphenytoin.[11]

This does not stop the activity. What next?

I would go to a "third-line" drug but also be prepared for intubation and the infusion of a continuous drug. Phenobarbital has been the standby third-line drug, although we have employed levitiracetam 20 mg/kg IV bolus due to its ease of access and low complication profile. We would intubate and begin an anesthetic drip—usually propofol (again due to the ease of access) although midazolam is often used.[11] I would ask my anesthesia and neurology colleagues for assistance here. We would initiate continuous EEG monitoring. As soon as it was deemed safe to transport the patient, I would want a CT scan of the brain to rule out a new structural intracranial event.

While intubated the patient becomes profoundly hypotensive. What are the main types of shock?

Classically, cardiogenic, hypovolemic, anaphylactic, septic, and neurogenic. Newer classification systems list distributive (vasodilation as in septic shock), cardiogenic (pump failure), hypovolemic (loss of intravascular volume), obstructive (obstruction of blood flow), and combined.[12]

What is the action of Dopamine?

Beta1 ionotrope at doses 2–10 mcg/kg/min. In doses greater than 10 mcg/kg/min metabolites significantly increase alpha vasoconstriction.

Phenylephrine?

Pure alpha sympathomimetic. Not recommended in spinal cord injuries.

Norepinephrine?

Alpha 1, 2 more than beta1 resulting in vasoconstriction.

Synthetic Human Angiotensin II?

Vasoconstrictor and increased aldosterone release. Binds with type II angiotensin receptors causing vascular smooth muscle constriction.[13]

The following day, the patient is markedly hypertensive. What is the action of Fenoldopam?

Vasodilation via peripheral D1 receptors. Rapid onset of action. Short duration. May increase renal blood flow.

Enalaprilat?

An ACE inhibitor. Prevents angiotensin II vasoconstriction. Acts within 15 minutes of IV administration.

Esmolol?

A selective Beta 1 blocker. Fast acting, short duration. Used for rapid heart rate arrhythmias but may be employed when tachycardia is associated with hypertension.

CASE 5

HISTORY AND
PHYSICAL EXAMINATION

A 25-year-old woman in good health runs into a telephone pole with her car. She arrives at your center awake but with left hemiparesis. She is conversant but amnestic of the accident. She has facial abrasions and a "seat-belt" abrasion across her chest. Preliminary trauma evaluation is negative for major injuries. She is alert. Her speech and cranial nerve functions are intact. Her right-sided function is normal.

IMAGING STUDIES

CT scan of the brain reveals a 4 × 5 × 3 cm. intraparenchymal hematoma in the deep frontal lobe with some associated

Case # 5- IPH from avm

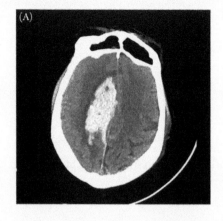

(A)

Case # 5- IPH from avm

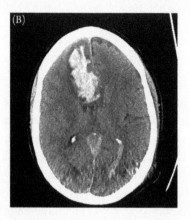

(B)

Case # 5- IPH from avm

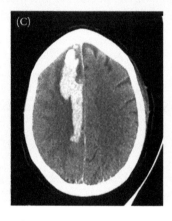

(C)

Case # 5- IPH from avm

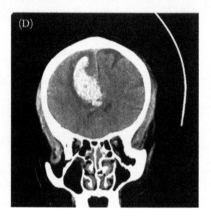

(D)

Figure 8.5 A–D. CT scan of the brain in a 25-year-old who is awake but hemiparetic after a motor vehicle accident.

intraventricular blood. There is local mass effect and 1mm of midline shift (Figure 8.5).

ANALYSIS OF CARE AND TREATMENT PLAN

This is presented as a trauma case but does not have to be. The examiners may want to make sure that you understand that not every presentation is straightforward. The classical case is a similar story with a CT scan that shows a sub-arachnoid hemorrhage very consistent with an aneurysmal hemorrhage. The motor vehicle accident may be a bit of a red herring—the patient experienced an intracranial event that caused her to run into a stationary object. The case presented here is not mounting up to be a surgical problem, and the hemorrhage is not in a classical trauma location, so keep your antenna up. Perhaps the patient sustained a

spontaneous intracerebral hemorrhage and ran into the telephone pole. She cannot remember if a headache or other symptoms preceded the collision.

SAMPLE QUESTIONS AND REASONABLE ANSWERS

So what do you want to do?

I would want to obtain more of a history. Does she remember anything before the accident? Had she ever had any previous syncopal events or seizures? What is her overall health status? Is she hypertensive? Does she take any medications or illicit drugs? I would obtain a drug screen. Although this hematoma may be of traumatic origin, I would have to worry about a spontaneous intraparenchymal hemorrhage precipitating her motor vehicle collision. I would want a vascular study, probably a CT angiography to begin with, but I might eventually want a full four-vessel angiogram.

What criteria would lead you to surgery in a patient with a traumatic intraparenchymal hemorrhage?

Guidelines (Level III evidence) suggest that surgical evacuation of traumatic intraparenchymal hematoma would be indicated for patients with neurological deterioration and a hematoma with mass effect or a hematoma volume of greater than 50 cm³ volume. Surgery is also considered if the patient has a GCS score of less than 8 and a hematoma larger than 20 cm³ with a midline shift greater than 5 mm and with or without compression of the basilar cisterns.[14] For spontaneous intraparenchymal hemorrhages, there is some conflicting notions coming out of the STICH and STICH 2 trials. These trials do not address traumatic hemorrhages or hemorrhages due to structural pathologies, but they do fail to show significant advantage to surgical hematoma evacuation in stable, conscious patients, particularly with deep hemorrhages. Further analysis, however, suggests that patients with initially poor prognoses and patients who deteriorate neurologically, particularly with superficial hematomas, do better with surgical evacuation.

How common is delayed traumatic intracerebral hemorrhage?

This is not an overly common phenomenon (estimated to occur in 10% to 20% of severe head injury patients) but can occur within the first few days of hospitalization. Delayed hemorrhage can result in the need for surgical evacuation and can occur spontaneously or in a region of previous hematoma or contusion. Because of the risk for delayed hemorrhage, most patients with severe head injuries, particularly those with intracranial findings on original CT, undergo delayed CT scans 1 to 3 days into their hospitalizations. Patients with deterioration on their neurological examination should also undergo a repeat CT to evaluate for this phenomenon.

What are the most common causes of spontaneous intracerebral hemorrhage in a nonhypertensive patient of this age?

Arteriovenous malformation, aneurysm rupture, illicit drug use, and tumor.

What if the hemorrhage was quite peripheral near a sinus?

I would suspect possible venous sinus thrombosis.

How do you treat sinus thrombosis?

Judicious anticoagulation, hydration, and close observation would be the initial treatment of sinus thrombosis. Interventional endovascular methods are available for extreme cases but have limited outcomes.

COMPLICATIONS

*This patient turned out to have an arteriovenous malformation and after a couple of hard seizures was started on phenytoin (Dilantin). Electrolyte evaluation documented a sodium of 120 mEq/L. What are the classifications of hyponatremia?

Hypovolemic, euvolemic, and hypervolemic hyponatremia, with subclassification into hypotonic, isotonic, and hypertonic groups.

*Differentiate hyponatremia secondary to SIADH and that secondary to cerebral salt wasting.

The exact cause of cerebral salt wasting is not well understood but may have to do with sympathetic tone and natriuretic factors and involves loss of salt from the kidneys with attendant loss of free water and thus a reduction in plasma volume. SIADH results in lack of release of free water at the kidneys and thus potentially increased plasma volume. Both result in a hypotonic hyponatremia.

*What lab values are important in evaluating hyponatremia?

The three most important would be serum osmolality, urine osmolality, and urine sodium concentration. (Be prepared to discuss how these might clarify things.)

*What parameters do you use to correct symptomatic severe hyponatremia?

Guidelines recommend 100 ml of 3% NaCl solution over 10 minutes up to 3 times if risk of cerebral herniation is high. If symptoms are less severe, 3% NaCl infused at 0.5 to 2 ml/kg/hr. Rapidity of serum sodium correction should be less than 8 mmol/L in any 24-hour period in patients with high risk of central pontine myelinolysis (CPM); 10 to 12 mmol/L in any 24-hour period, 18 mmol/L in any 48-hour period, in patients with normal risk of CPM.[15]

She ends up doing well, but 2 weeks later you are called to your emergency room because she is confused, ataxic, and has nystagmus. What is going on?

These are signs of Dilantin toxicity. I would hold her Dilantin and obtain a serum level. I would not necessarily obtain an emergent CT scan if her level is high (over 20 ug/ml).

*She presents again to your emergency department a month later with fatigue, fever, and a sore throat. On inspection, she has ulcers and vesicular lesions of her mucous membranes. She has a diffuse red purple rash on her trunk and extremities. Is this the flu?

This sounds like Stevens-Johnson syndrome (SJS).

*Tell me more about SJS.

SJS is on a spectrum with toxic epidermal necrolysis. It involves a potentially fulminant reaction of the skin and mucous membranes, generally to a medication such as Dilantin. It generally starts with a fever and flu-like symptoms. Within a few days, a red-purple rash that may blister and peel may cover substantial portions the face and torso and various mucous membranes. The rash may worsen for 2 or more weeks. The disorder must be aggressively managed because, although self-limited, it can be fatal.

*How is SJS managed?

Predominantly via supportive measures in an ICU setting. The offending medication must be stopped immediately and dermatology should be consulted. Skin lesions are treated much like burns, and patients with severe involvement should be transferred to a burn unit. The use of corticosteroids and immunosuppressants is not well supported in the literature.

CASE 6

HISTORY AND PHYSICAL EXAMINATION

A 30-year-old female equestrian in good health falls from her horse without a helmet. She is temporarily knocked unconscious but has a GCS of 14 on presentation. She has a comminuted tibia plateau fracture and a curved laceration over her right parietal region but no other major injuries. Orthopedics feel she will require a complex repair

sometime in the next few days. The scalp laceration edges appear dirty and a bit macerated.

IMAGING STUDIES

CT scan of the brain reveals a 4 × 5 cm region of comminuted skull fracture in the right parietal region (Figure 8.6). The greatest depth of infolded fragments is 2 cm. There is a small amount of intracranial pneumocephalus and some surrounding contusion of the brain without any midline shift.

ANALYSIS OF CARE AND TREATMENT PLAN

This is an open depressed skull fracture. Like most trauma scenarios, there is a range of options available in the general treatment of depressed skull fracture—be prepared to discuss them in adults and children. Do not guess what the examiner wants—go with what you would do and have a reason why. Open depressed skull fractures will likely require some level of cleaning up and repair. You will have to take it from there!

SAMPLE QUESTIONS AND REASONABLE ANSWERS
So what do you want to do?

I think this case requires surgery. Guidelines support surgery for open depressed skull fractures particularly if the depression is greater than 1 cm, there is evidence of dural laceration, and there is the potential for gross contamination. Other criteria not involved in this case might be

Case # 6 – Open depressed skull fracture

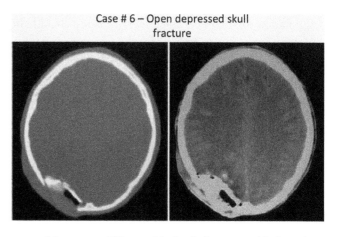

Figure 8.6 Noncontrast CT scan of the head of a 30-year-old who is alert after being kicked in the head by a horse.

significant associated hematoma, frontal sinus involvement, and significant cosmetic deformity.[16]

How would you perform the surgery?
(We do not need to hear about positioning, time out, and preparation.)

I would try to incorporate the laceration into my incision and would give myself a width of skull around the fracture site. I would inspect the site and check for mobility of the fragments. If they cannot be mobilized, I would make an adjacent burr hole and would slide a Penfield dissector under the fragments and deliver them up to curettes or grasping instruments. I might have to drill further along the periphery of the fracture to affect full mobilization. I would soak the fragments in bacitracin solution although there are discussions in the literature of soaking them in betadine. After the fragments were clear, I would inspect the underlying dura which I presume is lacerated. I would open the dura further so that I could evaluate the underlying brain. I would want to conservatively debride clearly macerated tissue and any contaminants in the field. I would ensure meticulous hemostasis. I would then irrigate profusely with bacitracin. I often use Surgicel on the injured brain for hemostasis and its bactericidal and static qualities. I would close the dura and tack it up circumferentially with 4-0 Neurolon sutures. I would then determine whether the bone fragments could be reconstructed with simple microplating. If not, or if they appeared hopelessly contaminated, I would discard them and close after further thorough irrigation.

So you would consider replacing the comminuted bone. What about infection?

There appears to be no increased risk for infection in replacing the fractured bone compared with discarding the bone. Using the bone would therefore potentially obviate a second surgery. Nonetheless, when the bone is grossly contaminated or severely comminuted, I would discard it.[16]

Would you use antibiotics?

Level III evidence suggests that antibiotics should be used for open depressed skull fractures. I generally employ a broad-spectrum antibiotic for 1 week to 10 days.

When should the surgery be carried out?

The sooner the better—I generally classify it as a non-life-threatening emergency and should be ideally completed within 24 hours of admission.[16]

Are your indications for surgery the same for closed depressed skull fractures?

I tend to be more conservative and limit surgery to cases of significant cosmetic deformity, deep laceration of the dura and brain, significant associated brain injury or hemorrhage, and/or deficits.

How about in a child?

Depressed fractures in young children will often smooth out as the skull grows so deformity is even less of a driver.

What about the propensity for seizures?

There is no evidence that elevation of depressed skull fractures will reduce the incidence of seizures. It is not an indication for surgery.

What about a "ping-pong" ball depressed fracture?

These usually occur in very young children and will usually smooth out spontaneously over time. In general, these are "greenstick" fractures and should not have bone shards to lacerate the dura. If there were lacerated dura and CSF leak or associated neurological deficit, the fracture could be elevated.

If you did have to elevate a ping-pong ball fracture, how would you do it?

Traditional descriptions involve making a small burr hole adjacent to the depression and then "popping" the depression back out with a Penfield-like dissector under the depression. We have used a technique in which a small cranial fixation screw is placed into the middle of the depression and pulled on—elevating the depression. The screw is then removed.

*In a head-injured patient in coma, what is your nutritional management?

Guidelines support initiation of feeding of these patients to a basal caloric replacement level by the fifth post-injury day to reduce mortality (Level IIA). They also support the use of transgastric jejunal feeding to reduce ventilator associated pneumonia (Level IIB).[1] There has been more aggressive recommendations made for military severe head injuries, including initiation of nutrition within 24 hours of injury bearing substantial protein loads of 1 to 1.5 g/kg.[17]

There is inconclusive evidence on glycemic control, nutritional makeup, and the use of vitamins and supplements.

COMPLICATIONS

What if you have a depressed fracture over the sagittal sinus?

I generally would take a more conservative approach to such a fracture. Unless there is a strong indication for surgery, elevating a fracture over the sinus incurs increased risk for substantial bleeding, sinus occlusion, and cortical vein injury.

What if there was a "strong" indication for surgery such as a CSF leak or associated compressive neurological deficit?

I would then approach the problem very judiciously with a wide-open exposure and preparation for potential sinus repair. This would include blood ready for transfusion; large bore intravenous lines, and a central line. A Fogerty catheter should be available for temporary occlusion. Ideally, I would isolate the bone over the sinus away from the remainder of the depressed fragments and could potentially leave the fragments over the sinus alone and elevate the remainder of the fracture separately.

*The patient is extubated after surgery. She is slow to awaken but remains nonfocal. The next morning, she is difficult to arouse, she is hypoxic and tachypneic, and she has a new diffuse petechial rash. Thoughts?

(Wow, this is rather open ended, but they gave you a constellation of problems—for a reason. Try to process the information at hand. Remember the long bone fractures. Although many things could be happening, let us offer up the possibility of a fat embolism.)

*What MRI appearance would you expect for a cerebral fat embolism?

There is no pathognomonic constellation but you might see a "starfield pattern" of high signal on DWI, many scattered small spots of increased signal on T2, multiple small hypointense spots on SWI indicating tiny petechial hemorrhages. Generally, the more numerous and pronounced lesions seen on MRI, the worse the clinical syndrome.[18–20]

*What treatment would you advocate?

Treatment is principally supportive. There is evidence that early stabilization of the fracture reduces further embolization. Otherwise, all systems should be supported. The use of steroids, anticoagulants, and/or hyperbaric oxygen have been advocated by some.[18–20]

REFERENCES

1. Brain Trauma Foundation. Guidelines for the Management of Severe Traumatic Brain Injury.4th ed. https://braintrauma.org/uploads/13/06/Guidelines_for_Management_of_Severe_TBI_4th_Edition.pdf. Published September 2016. Accessed July 16, 2019.
2. Trinka E, Leitinger M. Which EEG patterns in coma are nonconvulsive status epilepticus? *Epilepsy Behav.* 2015;49:203–222.
3. Edwards P, Arango M, Balica L, et al. Final results of MRC CRASH, a randomised placebo-controlled trial of intravenous corticosteroid in adults with head injury-outcomes at 6 months. *Lancet.* 2005;365(9475):1957–1959.
4. Hutchinson PJ, Kolias AG, Timofeev IS, et al. Trial of decompressive craniectomy for traumatic intracranial hypertension. *N Engl J Med.* 2016;375(12):1119–1130.
5. Tunkel AR. Initial therapy and prognosis of bacterial meningitis in adults. https://www.uptodate.com/contents/initial-therapy-and-prognosis-of-bacterial-meningitis-in-adults#H21. Published March, 2019. Accessed July 16, 2019.
6. Tunkel AR, Hasbun R, Bhimraj A, et al. 2017 Infectious Diseases Society of America's clinical practice guidelines for healthcare-associated ventriculitis and meningitis. *Clin Infect Dis.* 2017;64(6):e34–e65.
7. Alvis-Miranda HR, A MR, Agrawal A, et al. Craniocerebral gunshot injuries; a review of the current literature. *Bull Emerg Trauma.* 2016;4(2):65–74.
8. Flower O, Hellings S. Sedation in traumatic brain injury. *Emerg Med Int.* 2012;2012:637171.
9. Bullock MR, Chesnut R, Ghajar J, et al. Surgical management of acute epidural hematomas. *Neurosurgery.* 2006;58(3 Suppl):S7–S15; discussion Si–Siv.
10. Asehnoune K, Roquilly A, Cinotti R. Respiratory management in patients with severe brain injury. *Crit Care.* 2018;22(1):76.
11. Glauser T, Shinnar S, Gloss D, et al. Evidence-based guideline: treatment of convulsive status epilepticus in children and adults: report of the Guideline Committee of the American Epilepsy Society. *Epilepsy Curr.* 2016;16(1):48–61.
12. Vincent JL, De Backer D. Circulatory shock. *N Engl J Med.* 2013;369(18):1726–1734.
13. Kalil A. Septic shock medication. https://emedicine.medscape.com/article/168402-medication#2. Published January 2019. Accessed July 16, 2019.
14. Bullock MR, Chesnut R, Ghajar J, et al. Surgical management of traumatic parenchymal lesions. *Neurosurgery.* 2006;58(3 Suppl):S25–S46; discussion Si–Siv.
15. Verbalis JG, Goldsmith SR, Greenberg A, et al. Diagnosis, evaluation, and treatment of hyponatremia: expert panel recommendations. *Am J Med.* 2013;126(10 Suppl 1):S1–S42.
16. Bullock MR, Chesnut R, Ghajar J, et al. Surgical management of depressed cranial fractures. *Neurosurgery.* 2006;58(3 Suppl):S56–S60; discussion Si–Siv.
17. Institute of Medicine. Improving acute and subacute health outcomes in military personnel. In: Erdman J, Oria M, Pillsbury L,

eds. *Nutrition and traumatic brain injury*. Washington, DC: The National Academies Press; 2011:249–286.

18. Zhou Y, Yuan Y, Huang C, Hu L, Cheng X. Pathogenesis, diagnosis and treatment of cerebral fat embolism. *Chin J Traumatol*. 2015;18(2):120–123.

19. Bulauitan, CS. Fat embolism treatment & management. https://emedicine.medscape.com/article/460524-treatment#d9. Published March 2018. Accessed July 16, 2019.

20. Weerakkody Y. Cerebral fat embolism. https://radiopaedia.org/articles/cerebral-fat-embolism?lang=us. Accessed July 16, 2019.

9.

SPINE

Allan D. Levi

Spine cases form a significant component of neurosurgery procedures performed daily across the country. Using Medicare data sets, approximately 65% of all neurosurgical procedures involve the spine. In the oral board exam, you will encounter spine cases in your general session, whether you do 1 or 2 general sessions. A familiarity with the common cases is essential in preparing for this part of the boards. If you have a focused practice that involves spine in session 2, you will need to be prepared to discuss complex spine cases including deformity, high-grade spondylolisthesis, and radical resection of spinal cord and spine tumors. The bulk of the current spine chapter includes cases that might be seen in the general session of hour 1 or 2. To illustrate an example of a more complex spine case for spine-focused neurosurgical providers, case # 5 depicts a case of sagittal deformity correction.

Covering the gamut of spine is difficult in a single chapter of one reference text that prepares candidates for the board. Spine includes cases that span from the skull base to the sacrum. Degenerative, congenital, trauma, tumors, infections, and inflammatory pathologies are all important in the differential diagnosis. Pediatric spine conditions are unique, and some congenital conditions will present in adulthood, including congenital anomalies of the skull base, diastematomyelia, and lumbar spondylolisthesis due to a pars defect. Neurological disorders that can mimic neurosurgical spine and spinal cord conditions are also seen and include amyotrophic lateral sclerosis, Guillain-Barré syndrome, and multiple sclerosis.

Another component of spine includes an understanding of spine stability, as well as the use of spinal instrumentation. In some cases, spine instability is determined by the presenting pathology (e.g., bilateral cervical facet dislocation). At other times, the effects of the decompression on spine stability (e.g., removal of a tumor sacrificing posterior elements at the level of the thoracolumbar junction) must be considered in addition to the existing pathology.

Spine technologies and instrumentation continue to evolve. Twenty-five years ago, anterior cervical plating and pedicle screws were considered new technologies and likely not to be tested in detail in the Oral Board Examination. Now these instrumentation techniques are a standard part of the neurosurgical armamentarium. Current new technologies or approaches to the spine, whether minimally invasive techniques or surgery for deformity, are a growing part of standard neurosurgical practice and will continue to form a larger part of the Oral Board Examination.

CASE 1

HISTORY AND PHYSICAL EXAMINATION

An 18-year-old man fell while snow skiing and became paralyzed in the upper and lower extremities. He was transported on a board to a local hospital in a collar, and on examination he was diagnosed with a C 6 quadriplegia ASIA A. His motor exam demonstrated his bilateral wrist extensors are 4 on 5 with a sensory level of C6 but no motor or sensory function below that level. His neck was stabilized in a collar, and he was transferred to your institution and arrived 8 hours post-injury. His blood pressure is 90/60 and is heart rate is 45 beats per minute. His respiratory status is stable.

IMAGING STUDIES

The imaging studies included sagittal reconstructions of a computed tomography (CT) scan of the cervical spine (Figure 9.1). There are bilateral cervical locked facets at the C6C7 level with significant narrowing of the spinal canal. The superior articular process of C7 is locked behind the inferior articular process of C6. A magnetic resonance imaging (MRI) obtained immediately upon arrival

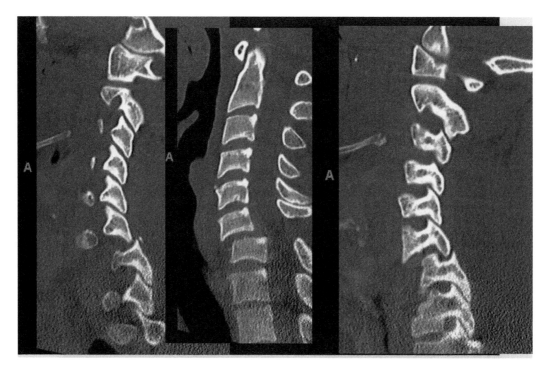

Figure 9.1 Sagittal reconstructed CT scans demonstrating bilateral C6–C7 locked facets. There is a high-grade anterolisthesis of C6 on C7.

demonstrated approximately 50% lysthesis of C6 on C7 with splaying of the interspinous processes, tearing of the ligamentum flavum, severe narrowing of the spinal canal, and edema of the spinal cord at that level. There is a combination of disc material versus hematoma behind the vertebral body of C6 (Figure 9.2).

ANALYSIS OF CASE AND SURGICAL PLAN

This case illustrates many of the common themes in the management of acute cervical spinal cord injury (SCI). The first is that in emergency management of such patients, it is important to recognize that the patient has a physiologically complete cervical SCI. It is common for these patients to have hemodynamic issues on presentation, including bradycardia and hypotension related to neurogenic shock. This is commonly seen in patients with SCI above the T6 level. The sympathetic plexus 2nd order neurons within the spinal cord reside in the interomediolateral cell column from T1 to L3. Spinal cord injuries above T6 injure enough of the sympathetic outflow to produce parasympathetic imbalance with unopposed vagal tone resulting in low blood pressure accompanied by a low heart rate. The management includes diagnosis of neurogenic shock, placement of an arterial line, replacement of volume with fluids, and at times the administration of vasopressors such as norepinephrine, dopamine, or phenylephrine. There is Level II evidence that

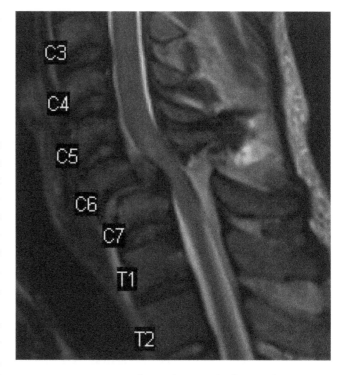

Figure 9.2 Demonstrates a mid-sagittal T2-weighted MR with a C6C7 with a 50% lysthesis of C6 on C7 with splaying of the interspinous processes, tearing of the ligamentum flavum, severe narrowing of the spinal canal, and edema of the spinal cord at that level. There is a combination of disc material versus hematoma behind the vertebral body of C6.

treating hypotension to achieve mean arterial pressures of 80 to 85 mm Hg can improve neurological outcomes after SCI.[1] Respiratory failure is also common, particularly after cervical SCI, because of loss of the accessory muscles of respiration. High cervical SCI at C4 and above can affect diaphragmatic function, and the physician needs to be ready to intubate with spinal precautions, including in-line traction or awake fiber optic intubation.

The next issues that are important to address after stabilizing the patient and evaluating his airway, breathing, and circulation (ABCs) are the use of additional imaging studies and the role of emergency reduction.

The role of intravenous (IV) steroids in these cases remains controversial. Clearly, there is no role for steroids in this patient who was transferred 8 hours after injury, because the upper time limit for administering steroids according to the National Acute Spinal Cord Injury Study II protocol is 8 hours.[2] In patients who are seen with SCI of less than 8 hours, neurological surgery guidelines now consider the use of steroids to be "not recommended," because the evidence for complications due to steroids is more evident than its benefits.[3] Because this is controversial, you should have a ready response, and if you use steroids as a neuroprotective strategy, you must be prepared to cite the dose (e.g., methylprednisolone [Solu Medrol]—5.4 mg/kg IV loading dose over 15 minutes followed by 30 mg/kg over 23 hours.

The timing of surgery for acute SCI has been debated for many years. The pendulum over the last decade in particular has swung towards early (< 24 hr) surgery.[4] This is particularly the case for cervical SCI, which tends to be somewhat lower velocity injuries with a better prognosis than thoracic SCI. In patients such as the one here, who present with SCI as an isolated injury, we will operate as soon as feasible and that would include performing surgery in the middle of the night.

The patient has bilateral C6C7 locked facets and has a complete cervical SCI. In this setting, it is more valuable to attempt an urgent closed reduction with cranial tongs to provide immediate decompression of the spinal cord, particularly when the patient is seen early on after the injury. In patients with bilateral cervical facet dislocations who present as AIS A neurologically complete, we now tend to do early manual reduction, and then once the reduction is successful, we can then obtain a postreduction cervical MRI. If a patient is incomplete (AIS B-D) or has a normal neurological exam (AIS E) and has a bilateral facet dislocation, we tend to do imaging first to rule out pathology that suggests a potential disc herniation with realignment, which has been rarely reported in the literature.[5,6]

In our practice, we do not use a protocol with ascending weights because of time considerations, and we prefer to use manual traction with fluoroscopy either in the trauma center or in the operating room. Sedation may enhance the reduction process and ultimately some patients will need general anesthesia. In an article by Grant et al.,[7] preoperative reduction in the awake patient with cranial tongs was shown to be safe.

In cases such as the one here, we will plan for reduction in the operating room either with manual traction just prior to anesthesia and intubation or more commonly plan for reduction after surgically removing the cervical disc via an anterior approach. This essentially reduces to zero the chance of a disc herniation with cervical facet reduction maneuvers. The technique for manual reduction consists of axial distraction via tongs followed by gentle flexion to allow the inferior articular process of the vertebra above to slide over the superior articular process of the vertebrae below.

Another surgical option in the unreducible cervical facet fracture is a posterior approach, where a portion of the facet joint (i.e., the superior articular process of C7 is drilled). As soon as a small amount of bone is removed, you will hear and see the facet dislocation "pop" back into alignment, and then the spinal fracture can be stabilized by posterior cervical instrumentation consisting of lateral mass screws at one or two levels above and below the injury level. The typical entry point for the lateral mass screws involve identifying the midpoint of the lateral mass and entering the bone 1 mm inferior and 1 mm medial to this point. Drill trajectory is upward and outward. Typical screw length particularly in an adult male would be 14 to 18 mm. Supplementing the instrumented fusion with bone graft, either local, auto, or allograft and possibly a bone extender would be important to ultimately obtain a bone fusion. A cervical collar after an instrumented fusion for a fracture is typically 6 to 12 weeks.

Many patients with bilateral cervical facet dislocation can undergo surgical reduction after an anterior approach and removal of the intervening disk.[8] This can be accomplished with either tong reduction or by using Caspar vertebral distraction pins or by placing a Cobb elevator, or a similar instrument and distracting. In approximately 92% of cases, the surgeon can obtain an anatomical reduction after an anterior approach.[9] If an anterior reduction was unsuccessful in reducing the fracture dislocation, an interbody graft can be placed; the patient can then be flipped posteriorly and the same procedure performed by drilling the superior articular process of C6. If the surgeon is successful in reducing the fracture from the anterior, then an interbody graft and plate can be placed to stabilize the fracture. Critical aspects of this portion of the procedure

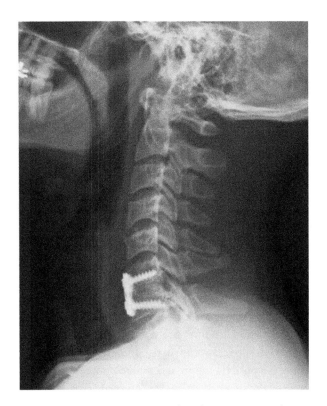

Figure 9.3 Demonstrates a postoperative lateral c-spine X-ray with an anterior plate fixating the vertebral bodies. Note the screws are almost bicortical and careful attention was placed in not oversizing the graft.

is not to oversize the graft potentially resulting in distraction of the facets and to place bicortical or near bicortical screws to maximize the strength of fixation (Figures 9.3 and 9.4).

COMPLICATIONS

Respiratory failure early on after a cervical SCI is incredibly common. With paralysis of the accessory muscles of respiration, vigorous chest physiotherapy and pulmonary toilet is critical. Bronchoscopy to remove mucous plugs is also important. Unfortunately, many patients fatigue and will require intubation and some a tracheostomy. The incidence of tracheostomy correlates with the level of injury.[10]

CASE 2

HISTORY AND PHYSICAL EXAMINATION

A 72-year-old woman presented with progressive bilateral lower extremity numbness and weakness. On neurological examination, she demonstrated generalized bilateral lower extremity weakness; most severe involvement was ankle dorsiflexion at 3 and 5 and the remainder was 4/5. She had hyper-reflexia at the knees and ankles at 3 to 4+/4, and she had up-going toes. She also had sensory level to pinprick at T10.

IMAGING STUDIES

The patient has a central thoracic disk herniation at the T10T11 level, which is ventral to the dural sac and calcified

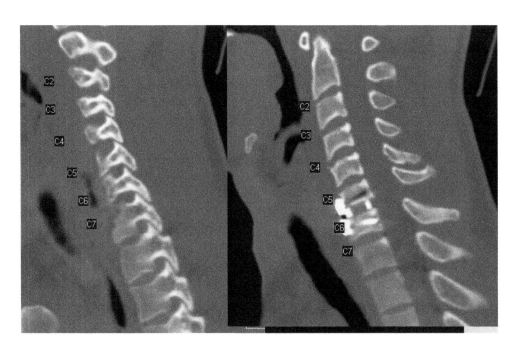

Figure 9.4 Demonstrates a sagittal CT scan with fibular allograft spanning the vertebral bodes of C6 and C7.

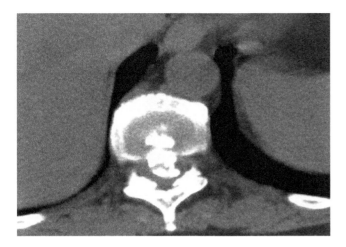

Figure 9.5 Demonstrates a thin cut CT scan with a large ventral thoracic calcified disc.

(Figure 9.5). It has significantly compressed the ventral spinal cord on MRI (Figures 9.6 and 9.7). The differential diagnosis includes a ventral calcified meningioma, but the absence of a dural tail and the presence of the lesion at the disk space make this much less likely.

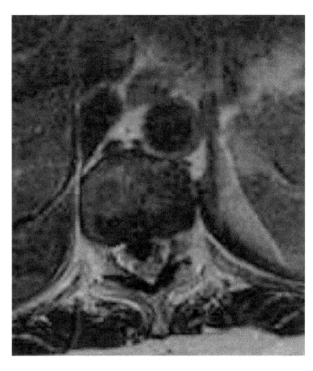

Figure 9.7 Demonstrates an axial T2-weighted image with the central disc seeing compressing the ventral spinal cord.

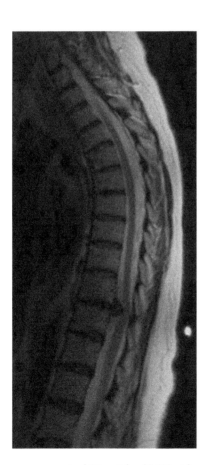

Figure 9.6 Demonstrates a sagittal T2-weighted MRI with severe ventral thoracic spinal cord compression with a calcified disc opposite the disc space.

ANALYSIS OF CASE AND SURGICAL PLAN

This is a classic Oral Board Examination question in which the examiners want to determine your surgical approach and safety. One of the clear-cut wrong answers is the performance of a mid-line thoracic laminectomy in the face of a central calcified disc. Please do not entertain this response.

The surgical options include a lateral approach sometimes referred to as an "anterior approach," which would consist of a thoracotomy. The thoracotomy can be done from the right or the left depending on whether the disk is eccentric to the right or the left, respectively. If it is central, and all things being equal, it is preferable to go on the left side because the thoracic aorta is easier to mobilize than the inferior vena cava. This often will require a rib resection (typically the 9th rib), which can be done through a full open or minimally invasive approach. After deflating the ipsilateral lung, it is critical to identify the 11th rib head because this will lead you to the location of the underlying 11th pedicle. You can then safely enter the lateral spinal canal by drilling away the pedicle. You can then proceed with a lateral discectomy and a partial corpectomy of T11 and T10 above and below the target disk level. You can then identify the ventral compression of the thecal sac by the calcified thoracic disk and empty the disk material into the decompression area, which was created by the partial corpectomy. It is not uncommon to have calcified disk that is adherent to the dura, which may result in an inadvertent cerebrospinal fluid (CSF) leak.

Another approach to this central calcified disk would be a "posterolateral approach," and this is very different from a laminectomy. This approach requires a transpedicular decompression, facetectomy, partial rib resection, partial corpectomy, and reaching somewhat blindly in front of the dural sac with reverse-angle curettes and decompressing the ventral disk into the corpectomy defect. This often is supplemented by a posterior instrumented pedicle screw fusion. A spinal fluid leak is not uncommon and requires further management with indirect repair and a CSF drain.

COMPLICATIONS

Correction of a CSF leak into the thoracic cavity can be problematic. It is very difficult to perform a direct repair of the dura after a thoracotomy and an anterior approach, but you can consider an indirect repair by placement of collagen dural substitute or glue. You can also consider placing either a lumbar or a cervical CSF drain to reduce the pressure head of the CSF leak on the dural repair. We usually place a number 28 or number 32 chest tube on suction and then switch to water seal in the subsequent 24 hours to prevent a CSF fistula into the chest cavity from forming.

Although intraoperative monitoring is not standard of care for every spine case, the use of intraoperative monitoring (Figure 9.8) for high-risk cases such as a calcified thoracic disk or an intramedullary tumor can be helpful. In this particular case, there was a decline of motor evoked potentials (MEPs) during the surgery on the contralateral side from where the disk was being removed, as rotation of the calcified disk fragment impinged on the right side of the spinal cord. This is a true-positive finding with a decline, reflecting an injury to the spinal cord. Additional bone removal allowed better access to the ventral dura, and we had to resect the dura along with the calcified disk to adequately decompress the spinal cord. By comparing Figure 9.8C and D, you can see that the lower extremity right MEPs to the quadriceps at 350 mA stimulation are now gone.

There are many reasons that intraoperative potentials can change during surgery. The first step would be to rule out spinal cord unrelated causes for the intraoperative changes. Low core body temperature, (e.g., hypothermia), can result in reduced somatosensory evoked potentials (SSEPs) but not MEPs; increased concentration of gas anesthetic, and hypotension are alternative etiologies of decreased MEPs

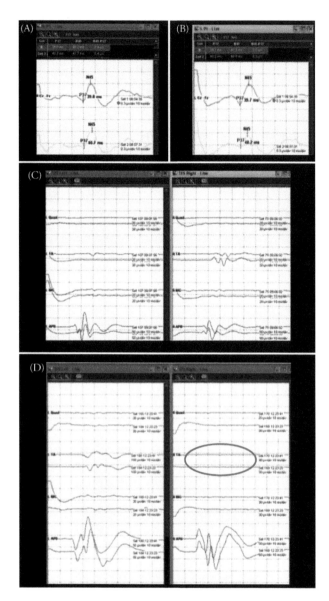

Figure 9.8 A–D is a baseline and intraoperative at SSEP and MEP. SSEPs to the left, MEPs to the right. One can see that on the right-sided MEPs, there is a decrement or absence of the quadriceps MEP at the time where the calcified disc was rotated into the cord.

(false-positive findings), and need to be ruled out. It is important to have a management algorithm when there are intraoperative changes in evoke potentials.

The patient ultimately returned with shortness of breath and worsening headache especially when upright. The chest x-ray (Figure 9.9) demonstrated a large left-sided pleural effusion and a significant left-sided chronic subdural hematoma (Figure 9.10).

The patient then required a repair of the ventral CSF leak through a repeat thoracotomy and placement of a cervical CSF drain for 5 days to reduce the pressure head at the repair site. Drainage of the subdural hematoma was not required because the patient was neurologically stable, and

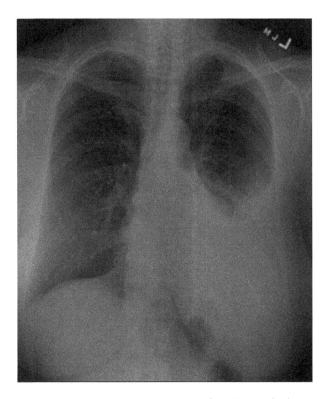

Figure 9.9 Demonstrates an anterior–posterior chest X-ray with a large left-sided plural fusion obscuring the heart shadow.

CSF leak repair resulted in disappearance of the subdural over a period of 12 weeks.

HISTORY AND PHYSICAL EXAMINATION

This is a 56-year-old man with a long-standing history of low back pain since adolescence. He now presents with low back pain and right greater than left leg pain that radiates down the lateral aspect of the legs. On examination, he is neurologically intact. Imaging studies are presented.

IMAGING STUDIES

The imaging studies demonstrate evidence of a grade I L5–S1 spondylolisthesis (Figure 9.11). The most common form of spondylolisthesis at this level is a congenital isthmic spondylolysis with subsequent spondylolisthesis. This can be diagnosed using oblique images in which a Scotty dog is seen, and typically the fracture line goes along or across the neck of

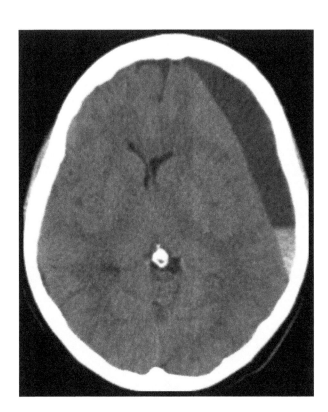

Figure 9.10 An axial CT scan of the brain showing a large acute on chronic subdural hematoma, with left-sided frontal with midline shift.

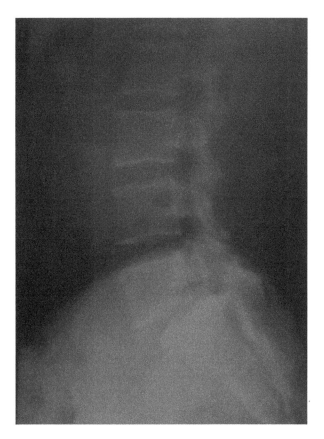

Figure 9.11 Demonstrates a grade I spondylolisthesis at L5–S1 due to a congenital isthmic spondylolysis.

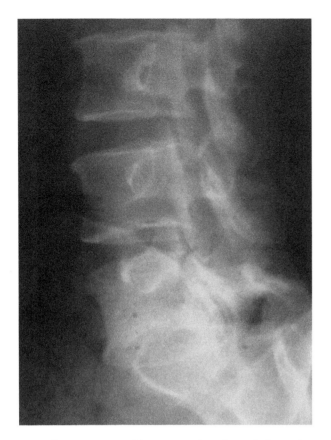

Figure 9.12 Demonstrates an oblique view with evidence of a Scotty dog appearance incorporating the L5 superior and inferior articular process.

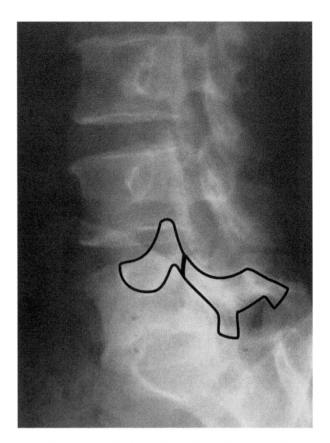

Figure 9.13 Demonstrates the Scotty dog outline with a fracture along the neck of the dog.

the Scotty dog (Figures 9.12 and 9.13). Similarly, a fine-cut CT scan shows the chronic pars fracture (Figure 9.14). The fracture is best appreciated on sagittal CT scans in which the superior and inferior articular process appears separated.

ANALYSIS OF CASE AND SURGICAL PLAN

Patients with isthmic spondylolysis typically have a chronic history of low back pain, and, as they age, they develop inflammatory or arthritic changes around the fracture with resultant lateral recess stenosis due to a combination of the slip, and the facet arthroplasty. They may eventually develop radiculopathy. In general, patients who present with radicular symptoms complain of pain and numbness along the L5 nerve root as it is entrapped and as it exits around the L5 pedicle.

In these conditions, it is always important to initially advocate for conservative treatments, such as physical therapy, epidural injections, anti-inflammatory drugs, and the like.

Ultimately, patients often require surgical intervention. There are a number of surgical approaches that can be considered. From a historical perspective, a L5 laminectomy

alone or a Gill procedure (named after the initial surgeon who described it) is a historical option. The most common or favored options are those that involve a laminectomy and fusion.

The fusion options would include a laminectomy of L5 and posterolateral fusion at L5–S1, a laminectomy with

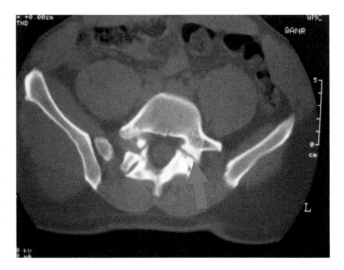

Figure 9.14 Demonstrates an axial CT scan of L5 where the arrows point to the pars fracture. The L5S1 joint is also seen posteriorly.

posterolateral fusion with pedicle screws, or a laminectomy with interbody fusion and pedicle screw instrumentation.

The advantage of an interbody graft for this procedure is that the placement of such grafts will allow you to distract the disk space, thereby indirectly decompressing the L5 nerve root underneath the pedicle as it exits the foramen, as well as enhancing the overall fusion rate for these conditions. One of the most difficult levels to fuse is the L5–S1 interspace, and the interbody graft will substantially increase the fusion rate. This should be supplemented by a placement at L5–S1 pedicle screw instrumentation (Figures 9.15 and 9.16). Typically, when we place pedicle screws, we identify the mamillary tubercle of L5, and use a gear shift followed by a tap, and then placement of the pedicle screws, which measure from 5 to 7.5 mm in width. One can consider monitoring, fluoroscopy, or both to improve the accuracy of placement of the screws. Impedance monitoring typically produces a current to the pedicle screw, and if there is a breach in the medial pedicle screw wall, one can detect a lower impedance (<20 mA). Similarly, anteroposterior and studies lateral fluoroscopy images can help localize the pedicle screw within the pedicle.

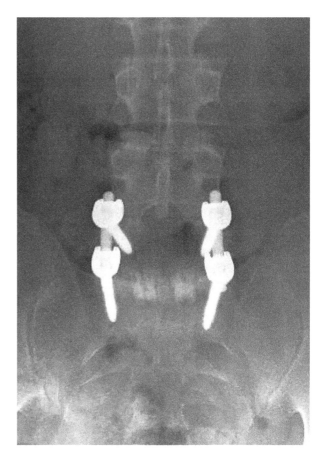

Figure 9.16 Demonstrates a 2-week postoperative incision with evidence of purulent drainage from the wound.

COMPLICATIONS

The patient awakens with severe paresthesias, burning, and an incomplete unilateral foot dorsiflexion weakness after surgery. The differential diagnosis includes a retraction injury to the L5 nerve root when placing the interbody grafts, a malpositioned pedicle screw at L5, and a hematoma or retained disk fragment. These various possibilities can be ruled out with postoperative CT and MRI. Should the investigations fail to reveal a structural cause for the L5 radiculopathy, the pain can be treated with medications such as gabapentin. The most common side effects of gabapentin in adult patients include dizziness, fatigue, drowsiness, weight gain, and peripheral edema.

Another potential complication with these cases is the development of a postoperative deep wound infection. The infection rate after spinal instrumentation ranges anywhere from 1% to 8%.[11] Should these infections develop, it typically occurs some 1 to 4 weeks postoperatively. These cases present with a wound that fails to heal and egress of turbid fluid (Figure 9.17) systemically with fever, chills, and malaise. Additional studies that can help support the diagnosis includes a white blood cell count, ESR and CRP. These

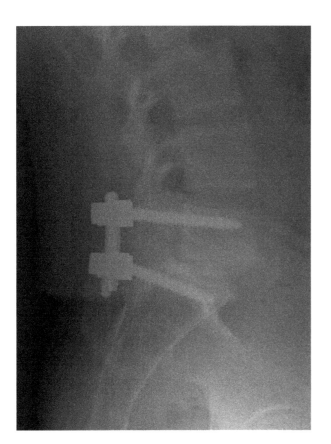

Figure 9.15 (A) Demonstrates the presence of bilateral pedicle screws at L5 and S1 with an interbody graft at L5S1 that results in an increase of disc space height and (B) demonstrates an anterior–posterior view of the lumbar spine with bilateral paired pedicle screws and 2 interbody grafts.

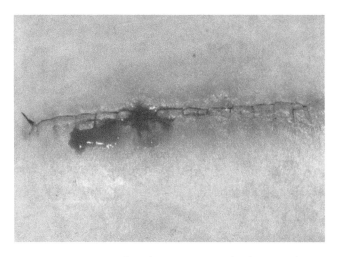

Figure 9.17 Demonstrates a lateral C spine X-ray with a destructive lesion involving the C6 vertebral body.

patients require a return to the operating room and formal irrigation and debridement (I and D) procedure under general anesthesia. Removal of any obviously infected bone graft or dead necrotic tissues, irrigation of the wound, placement of drains, and then primary closure. Identification of the bacterial pathogen is key. One can obtain a diagnosis with blood cultures if the patient is septic, as well as intraoperative cultures. We can then tailor the IV antibiotics according to the cultured organism. The patient generally receives 6 weeks of IV antibiotics or treatment until the ESR normalizes for any deep-seated infection with spinal instrumentation. In the setting of an acute infection, the spinal instrumentation may be maintained in place. With chronic infections that go on to develop osteomyelitis—the instrumentation is frequently removed.

CASE 4

HISTORY AND PHYSICAL EXAMINATION

A 56-year-old man presents with a history of severe and incapacitating neck pain that is worse at night or when upright over a period of 4 weeks. In addition, he complains of weakness in his hands and gait instability.

On examination, he is hyper-reflexic in both the upper and lower extremities with bilateral intrinsic muscle weakness in the hands.

IMAGING STUDIES

Imaging shows a lateral cervical-spine x-ray with destruction of the vertebral body of C6. The end plates of C5 and C7 are

relatively intact (Figure 9.18). The appearance is most suggestive of a metastatic lesion and less likely a primary tumor or tuberculoma (which also tends to preserve the end plates above and below). CT scan demonstrates a destruction of the C6 vertebral body (Figures 9.19 and 9.20). The facet joints and posterior elements are relatively intact. There is some prevertebral soft tissue swelling consistent with the tumor.

The next logical test to be ordered would be MRI of the cervical spine with gadolinium. MRI demonstrates a tumor that involves the C6 vertebral body with significant bilateral anterior/ventral epidural compression and deformation of the spinal cord (Figures 9.21 and 9.22).

ANALYSIS OF CASE AND SURGICAL PLAN

The initial question is always whether this is a primary or a metastatic bone lesion. The patient's advanced age and short duration of presentation are more suggestive of a metastasis. In trying to ascertain the diagnosis, it would be prudent to order further imaging studies, including a metastatic survey; which would include a bone scan; CT of the chest, abdomen, and pelvis; prostate specific antigen; and multiple myeloma markers.

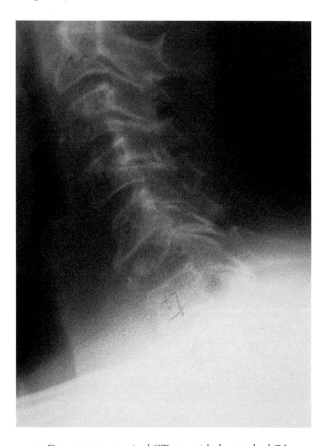

Figure 9.18 Demonstrates a sagittal CT scan with the vertebral C6 vertebral body destruction.

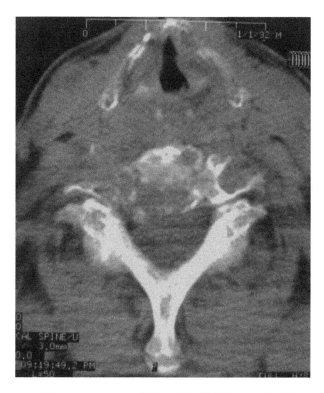

Figure 9.19 Demonstrates an axial T2-weighted MRI scan with soft tissue tumor along with vertebral body destruction at C6 with ventral cord compression.

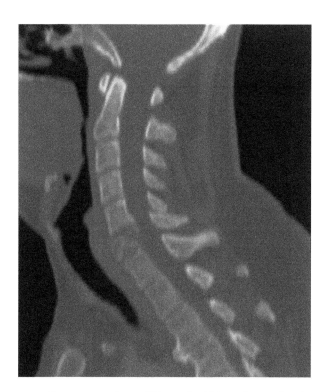

Figure 9.20 Demonstrates the axial T2-weighted MR with ventral cord compression by the tumor.

In patients with emergency department presentation of a pathological spine fracture, new neurological deficit, and no history of a primary tumor, multiple myeloma is one of the most frequent diagnoses. This diagnosis would be supported if multiple lytic lesions were seen on the skeletal survey. That was not the case here.

The medical management of this patient who has severe pain that appears to be position dependent, as well as cord compression and neurological deficit, would include the application of a rigid cervical collar. The patient should be started on IV steroids. A study by Slatkin and Posner[12] recommended high doses of dexamethasone (Decadron): 100 mg IV loading dose,[13] followed by 10 mg 4 times daily. This dosage is relatively large, but steroids certainly will provide the patient both pain relief and the possibility of neurological improvement.

The additional imaging studies were negative. Therefore, this appears to be a solitary vertebral lesion, and the question becomes what additional treatment is required. The options always are surgery, radiation, and chemotherapy. The indication for surgery in this case is quite strong:

1. To obtain a pathological diagnosis

2. To treat severe and intractable neck pain secondary to the pathological fracture

3. Spinal cord decompression to improve neurological function

Other indications for surgery that this patient does not have as of yet are spinal deformity and failure of other forms of adjuvant treatment, such as chemotherapy or radiation.

The simplest way to reach this tumor would be from an anterior approach to perform a C6 corpectomy and

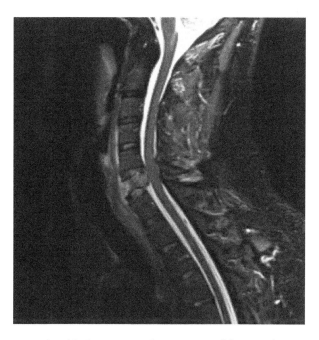

Figure 9.21 A and B. Demonstrates the appearance of the cervical spine after a C6 corpectomy, placement of methyl methacrylate and Steinman pins and an anterior cervical plate from C5–C7.

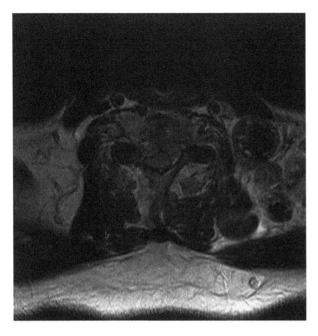

Figure 9.22 An axial CT scan after IV contrast, which demonstrates an abscess in the prevertebral space just posterior to the esophagus.

reconstruction. There are many different options for the reconstruction material, including iliac crest structural autograft, allograft, expandable or stackable cages, or what was done here from this relatively old slide, but a very tenable solution is cement and Steinman pins. Any of these interbody options should be supplemented by an anterior plating system (Figure 9.23).

After the patient's incisions are well healed, adjuvant therapy certainly can be considered depending on the pathology. In this case, the patient was found to have adenocarcinoma with an unknown primary tumor, and he received adjuvant radiation therapy.

COMPLICATIONS

The patient presented 2 weeks later with fever, difficulty swallowing, and pustulous discharge from the wound. When such a patient is seen in the emergency department with this presentation; the most likely diagnosis is an infection. A wound infection after an anterior cervical spine surgery is secondary to an esophageal injury until proved otherwise. This is almost always secondary to an unrecognized perforation during the initial dissection or reconstruction. The frequency is increased with anterior revision surgery. Lateral radiography and contrast esophagography remains the "gold standard" for the diagnosis of a perforation, but they lack sensitivity. A CT scan of the neck (Figure 9.24) to look for swelling or free air within the neck is useful. Although flexible esophagoscopy can be used to assess mucosal integrity, rigid esophagoscopy is more sensitive in assessing a perforation but may not be possible if the spine is deemed "unstable." We often perform a combination of these diagnostic modalities to establish the diagnosis.

In addition to broad-spectrum antibiotics to include anaerobe coverage, successful management of an esophageal

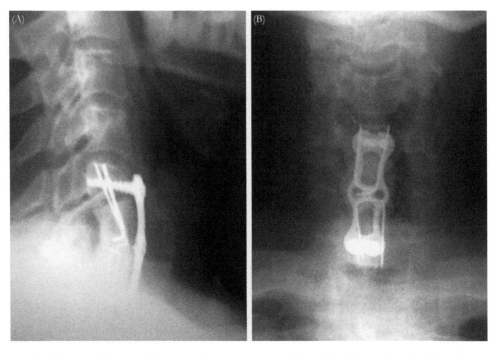

Figure 9.23 Demonstrates the placement of a sternocleidomastoid flap to repair an esophageal fistula flap.   Republished with permission of Wolters Kluwer Health, from Navarro R, Javahery R, Eismont F, Arnold DJ, Bhatia NN, Vanni S, Levi AD. The role of sternocleidomastoid muscle flap for esophageal fistula repair in anterior cervical spine surgery. *Spine.* 2005; 30(20): E617–622.

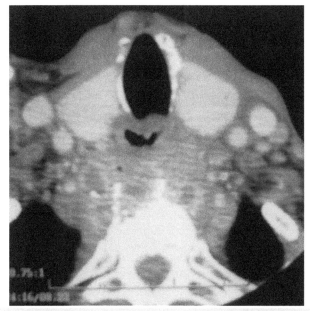

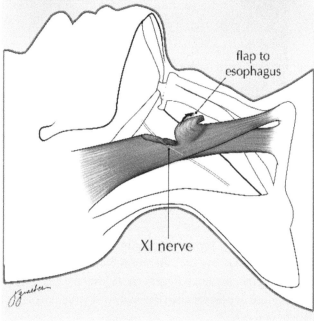

Figure 9.24 and 9.25 Plain X-rays demonstrate evidence of sagittal imbalance with her pelvic incidence (PI) = 45 degrees, lumbar lordosis (LL) – 32 degrees and the PI – LL = 77 degrees. The SVA measures 19.5 cm.

muscle flap (Figure 9.25). The muscle functions as a bolster for the repair; it provides a layer of separation between the esophagus and the graft and/instrumentation, and it increases the antibiotic delivery because of its vascularized nature. The SCM muscle is a useful tool in these cases because of its pliable nature, its multifocal blood supply, the ease with which it is raised and can be brought in to the esophageal defect, good cosmetic result, and the lack of significant donor site morbidity. Other flaps have also been used, such as a sternohyoid muscle, sternothyroid muscle, pectoralis muscle, and free omentum. A primary repair without reinforcement can take a long time to heal, preventing the patient from starting oral feedings. In addition, direct primary repair has a significant failure rate. In our series,[14] all the SCM-reinforced esophageal repairs were successful, and the time for return to oral feedings was significantly shorter (mean of 59 days) than when a primary repair was attempted (mean of 153 days).

CASE 5

HISTORY AND PHYSICAL EXAMINATION

An 81-year-old female presents to you with a 2-year history of progressive low back pain, as well as leg pain and paresthesias made worse by walking more than 1 block. While that is a major problem—her most troubling issue is her complaint of her "inability to stand up straight." Her past medical history is significant for hypertension and prior surgical history of a L1 laminectomy. On examination, she has hyporeflexia in the lower extremities, as well as some gait imbalance. Plain x-rays demonstrate evidence of sagittal imbalance with her pelvic incidence (PI) = 45 degrees, lumbar lordosis (LL)–32 degrees and the PI – LL = 77 degrees. The sagittal vertical axis (SVA) measures 19.5 cm (Figures 9.26 and 9.27 and Table 9.1).

The CT scan done in the supine position continues to demonstrate loss of lumbar lordosis without evidence of spontaneous fusion at the disc levels. The sagittal MR demonstrates an element of severe spinal stenosis at L1–L2 (Figures 9.28 and 9.29).

ANALYSIS OF CASE AND SURGICAL PLAN

The differential diagnosis is not at question in this case—this is a surgical management dilemma. The patient has evidence of spinal stenosis and neurogenic claudication—however, a

perforation has to fulfill the following conditions: functional closure of the perforation (patient is able to eat), control or prevention of infection (local abscess, spondylodiscitis, septicemia, and mediastinitis), and stabilization of the cervical spine. In general, a fistula is most likely to close when a patient's nutritional requirements are met and no obstruction exists below the leak.

Our general bias is toward cervical exploration, repair of the esophageal perforation with inverted sutures, and reinforcement with a rotational sternocleidomastoid (SCM)

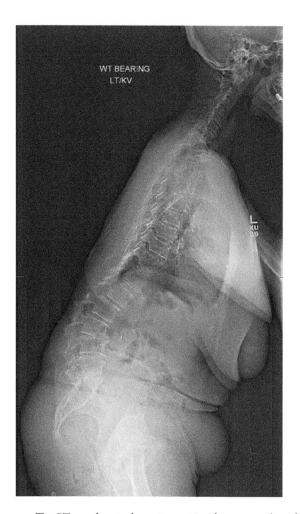

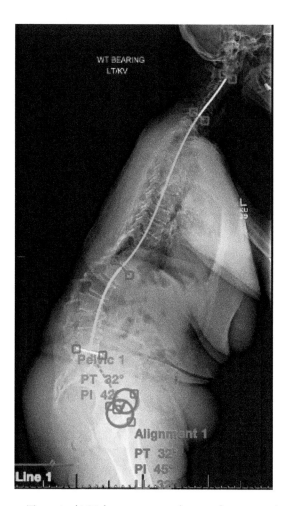

Figures 9.26 The CT scan done in the supine position demonstrates loss of lumbar lordosis without evidence of spontaneous fusion at the disc levels.

Figure 9.27 The sagittal MR demonstrates an element of severe spinal stenosis at L1–L2.

simple laminectomy is not the answer. A laminectomy and fusion without sagittal balance correction will result in a poor outcome. It is *critical* to recognize that a sagittal balance problem also exists. The clues include a history that the patient cannot stand straight. However, a detailed analysis of sagittal parameters establishes that the patient is out of balance. The most important sagittal balance measurements include the SVA. It is measured as the distance from the plumb line from the center of C7 vertebral body to the posterior edge of the upper sacral endplate surface. In this patient—the SVA is 19.5 cm and while in part age, sex, and ethnic dependent, in general should be <5 cm. Similarly, the mismatch between PI – LL—measuring 75 degrees demonstrates the patient is grossly out of balance. This PI – LL should be approximately about 10 degrees. This calculation not only confirms a sagittal imbalance issue but dictates the degree of sagittal balance correction required—about 75 – 10 degrees or "65 degrees." There are many options to obtain that correction, and a general knowledge of what spinal operative correction will accomplish is critical in

developing an operative plan. Examples include a pedicle subtraction osteotomy that typically provides 30 degrees of correction versus a ponte osteotomy, which typically gives 5 to 10 degrees per level. In general, sagittal balance correction is more important than coronal correction in terms of patient outcomes.

A detailed discussion regarding how to prepare for surgery is important as is the knowledge of the complications. Intraoperative electrophysiologic monitoring is critical in these cases to help determine the safety of the correction, and again knowing what to do in advance of any changes in either SSEPs or MEPs must be considered (see Case 3).

Table 9.1. **PREOPERATIVE SAGITTAL BALANCE MEASUREMENTS**

PI	45 degrees
LL	32 degrees
PI – LL	77 degrees
SVA	19.5 cm

Note: PI = pelvic incidence; LL = lumbar lordosis; SVA = sagittal vertical axis

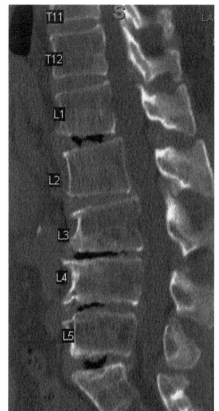

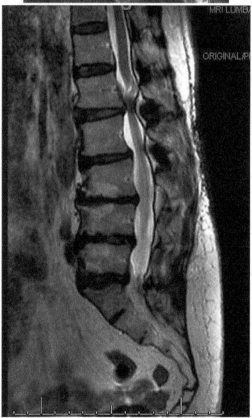

The surgery should be done initially in the supine position with an inflatable device or an IV bag of saline behind the small of the back to increase lordotic posture. The anterior approach to L5–S1 and L4–L5 with anterior lumbar interbody fusion and placement of a lordotic femoral ring allograft typically provides 15 to 20 degrees of correction per level. Finally, a lateral mini-open approach with anterior release via a section of the anterior longitudinal ligament and placement of a 30-degree lordotic cage was done. It should be noted that this differs dramatically from a simple lateral discectomy and interbody fusion (e.g., XLIF/DLIF procedure), which does not provide any significant sagittal correction. This anterior and lateral approach was then followed by a posterior decompression and long segment instrumented fusion from T10 to the pelvis. This was supplemented by ponte osteotomies to obtain another 5 degrees per level. This approach will provide with a more than adequate sagittal balance correction (Figures 9.30, 9.31, 9.32, and Table 9.2).

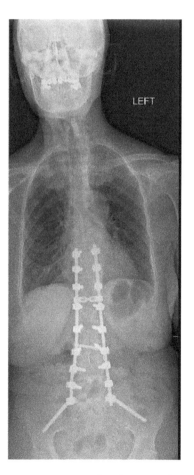

Figure 9.30 Demonstrates post-operative lateral images with anterior lumbar interbody fusion at L4–L5 and L5–S1: an anterior release with a hyperlordotic graft placed at L3L4 and posterior segmental instrumentation from T10 to the pelvis with superimposed marks to determine (PI) = 37 degrees; lumbar lordosis (LL) = 20 degrees; and the PI – LL = 17 degrees. The SVA measures 4.6 cm.

Figures 9.28 and 9.29 Demonstrates postoperative images (anterior–posterior and lateral and with anterior lumbar interbody fusion at L4–L5 and L5–S1) an anterior release with a hyperlordotic graft placed at L3–L4 and posterior segmental instrumentation from T10 to the pelvis.

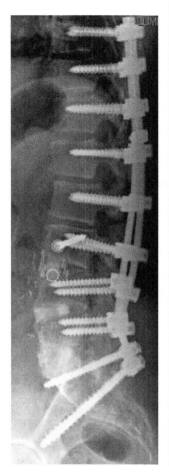
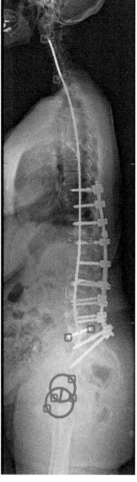

Figuress 9.31 and 9.32 Demonstrates a postoperative standing sagittal x-ray with anterior lordotic grafts placed at L3–L4, L4–L5, L5–S1 and posterior instrumentation from T10 to the pelvis. Her pelvic incidence (PI) = 37 degrees, lumbar lordosis (LL) – 20 degrees and the PI – LL = 17 degrees. The SVA measures 4.6 cm. The SVA is markedly improved as well as her symptoms of inability to stand straight and her complaints of leg pain with walking.

INDICATIONS

Indications for a long segment fusion from T10 to the pelvis clearly exist, and this case example provides a rather robust illustration of a solid indication for this surgery and what can be achieved in regards to sagittal balance correction.

Table 9.2. POSTOPERATIVE SAGITTAL BALANCE MEASUREMENTS

PI	37 degrees
LL	−20 degrees
PI – LL	17 degrees
SVA	4.6 cm

Note: PI = pelvic incidence; LL = lumbar lordosis; SVA = sagittal vertical axis

Unfortunately, individual case reviews of candidates submitted data have demonstrated indications such as painful, multilevel degenerative disc disease, prevention of kyphotic deformity, preventative maintenance, or "my partners perform similar procedures." These proposals will be difficult to defend on the oral boards.

COMPLICATIONS

Complications are incredibly common with this type of surgery—probably as high as 50%. These include at the acute stage—infection, bleeding, seroma, cerebrospinal fluid leak, nerve or SCI, hernia, vascular or visceral injury. In the long run, one must be aware of failed fusion, instrumentation failure/fracture/pseudoarthrosis, and post junctional kyphosis as real possibilities.

REFERENCES

1. Vale FL, Burns J, Jackson AB, Hadley MN. Combined medical and surgical treatment after acute spinal cord injury: results of a prospective pilot study to assess the merits of aggressive medical resuscitation and blood pressure management. *J Neurosurg.* 1997;87(2):239–246.
2. Bracken MB, Shepard MJ, Collins WF, et al. A randomized, controlled trial of methylprednisolone or naloxone in the treatment of acute spinal-cord injury. results of the Second National Acute Spinal Cord Injury Study. *N Engl J Med.* 1990;322(20):1405–1411.
3. Hurlbert RJ, Hadley MN, Walters BC, et al. Pharmacological therapy for acute spinal cord injury. *Neurosurgery.* 2015;76(Suppl 1):S71–S83.
4. Fehlings MG, Vaccaro A, Wilson JR, et al. Early versus delayed decompression for traumatic cervical spinal cord injury: results of the Surgical Timing in Acute Spinal Cord Injury Study (STASCIS). *PLoS ONE.* 2012;7(2):e32037.
5. Doran SE, Papadopoulos SM, Ducker TB, Lillehei KO. Magnetic resonance imaging documentation of coexistent traumatic locked facets of the cervical spine and disc herniation. *J Neurosurg.* 1993;79(3):341–345.
6. Eismont FJ, Arena MJ, Green BA. Extrusion of an intervertebral disc associated with traumatic subluxation or dislocation of cervical facets. Case report. *J Bone Joint Surg Am.* 1991;73(10):1555–1560.
7. Grant GA, Mirza SK, Chapman JR, et al. Risk of early closed reduction in cervical spine subluxation injuries. *J Neurosurg.* 1999;90(1 Suppl):13–18.
8. Theodotou CB, Ghobrial GM, Middleton AL, Wang MY, Levi AD. Anterior reduction and fusion of cervical facet dislocations. *Neurosurgery.* 2019;84(2):388–395.
9. Razack N, Green BA, Levi AD. The management of traumatic cervical bilateral facet fracture-dislocations with unicortical anterior plates. *J Spinal Disord.* 2000;13(5):374–381.
10. Harrop JS, Sharan AD, Scheid EH, Jr., Vaccaro AR, Przybylski GJ. Tracheostomy placement in patients with complete cervical spinal cord injuries: American Spinal Injury Association Grade A. *J Neurosurg.* 2004;100(1 Suppl Spine):20–23.
11. Levi AD, Dickman CA, Sonntag VK. Management of postoperative infections after spinal instrumentation. *J Neurosurg.* 1997;86(6):975–980.

12. Slatkin NE, Posner JB. Management of spinal epidural metastases. *Clin Neurosurg.* 1983;30:698–716.

13. Greenberg HS, Kim JH, Posner JB. Epidural spinal cord compression from metastatic tumor: results with a new treatment protocol. *Ann Neurol.* 1980;8(4):361–366.

14. Navarro R, Javahery R, Eismont F, et al. The role of the sternocleidomastoid muscle flap for esophageal fistula repair in anterior cervical spine surgery. *Spine.* 2005;30(20):E617–E622.

10.

PERIPHERAL NERVE

Robert J. Spinner

- History

  - Ask about 3 things: motor, sensory, and pain. An important question is: where does the pain start?

- Physical examination

  - Examine for 3 things: motor, sensory, and pain. Motor testing includes an examination of strength (Medical Research Council grading 0 to 5/5), atrophy, and tone. Sensory testing can include pin-prick, light touch, and two-point discrimination. Pain can be assessed by a provocative test (such as the presence of Phalen's sign, a positive elbow flexion test, or a thoracic outlet maneuver); the presence of percussion tenderness (a so-called Tinel's sign) can help localize the site of a peripheral nerve lesion. The major differential diagnosis is often peripheral versus spinal. For peripheral nerve lesions, one would typically find a positive sign in the periphery and a negative one at the spine level (e.g., Spurling's test, straight-leg raise test). For spinal sources, one would typically not find a provocative sign in the periphery but would find one at the spine level.

- Electrodiagnostic studies

  - Electromyography (EMG)

  - Nerve conduction study (NCS)

- Imaging: ultrasound (US) or magnetic resonance imaging (MRI) and nerve blocks where applicable

  - Image nerves at unusual sites of compression (localized clinically, such as with percussion tenderness) to rule out an undiagnosed mass lesion with high-resolution US or MRI.

- Nerve blocks may be done for diagnostic purposes (local agents) and may provide transient relief of pain. They do not define the exact site of the problem but may block the pathway. Therapeutic blocks (with steroids) can also be considered.

An analogy would be the four legs of a table–the more legs (i.e., "positives" of the four parts of the evaluation) the more stable the table.

CASE 1

HISTORY

A 45-year-old woman presents with a 6-month history of right calf pain with dysesthesias radiating into the plantar aspect of the right foot. She has no low back pain and no weakness. She is otherwise healthy.

PHYSICAL EXAMINATION

The patient has normal strength in the lower limb. She has normal sensation in the leg and foot. She has a negative straight leg raise (SLR) test.

DIFFERENTIAL DIAGNOSIS

The differential diagnosis is tibial neuropathy versus S1 radiculopathy.

ADDITIONAL INFORMATION

Physical examination would reveal pain on percussion in the proximal posterior leg, which would reproduce her symptoms. No mass could be appreciated.

An EMG/NCS was normal. Outside MRI of the lumbar spine also was unrevealing.

Because the proximal leg is an unusual site of nerve compression, MRI (or US) of the proximal leg should be considered. This would reveal a mass lesion within the tibial nerve (Figure 10.1). T2-weighted imaging shows an approximately 2-cm hyperintense well-encapsulated round lesion with a speckled appearance (target sign).

HOW SHOULD THIS CASE BE MANAGED?

The clinical and radiologic features would be consistent with a benign nerve sheath tumor (contrast those of a malignant peripheral nerve sheath tumor [MPNST]). Further questioning would reveal no history or family history suggestive of multiple nerve sheath tumors (such as schwannomatosis or neurofibromatosis). Surgical resection is generally safe. For a schwannoma (the most common benign nerve sheath tumor found in a nonsyndromic patient), the mass can typically be removed at a fascicular level (Figure 10.2). In this case, the lesion, although relatively small, is sufficiently symptomatic to warrant surgical resection. Alternatively, this may be observed with clinical and radiologic follow-up.

At operation, a posterior approach to the proximal leg is performed with the patient in the prone position. Preoperative localization with US can help focus the incision. The nerve is accessed through a longitudinal incision from the popliteal crease distally, centered on the region of pain. The interval between the 2 heads of the gastrocnemius muscles is opened. Proximal and distal control of the tibial nerve is obtained (Figure 10.3A). The nerve tumor is seen. Major branches to the gastrocnemius and soleus muscles are protected. Mapping of the tumor can be performed using a portable electrical stimulator. Nerve stimulation allows one to determine that the fascicle of origin is nonmotor. Typical stimulation parameters are 1 to 2 mA. A longitudinal incision is made in the bare area on the top surface of this image, and the fascicles are swept away. A single entering fascicle and 2 exiting fascicles are identified (Figure 10.3B). Stimulation of these fascicles does not produce any muscle contraction (or nerve action potentials [NAPs] if this technique was used). The lesion is resected (Figure 10.3C). Histologically, it is a schwannoma.

One of the critical aspects of any Oral Board Examination case involving a peripheral tumor is to ensure before surgery that it does not represent a malignant lesion such as an MPNST. Clinical factors that favor this diagnosis are a history of neurofibromatosis type 1 (NF-1), rapid growth over weeks or months, increased refractory pain, large size, and, most important, significant motor deficits at presentation. Most benign tumors present like the current case with paresthesias and pain that is less severe. Radiologic features that may support the diagnosis of an MPNST would include irregular borders, irregular enhancement, necrosis on MRI, and increased avidity on positron emission tomography/computed tomography (PET/CT)—typically with an SUV of greater than 5.2.

COMPLICATIONS

One hour after surgery, while the patient is in the recovery room, you get a call that she is experiencing severe calf pain that has been refractory to medical treatment. Plantarflexion and toe flexion are quite weak (and painful). She is numb on the plantar aspect of the foot.

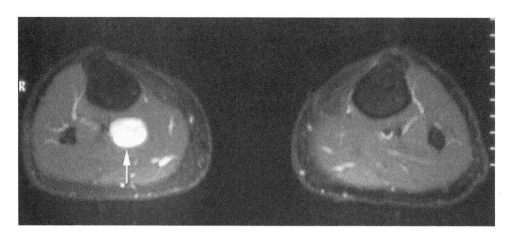

Figure 10.1 A mass lesion (*arrow*) within the tibial nerve. T2-weighted MRI shows an approximately 2-cm hyperintense, well-encapsulated round lesion with a speckled appearance (*target sign*).

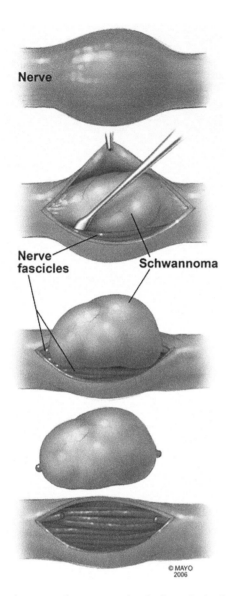

Nerve

Nerve fascicles

Schwannoma

© MAYO
2006

Figure 10.2 A schwannoma being removed at the fascicular level.

The history and the presence of a new (*evolving*) neurologic deficit would be diagnostic with a tibial neuropathy likely from an expanding hematoma (rather than nerve injury from the surgical manipulation). Removal of the dressing would reveal a large hematoma in the posterior calf. This should be evacuated emergently.

BENIGN NERVE SHEATH TUMORS

Benign nerve sheath tumors may include the following:

- Schwannoma

- Neurofibroma (may rarely transform into malignancy)

    - Most are solitary and conventional globular masses

- If multiple, suspect syndromes (know features and genetics)

    - NF-1 (neurofibromas in periphery); NF-2 and schwannomatosis (schwannomas in periphery)

- Resect symptomatic or large conventional lesions. Typically, tumors can be resected at the fascicular level, sparing most of the nerve with good to excellent outcomes 80% to 90% of the time in skilled hands.

- Treat plexiform lesions (especially those with NF-1 and NF-2) with respect (observe in most cases; perform subtotal debulking of the predominant nodule on occasion for worsening symptoms, growth, or concern about malignant transformation of a plexiform neurofibroma).

OTHER BENIGN LESIONS

- Intrinsic mass—intraneural ganglion cyst (cyst within the epineurium)

This typically occurs within the common peroneal nerve near the fibular neck. It produces a predominant deep peroneal nerve palsy (foot and toe drop and strong eversion). EMG scan help localize the mass. Imaging reveals a cystic lesion. Cyst is derived from a neighboring joint (for common peroneal nerve, the origin is from the anterior aspect of the superior tibiofibular joint). Intraneural ganglion cyst is formed by propagation along the articular branch with extension into the parent nerve (common peroneal nerve). The main goal of surgery is to disconnect the articular branch connection and decompress the cyst.

- Extrinsic mass—may compress neighboring nerve by mass effect

Protect the nerves first, and then remove the tumor. Examples include extraneural ganglion cysts and lipomas.

MALIGNANT PERIPHERAL NERVE SHEATH TUMOR

An MPNST may form spontaneously, occur after radiotherapy, or appear in patients with neurofibromas and NF-1. If a lesion were suspicious for malignancy based on

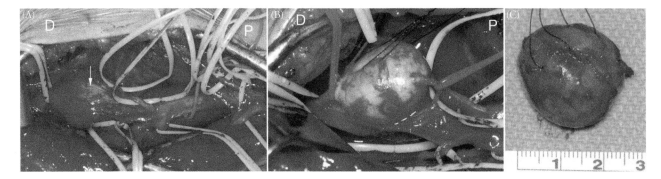

Figure 10.3 Open interval between the gastrocnemius muscles. A: Proximal (P) and distal (D) control of the tibial nerve is obtained with nerve tumor (*arrow*) shown. B: A single entering fascicle and two exiting fascicles are identified. C: Resected schwannoma.

clinical and radiologic features (see case discussion), then percutaneous (image-guided) or limited open biopsy and staging would be performed. Most surgeons prefer wide resection after nerve tumor resection after a definitive diagnosis has been made. This approach is often combined with radiotherapy. The 5-year survival rate is about 50%. Do not perform aggressive resection based on intraoperative histology because the frozen section may be incorrect.

CASE 2

HISTORY

A 40-year old man sustained an accidental self-inflicted machete injury to the left popliteal fossa during a fall while he was deer hunting. He had an immediate foot drop and presented to the local emergency room. A 2-inch laceration was primarily closed at that time. A referring physician calls you 4 days later with the referral.

DIAGNOSIS

The likely diagnosis is a transected common peroneal nerve in the popliteal fossa (proximal to the fibular neck). One should try to ensure that there is no associated tibial nerve or vascular injury.

HOW SHOULD THIS CASE BE MANAGED?

A sharp neural injury should be managed acutely with nerve exploration and repair (if possible). Ideally, these types of nerve injury should be identified as early as possible, within 3 days or so. Observation is not appropriate if a transection is suspected. Cut ends of a nerve will not repair themselves. While compression is theoretically possible from an evolving hematoma, in this case scenario the mechanism (of the

machete injury) and the immediate foot drop would be consistent with a sharp injury (an ensuing nerve transection) and an immediate neural deficit.

The patient should be sent to you immediately NPO for surgical exploration.

PHYSICAL EXAMINATION

The oblique laceration is showing signs of good healing without infection. There is a complete loss of foot dorsiflexion, toe and big toe extension and eversion (Figure 10.4). Plantar flexion, toe flexion, and inversion are normal. There is decreased sensation on the dorsum of the foot, including the first dorsal web space and preserved sensation on the plantar foot. There is a pain on percussion just proximal to the incision that causes paresthesias on the dorsal foot. There are good pedal pulses.

TESTING

No additional testing per se is needed. EMG/NCS would not change management. At this early time, EMG would

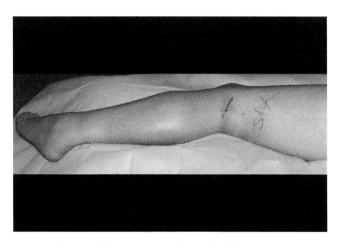

Figure 10.4 The site of the laceration in the popliteal fossa is seen in this patient with a complete footdrop.

not show evidence of denervation. Imaging may be considered but is not mandated. Ultrasound in the hands of an experienced examiner will show the nerve in discontinuity. This study would be preferable to MRI in an emergency room setting for a suspected transected nerve.

WHAT SHOULD BE DONE?

The patient should be counseled regarding nerve exploration, nerve repair, and possible nerve grafting using sural nerve (if necessary). The patient should be placed in a lateral or prone position. The previous wound can be incorporated into a more extensile approach.

Reopening of the wound itself revealed the distal end of the nerve (Figure 10.5); this can be misleading as the proximal stump of the nerve was not evident (partially due to its retraction and coverage by hematoma) and the distal portion of the transected nerve if stimulated would cause muscle contraction in the leg (i.e., Wallerian degeneration would not have occurred yet).

More proximal exposure reveals the retracted proximal stump (Figure 10.6) and, in this case, a transected sural communicating branch of the common peroneal nerve (Figure 10.7) (note the tibial nerve would be more deeply and posteriorly located, and if stimulated would have caused contraction).

A direct repair should always be attempted, as results are better with end-end repair than with interpositional grafting. Proximal and distal stumps are mobilized circumferentially (Figure 10.7). Distally, the fibular tunnel is released. Nerve stumps are freshened up and good fascicular structure is noted. Direct end-end nerve repair can be done without tension (Figure 10.8). Gentle flexion of the knee can further prevent tension, if necessary.

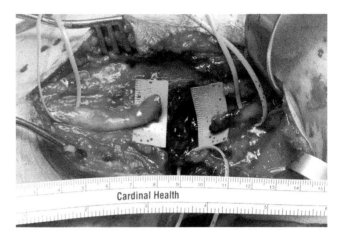

Figure 10.6 When further exposure is obtained by extending the incision proximal to the knee crease, the proximal stump of the common peroneal nerve is seen. A several centimeter gap is appreciated.

Nerve ends are aligned. Several 8-0 nonabsorbable sutures are placed microsurgically in the epineurium of the common peroneal nerve (and the sural communicating branch). Some reinforce repairs with fibrin glue.

If there were undue tension preventing a direct end-end repair after nerve mobilization, nerve grafting should be done. The sural nerve (even though it was transected) could still be used; several interpositional cable grafts could be placed.

The wound is closed in layers. The knee is immobilized in gentle flexion (30 to 45 degrees) for 3 weeks to protect the nerve repair. The patient can use crutches during this time.

FOLLOW-UP

The patient is seen back for routine wound examination. At 3 weeks, the patient can start ambulating as tolerated. He

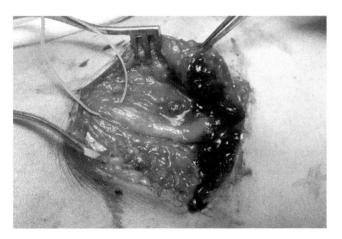

Figure 10.5 The distal end of the common peroneal nerve is seen. The distal stump is buried beneath hematoma. The proximal portion of the transected common peroneal nerve is not seen in this limited exposure.

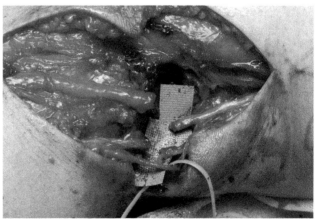

Figure 10.7 The proximal and distal ends of the common peroneal nerve have been mobilized. The laceration of the sural communicating branch from the common peroneal nerve is noted.

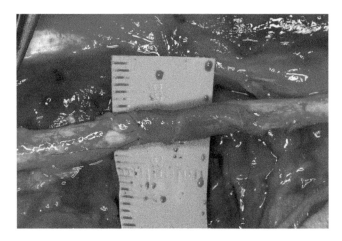

Figure 10.8 Direct end-end repair is done. There is good alignment without tension.

was fitted for an ankle foot orthosis (AFO) and instructed in keeping his heel cord supple. No formal physical therapy program is needed.

The patient would be followed up with serial clinical and electrophysiological testing. Early clinical or EMG recovery could be seen in 4 to 6 months and would improve over 18 months or so. Here the patient regained MCR Grade 4 ankle dorsiflexion and toe extension and eversion at long-term follow-up and was weaned from the AFO.

WHAT IF THERE WERE NO RECOVERY?

If recovery does not occur or is insufficient to allow useful ankle dorsiflexion, the patient could continue use of the AFO as needed. Alternatively, the patient can be referred to an orthopedic or plastic surgeon for consideration of a tendon transfer (the functioning posterior tibialis tendon can be relocated); this tendon transfer can be done electively at any time assuming the heel cord is supple.

CASE 3

HISTORY

An 18-year-old female high school senior presented with persistent paralysis of her left dominant upper limb affecting shoulder motion and elbow flexion. She was in a rollover bus accident 6 months previously. There were no other injuries at the time, and she was discharged from the hospital on the same day. She has not noted any improvement in her condition.

PHYSICAL EXAMINATION

The patient has no active shoulder abduction. She has no elbow flexion. There is no muscular contraction of shoulder abductors or elbow flexors. She has normal trapezius function. She has strong elbow extension as well as wrist and finger flexion and extension. She has decreased sensation in the proximal posterior arm and in the volar forearm and thumb. A Tinel's sign was demonstrated in the supraclavicular fossa.

TESTING

EMG demonstrates no activation and 3+ fibrillations in the biceps, deltoid, and infraspinatus muscles; the rhomboid and cervical paraspinal muscles are normal. Lateral antebrachial nerve conduction is absent on the left compared with a normal right-sided response. Chest radiograph is normal. CT myelogram (or high-resolution brachial plexus MRI) shows no evidence of pseudomeningoceles.

DIAGNOSIS

The diagnosis is an upper trunk (C5-C6) brachial plexopathy, posttraumatic (post-ganglionic).

HOW SHOULD THIS CASE BE MANAGED?

Surgical exploration would be indicated because there is no evidence of clinical or electrical improvement at an appropriate time— that is, 6 months after injury.

A supraclavicular approach would be done (know the basics). Either a transverse incision several fingerbreadths above the clavicle in the posterior triangle or a zig-zag approach along the posterior border of the sternocleidomastoid and clavicle could be used. The external jugular vein is mobilized. The omohyoid is typically divided. The fat pad is reflected laterally. The phrenic nerve is seen on the anterior scalene and can be traced to the C5 nerve. The upper trunk and the rest of the brachial plexus are found in the interscalene triangle. The trunks are lateral to the anterior scalene. The spinal nerves are beneath the anterior scalene, which can be divided to improve proximal exposure. The subclavian artery is caudad by the lower trunk.

A neuroma-in-continuity of the upper trunk is found.

WHAT SHOULD BE DONE NEXT?

After external neurolysis, NAPs across the upper trunk lesion are recorded (Figure 10.9).

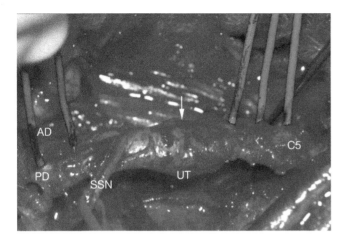

Figure 10.9 Nerve action potentials (NAPs) across the upper trunk (UT) lesion (*arrow*) present after external neurolysis. AD, anterior division of upper trunk; PD, posterior division of upper trunk; SSN, suprascapular nerve; 3 prong, stimulator; 2 prong, recorder.

No further surgical reconstruction would be necessary. The finding of preserved NAPs in this situation is an excellent prognosticator. Neurolysis alone yields an approximately 90% good or better recovery over 2 years. Recovery of proximal targets (shoulder and elbow) is better than that of more distal targets (below the elbow).

Nerve grafting or nerve transfers could have been considered if NAPs were not present in this postganglionic lesion. Details of nerve grafting or nerve transfer options are provided later in the discussion of preganglionic injury.

FOLLOW-UP

The patient made an excellent recovery over the following 2 years. There was mild atrophy of the deltoid and biceps, but the patient was able to return to full activity.

WHAT IF A PREGANGLIONIC INJURY WERE FOUND?

If a preganglionic C5-C6 lesion were presented instead, rhomboid and midcervical paraspinal muscles would typically have fibrillations on EMG, and the myelogram would have shown abnormalities involving the cervical roots at that level (absence or asymmetry compared with the other side) or pseudomeningoceles. Intraoperative electrophysiologic testing would reveal a preganglionic (rapid) NAP and absent evoked potentials. Nerve transfers would be performed to reconstruct shoulder function and elbow flexion (see later discussion). Neurolysis and nerve grafting would not be appropriate.

TIMING OF RECONSTRUCTION: RULE OF 3S + 1

- Less than 3 days—sharp injury, presumed laceration or transection (e.g., stab wound). If the patient presents later, then operate at the time of initial evaluation.

- At 3 weeks—blunt or jagged transection, rupture (e.g., propeller blade). This is controversial. Some surgeons prefer tagging nerve ends with slight tension (operation 1—immediately after injury) so that they do not retract and then reexploring and reconstructing the injured nerve subacutely about 3 weeks later (operation 2) when the zone of injury is better delineated. Others prefer performing the definitive operation immediately after injury and making a decision about the extent of injury based on the initial intraoperative appearance.

- At 3 to 6 months—closed injury, stretch, and gunshot wounds (note that most gunshot wounds do not transect nerve). If there is no clinical or electrophysiologic improvement, explore and perform NAP recordings (see later discussion).

- At 1 year—secondary surgery and reconstruction (e.g., other procedures, such as tendon transfers or joint fusions). Nerve (primary) surgery has the best results when performed by 6 months, but it typically does not work well after 9 months and especially after 1 year.

OPTIONS FOR NERVE SURGERY

Neurolysis

Circumferential dissection of nerve is done as the first part of the procedure. If an NAP is obtained across a neuroma-in-continuity, neurolysis alone is performed. In this situation, about 90% of patients obtain favorable outcomes at long-term follow-up.

Nerve Repair

Direct repair is performed to approximate nerve ends after transection or after a focal neuroma-in-continuity is resected (in the setting of an absent NAP). Mobilize stumps to obtain end-to-end repair if possible without tension. Techniques to shorten the nerve gap include mobilization of nerve ends by freeing them up proximally and distally; transposition of nerve to make a straighter line (such as for ulnar or radial nerves) when feasible; and gentle flexion of the joint and immobilization postoperatively in that position if necessary for several weeks. Early repair facilitates direct repair. Align fascicles as best as possible. Several fascicular or epineurial sutures are applied using microsurgical technique and 8-0 to 10-0 suture material. Immobilize for 3 weeks postoperatively to protect the integrity of the suture line. Results with nerve repair (1 suture line) are better than with nerve grafting (2 suture lines).

Nerve Grafting

If a gap exists after nerve stump retraction (following delay in treatment of transection or rupture) or after resection of a more lengthy neuroma-in-continuity (absent NAP), resect the neuroma back to normal nerve ends and good fascicular structure as gauged by visual inspection after sectioning or determined microscopically at frozen section. Estimate the gap between stumps and the number of cable grafts needed to fill the face of the nerves. Harvest an appropriate length of sural nerve from the leg. Be generous with the nerve harvest—err on taking more because nerve shrinks during surgery. Avoid tension in the repair. Sometimes, you will need or want an extra cable graft. Make an incision in the posterolateral leg obliquely from the ankle to popliteal fossa as necessary. The sural nerve is identified midway between the lateral malleolus and lateral edge of the Achilles tendon next to the lesser saphenous vein. You can obtain 30 to 40 cm of sural nerve from each leg if necessary. Donor morbidity includes an expected sensory loss in the dorsolateral foot and the possibility for neuropathic pain after harvest.

Techniques

Option 1: Suture each graft individually both proximally and distally.

Option 2: Use fibrin glue to form a cable of grouped grafts. Freshen up ends with a sharp knife. Suture cabled grafts as one unit.

Following either method, immobilize the limb for 3 weeks.

Nerve Transfer

Transfer of an expendable or redundant nerve, nerve branch, or fascicle may be done for preganglionic (avulsion) injury when standard nerve grafting techniques cannot be performed. An example in a patient with a severe brachial plexus injury would include intercostal nerve transfers used to obtain elbow flexion in brachial plexus reconstruction (usually 3 intercostal nerves from T3 to T5 are transferred

from the chest to the musculocutaneous nerve in the axilla). Because of encouraging results with nerve transfers, these techniques are being employed by some surgeons in patients with postganglionic injury as a substitute for nerve grafts (which could also be done). A new approach to an upper trunk (C5-C6) brachial plexus injury would be to transfer the distal portion of the spinal accessory nerve to the suprascapular nerve to try to regain some shoulder stability (abduction and external rotation), along with a branch of the triceps to the axillary nerve (for deltoid function—additional abduction), and transfer an expendable fascicle of the ulnar nerve in the proximal arm directly to the biceps branch of the musculocutaneous nerve (Oberlin procedure) to try to regain elbow flexion. These types of nerve transfers are done closer to the muscle end organs, and they speed up and often improve recovery.

CASE 4

HISTORY

A 35-year-old man presents with difficulty raising his right arm above his head for 6 months. He had received a tetanus shot into his right arm a few days before the onset of his shoulder symptoms. He had experienced severe right periscapular pain, which lasted for 10 days. The pain then resolved, and the weakness became apparent and has persisted.

PHYSICAL EXAMINATION

The patient is only able to abduct and forward-flex 90 degrees. He has strong deltoid and supraspinatus muscles. There is no sensory abnormality. He has prominent winging of the right scapula (Figure 10.10).

DIAGNOSIS AND DIFFERENTIAL DIAGNOSIS

The clinical scenario would be quite typical for Parsonage-Turner syndrome (idiopathic brachial plexopathy). Here the trigger was provided. If it is not obvious, ask about known immune or infectious-type associations (e.g., flu, flu shots or immunizations, recent surgery or trauma). Parsonage-Turner syndrome is well known to affect the long thoracic nerve by causing winged scapula (differentiate other causes of winged scapula from a spinal accessory nerve lesion—i.e., following posterior triangle of the neck operations, the trapezius is affected but not the sternomastoid, or

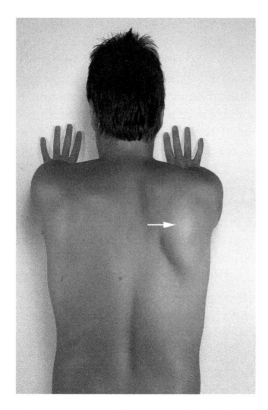

Figure 10.10 Prominent winging of the right scapula (*arrow*).

after dorsal scapular nerve injury, which is rare). Long thoracic neuropathy may also occur in combination with other nerves (e.g., suprascapular, axillary, and anterior and posterior interosseous nerves, which may have a predilection) as part of Parsonage-Turner syndrome, producing a more diffuse patchy neurological process (know how to differentiate this condition from a several-level spinal localization). The serratus anterior is innervated by C5-7 spinal nerves; a spinal level localization would not produce isolated serratus anterior paralysis; other C5-7 innervated muscles (e.g., deltoid, spinati, rhomboids, biceps, brachioradialis, brachialis, triceps, etc.) would also have to be affected.

Nerve injury could follow directly from a needle stick or indirectly from a hematoma and might be considered. However, the clinical picture and the timing of the neurological deficit would differ from this case.

ADDITIONAL TESTING

Electrophysiologic testing would confirm an isolated long thoracic neuropathy. In this case, fibrillations were present (indicative of denervation) along with several nascent units (indicative of reinnervation). Note that standard EMG examination would not ordinarily include needling the serratus anterior muscle. Cervical MRI would be normal but might show subtle pathology, such as mild central or foraminal stenosis at several levels of the cervical spine. Do not be fooled in to suggesting a multilevel anterior cervical discectomy and fusion, for example. Brachial plexus MRI could be considered and might show some subtle T2-weighted hyperintensity (i.e., nonspecific inflammatory) changes diffusely in the brachial plexus.

HOW SHOULD THIS CASE BE MANAGED?

Given the fact that there was some evidence of EMG recovery at 6 months, the patient would be treated with physical therapy. Pain management may be necessary. In general, the natural history is favorable; approximately 80% of patients make a good (although incomplete) recovery of function; rarely do patients have persistent problematic pain. Some surgeons have described decompression of the long thoracic nerve at the level of the middle scalene (supraclavicular) in suspected cases of entrapment, but this is controversial. There is no proven benefit of medications or even steroids, although frequently a short course may be tried empirically. Surgical decompression in my opinion was not recommended here given the early recovery. Maximal recovery may take up to 2½ years (note the long time for reinnervation, especially given the anatomic course of the long thoracic nerve). Patients should be counseled about the small risk for having a second attack or having a family member affected with an inflammatory neuropathy.

FOLLOW-UP

The patient noted slow improvement in shoulder active range of motion over the next 18 months. Mild scapular winging persisted at long-term follow-up but was asymptomatic.

A tendon transfer could be considered at approximately 2 years to stabilize the winged scapula for persistent symptoms (i.e., periscapular pain or loss of motion) or cosmetic concerns.

CASE 5

HISTORY

A 38-year-old man presents with a 3-year history of burning lateral thigh pain. He is unable to wear long pants due to hypersensitivity. He has no weakness in the lower limb and no history of back pain. He is taking multiple medications for pain control.

The patient is an obese man. He is numb and has allodynia in the lateral thigh. He has normal strength in the lower limb, including the quadriceps. His deep tendon reflex at the knee is normal. He has a negative SLR.

ADDITIONAL TESTS AND DIFFERENTIAL DIAGNOSIS

Percussion (over the lateral femoral cutaneous nerve) just medial to the anterior superior iliac spine over the inguinal ligament would be painful and produce radiating paresthesias in the lateral thigh (Figure 10.11A).

Blood tests (such as glucose or hemoglobin A_{1C}) would be normal and would be a good consideration for a diabetic neuropathy.

Routine electrophysiologic testing would be normal and would differentiate a lumbar radiculopathy. Specifically, NCS of the lateral femoral cutaneous nerve (not ordinarily done) can show an asymmetrical or absent response compared with the opposite limb. However, technical issues, especially with an obese patient, might limit the utility.

Multiple imaging studies had been done. The patient presented with stacks of lumbar MRI results that were repeatedly normal. US or high-resolution MRI of the lateral femoral cutaneous nerve could show a subtle nerve abnormality.

The major differential diagnosis is a lumbar radiculopathy. Pain would start in the back and radiate distally to the lower limb. For upper lumbar radiculopathies, pain may radiate to the groin. L3 radiates to the anterior thigh. L4 goes below the knee. Physical examination, including provocative maneuvers, would also differ for a spine rather than a peripheral origin (see earlier discussion of the systematic approach to patients with peripheral nerve problems).

US-guided diagnostic (local) block could be considered and would produce transient block and pain relief. A local block also would afford the patient the opportunity to experience the expected numbness if a neurectomy is being considered.

HOW SHOULD THIS CASE BE MANAGED?

Weight reduction was recommended without benefit. The patient avoided compressive objects (e.g., tight belts). In

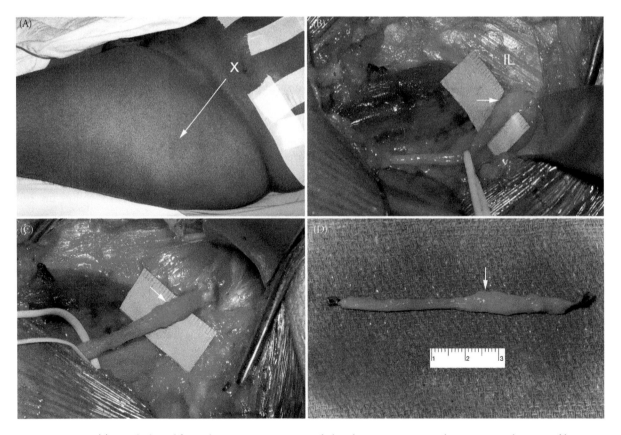

Figure 10.11 A: Percussion (x) over the lateral femoral cutaneous nerve just medial to the anterior superior iliac spine over the inguinal ligament (IL) causes paresthesias in the lateral thigh (*arrow*). B: The lateral femoral cutaneous nerve found beneath the fascia overlying the sartorius muscle just distal to the IL. C: The nerve is compressed at the leading edge of the inguinal ligament (*arrow*). The ligament is released laterally. D: Lateral femoral cutaneous nerve resected with neuroma (*arrow*).

my experience, an US-guided therapeutic block (using steroids) does not often produce lasting results. Pain management was unsuccessful.

Surgery was offered. A transverse incision was made in one of Langer's lines just medial to the anterior superior iliac spine. (This is preferred over a longitudinal incision, which has more wound-related problems in the groin.) The lateral femoral cutaneous nerve (Figure 10.11B) is a relatively large cutaneous nerve that is found beneath the fascia overlying the sartorius muscle just distal to the inguinal ligament. The nerve can be difficult to locate, and some surgeons favor using US to assist. The nerve is compressed at the leading edge of the inguinal ligament; a pseudoneuroma is frequently identified. The ligament is released laterally (to avoid a postoperative hernia) (Figure 10.11C). Some surgeons favor neurectomy (Figure 10.11D) rather than decompression and allow the proximal stump to retract into the pelvis.

FOLLOW-UP

This patient underwent neurectomy and noted instantaneous improvement. The hypersensitivity was gone in the recovery room. He resumed wearing long pants and stopped pain medications (Figure 10.12). At last evaluation, 5 years after surgery, he had complete relief.

CASE 6

HISTORY

A 57-year-old man underwent open carpal tunnel release 2 months ago. He has had nocturnal paresthesias in the thumb, index, middle, and radial side of the ring finger that were relieved by shaking his hands. Symptoms were exacerbated by driving and wrist position. EMG and NCS confirmed mild carpal tunnel syndrome (CTS).

The patient presents with severe pain and dense numbness in the radial 3½ digits and new weakness in the thumb, which he noted immediately after the surgery.

EXAMINATION

The patient had a healed wrist-level incision (Figure 10.13). He has paralysis of the abductor pollicis brevis muscle. Other finger, thumb, and wrist flexors are of normal strength. He has severe loss of sensation to light touch and no two-point discrimination in the thumb, index, middle, and radial side of the ring fingers.

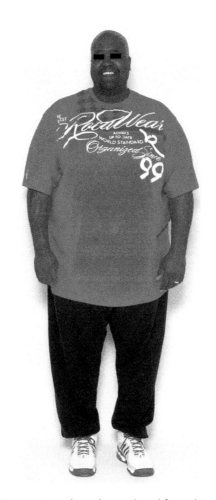

Figure 10.12 Happy patient who underwent lateral femoral cutaneous neurectomy and was able to resume wearing long pants and stop pain medications.

TESTS

Electrodiagnostic Studies

Electrodiagnostic studies showed a severe complete median neuropathy at the level of the wrist. EMG revealed fibrillations and no motor units in the abductor pollicis brevis. There was no motor or sensory conduction in the median nerve across the wrist. The preoperative study was compared with the postoperative study. The neurologist confirmed the original diagnosis and localization but documented a new, severe lesion after surgery.

Imaging Studies

Either MRI or US could be considered to determine a possible structural or anatomic cause for the postoperative worsening.

MRI (Figure 10.14) showed a severely flattened and hyperintense median nerve at the distal site of the carpal

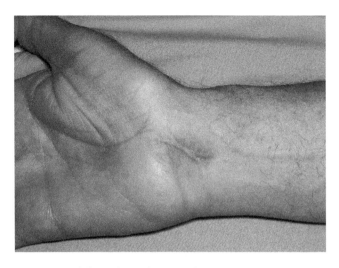

Figure 10.13 Healed carpal tunnel incision above wrist crease.

tunnel by the incompletely divided transverse carpal ligament. The nerve was compressed but in-continuity.

The benefit of imaging in this case is that it excluded the possibility of an iatrogenic transected nerve.

DIAGNOSIS

The diagnosis in this patient is severe compression of the median nerve at the distal edge of the carpal tunnel,

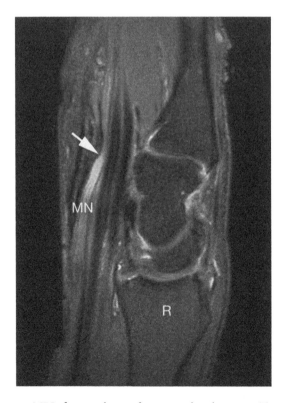

Figure 10.14 MRI of a sagittal view of compressed median nerve. The T2-weighted image shows a severely flattened and hyperintense median nerve (MN) at the distal site of the carpal tunnel by the incompletely divided transverse carpal ligament (*arrow*). R, radius.

presumably due to incomplete release of the transverse carpal tunnel.

The entire median nerve at the level of the wrist is affected. Motor loss of thenar muscles is present, although more proximal innervated muscles (wrist, finger, and thumb flexors) are spared. Sensory loss in the radial 3½ fingers is present, but sensation in the palmar cutaneous nerve distribution is normal.

HOW SHOULD THIS CASE BE MANAGED?

Surgical exploration would be indicated because this is a new (iatrogenic) and complete lesion.

The prior incision would be lengthened to facilitate identifying the median nerve in the normal proximal zone. The incision would also be lengthened distally into the palm. Note that the original skin incision (which did not extend into the palm) may not have been optimum to allow full visualization of the median nerve in the region of the carpal tunnel.

At the revision surgery, the median nerve would be circumferentially mobilized through the area, ensuring complete decompression.

Under tourniquet control, the median nerve was identified in the distal forearm and traced through the palm (Figure 10.15A). The transverse carpal ligament had not been completely released. The distal edge of it was compressing the median nerve (see Figure 10.15A). When the edge was divided, an abnormal indentation of the nerve was seen (Figure 10.15B). The median nerve was mobilized to the level of the digital nerves (note the recurrent motor branch). The median nerve appeared well decompressed.

When the tourniquet was released (Figure 10.15C and D), abnormal vascular markings were seen in that area of compression.

If imaging had not been done preoperatively, one would have needed to be prepared for the possibility of finding a transected nerve and performing nerve grafting (see information on nerve grafting in earlier discussion of nerve injury).

FOLLOW-UP

When in the recovery room, the patient noted improvement in his pain and resolution of the hypersensitivity in the radial 3½ digits.

At the first postoperative visit, two weeks later, his wound had healed (Figure 10.16A shows the healed incision, which now extends to the palm). He had regained some degree of opposition already (Figure 10.16B). He made a steady and full recovery over 9 months.

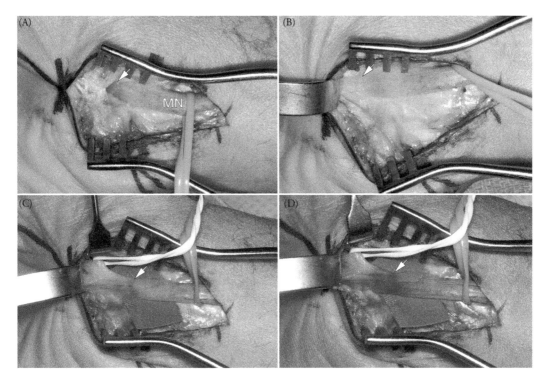

Figure 10.15 A: Median nerve (MN) identified in the distal forearm and traced through the palm, with the distal edge of the transverse carpal ligament not completely released and compressing the MN (arrow). B: Abnormal indentation of the nerve seen when the edge was divided (arrow). C, D: Abnormal vascular markings seen in area of compression (arrow) when the tourniquet was released.

COMMON NERVE ENTRAPMENT SYNDROMES

Carpal Tunnel Syndrome

In CTS, pain radiates from the wrist to the radial 3½ digits and sometimes proximally into the forearm and arm. Symptoms worsen with wrist flexion and extension. Classical provocative features include symptoms that occur with driving or sleeping but that are improved with shaking hands. Atrophy in the thenar eminence is a late finding. Palmar sensation is normal. Tinel's sign (percussion tenderness) is noted when tapping over the wrist crease; Phalen's and reverse Phalen's signs and compression test are also positive. EMG and NCS confirm the diagnosis of CTS. Beware of false-positive results; false-negative results also occur on occasion. In these cases, US or MRI can support the clinical diagnosis.

Know how to distinguish CTS from other, more proximal median nerve compression syndromes (commonly tested on Oral Board Examinations); these include anterior interosseous nerve (AIN) syndrome (discussed later); entrapment by a supracondylar spur or process, which can

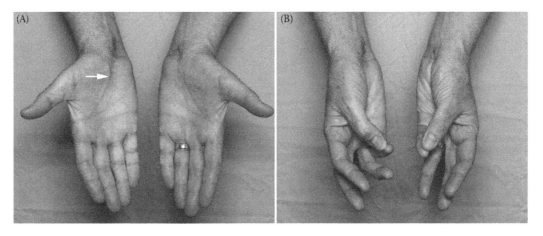

Figure 10.16 A: Healed incision that extends to the palm (*arrow*). B: Some degree of opposition regained.

be palpated or identified on imaging (found in 0.5% of the normal population, 6 cm above the elbow; the bony spur is found in association with the ligament of Struthers, creating a "tunnel," in which the median nerve and brachial artery might be compressed); and cervical radiculopathies (e.g., C6 or C7).

Surgery

Surgery is performed in patients with persistent symptoms of CTS after nonoperative trial (avoidance of exacerbating activities, splinting with the wrist in relatively neutral position) or steroid injection and in those with severe findings. Know the anatomic landmarks for incisions. Most neurosurgeons perform open release through a standard palmar incision: one needs to release the ligament so that the surgeon sees fat distally and decompresses the nerve proximal to the distal wrist crease. Some use endoscopic techniques (1 vs. 2 portals). Open and endoscopic techniques have similar results after 3 months. The endoscopic technique may have slight advantage in the initial 3 months after surgery in terms of return to work and grip strengths; results at longer follow-up after open and endoscopic techniques are comparable. Meta-analyses have shown a slight increased neurological risk with the endoscopic technique. Note, as a practical point, that there is a learning curve to the endoscopic technique. New ultrasound guided techniques are currently being used.

Ulnar Nerve Entrapment at the Elbow (Cubital Tunnel Syndrome)

In cubital tunnel syndrome, elbow pain radiates into the ulnar 2 digits of the hand. Symptoms often worsen with elbow flexion. Sensory abnormality occurs on the palmar (ulnar 1½ digits) and dorsoulnar aspects of the hand (dorsal cutaneous branch arises 6 cm above the wrist); weakness occurs in extrinsic (forearm) and intrinsic (hand) ulnar-innervated muscles. Tinel's sign is found at the elbow, and the elbow flexion test is positive, Spurling's sign is negative, and thoracic outlet maneuvers are negative. EMG and NCS confirm the diagnosis. MRI or US of the elbow also can confirm the diagnosis but are not routinely done.

Surgery

Surgery is performed in patients with persistent symptoms after nonoperative trial (avoidance of exacerbating activities such as elbow flexion, splinting with the elbow mildly flexed) and in those with severe findings. Surgical options include in situ decompression and transposition (subcutaneous, intramuscular, or submuscular). Few neurosurgeons perform a medial epicondylectomy. Recently published studies show no significant differences in outcomes for primary cases between various surgical options; transposition has higher complications (infection, hematoma). Submuscular transposition is generally performed for secondary cases.

Peroneal Nerve Palsy

Peroneal nerve compression may occur at the level of the fibular tunnel by a fibrous band beneath the peroneus longus.

Know how to distinguish L5 radiculopathy and peroneal nerve palsy, which are the most common causes of foot drop. If the posterior tibialis is abnormal, then the foot drop is not from peroneal nerve palsy. To test the posterior tibialis, have patient position the foot down and in (innervated by L5, tibial nerve). EMG can help localize peroneal nerve lesions. The short head of the biceps is the only peroneal-innervated muscle above the fibular head and neck region. Fibrillations in the short head of the biceps on EMG confirm a more proximal lesion (such as in the peroneal division of the sciatic nerve in the thigh or buttock).

The foot drop differential diagnosis is broad and can also occur from upper motor neuron causes (brain or spine) or from other lower motor neuron causes (sciatic neuropathy or lumbosacral plexopathy).

UNUSUAL ENTRAPMENT SYNDROMES

Ulnar Nerve Entrapment at the Wrist (Guyon's Canal Syndrome)

In Guyon's canal syndrome, wrist pain radiates into the ulnar digits of the hand. Symptoms worsen with wrist flexion (often seen in cyclists and mechanics, for example) and may affect the deep branch only, producing isolated motor findings. (An important differential diagnosis would be amyotrophic lateral sclerosis [ALS], so you should know about ALS, i.e., features of an upper and lower motor neuron lesion, tongue fasciculations, etc.) Guyon's canal syndrome also may affect superficial branch only, producing sensory symptoms only, or the parent ulnar nerve, producing motor and sensory symptoms. Sensory abnormalities occur only on the palmar side, not dorsally. Extrinsic muscles (flexor carpi ulnaris and flexor digitorum profundus to the little and ring fingers) are normal clinically and electrophysiologically. EMG is helpful in localizing and ruling out other pathology. MRI may reveal a mass lesion. In general, ulnar nerve entrapment at the wrist accounts for only 1% of all cases of ulnar nerve entrapment—other cases are nearly all at the cubital tunnel (see earlier discussion of common nerve entrapment syndromes).

Neurogenic Thoracic Outlet Syndrome

One must be able to distinguish ulnar nerve pathology from thoracic outlet syndrome (TOS) (symptomatic and neurogenic forms) as well as plexopathy from a Pancoast tumor or a C8 or T1 radiculopathy. In neurogenic TOS, patients may have clinical and electrophysiologic findings of a lower trunk plexopathy. In neurogenic TOS, the hand would have both thenar (median-innervated) and hypothenar (ulnar-innervated) motor weakness producing a Gilliatt-Sumner hand. EMG would show changes in muscles of C8 and T1 (beyond ulnar nerve distribution). A chest radiograph could show a cervical rib or an elongated transverse process for neurogenic TOS, or an apical lung mass lesion (in which case, additional imaging with MRI or CT scans would be done). In cases with neurogenic TOS, MRI (or US) of the brachial plexus could help localize the lesion. MRI of the spine would rule out a C8 or T1 radiculopathy. Surgery on neurogenic TOS could be done supraclavicularly or by the transaxillary route; most surgeons would perform scalenectomy (and removal of the cervical rib or elongated process); some would also perform first rib resection. Pathology usually affects C8 and T1 or the lower trunk near the foramina. Four unusual entrapments must be distinguished from Parsonage-Turner syndrome, or brachial plexitis: anterior interosseous nerve syndrome, posterior interosseous nerve syndrome, suprascapular nerve entrapment, and long thoracic neuropathy (previously discussed in Case 3).

Anterior Interosseous Nerve Syndrome

In AIN syndrome, the flexor pollicis longus, flexor digitorum profundus (index and middle fingers), and pronator quadratus are weak. There is no cutaneous innervation by the anterior interosseous nerve. The patient cannot make an "O" sign, which results in a "square pinch."

Posterior Interosseous Nerve Syndrome

In the posterior interosseous nerve syndrome, the wrist can dorsiflex strongly in radial deviation but cannot dorsiflex in a neutral position because of the lack of extensor carpi ulnaris. The patient has finger drop, but no sensory loss. (Contrast PIN palsy at the arcade of Frohse in the proximal forearm with wrist and finger drop characteristic of a radial nerve palsy

from Saturday night palsy, which occurs at the spiral groove at the mid-arm level and is usually due to compression on the arm, such as occurs from nonphysiologic sleeping, e.g., due to coma or drug or alcohol use. In typical radial nerve palsy, the patient has normal triceps strength.) Fortunately, most patients with so-called Saturday night palsy recover quickly (within days or weeks) because of neurapraxia (conduction block); those patients with a history of Saturday night palsy who do not show the expected recovery should have baseline EMG and NCS testing at 3 to 6 weeks.

Suprascapular Nerve Entrapment

Suprascapular nerve entrapment presents with weakness of the supraspinatus (shoulder abduction) and infraspinatus (external rotation) muscles. It typically occurs at the transverse scapular ligament. MRI may show a ganglion cyst from the shoulder joint. The differential diagnosis includes C5 radiculopathy and rotator cuff pathology.

Nine Photographs You Need to Know for the Boards

Figure 10.17 displays nine photographs that you will need to be familiar with when taking the Oral Board Examination.

A. Thenar Atrophy

In thenar atrophy, median nerve loss causes intrinsic muscle weakness, such as the abductor pollicis brevis or opponens pollicis. This patient had severe CTS (proximal median innervated muscles, such as wrist, finger, and thumb flexors, would be normal).

B. Anterior Interosseous Nerve Palsy

The patient is trying to make an "O" (the OK sign) but is unable because of paralysis of the terminal phalanges in the thumb (flexor pollicis longus) and index finger (flexor digitorum profundus). Note that the flexion at the proximal interphalangeal joint of the index finger is functioning because it is supplied more proximally from a branch of the median nerve (not the AIN).

C. High Median Nerve Palsy

The patient is attempting to make a fist but is unable to because of paralysis of the finger flexors. Contrast with the patient who has AIN palsy in B. Note the paralysis of the flexor digitorum superficialis, which is supplied by the median nerve proximal to the AIN. The middle, ring, and little fingers flex through the ulnar-innervated flexor digitorum profundi. This person would also have paralysis of the pronator teres, flexor carpi radialis, palmaris longus, and

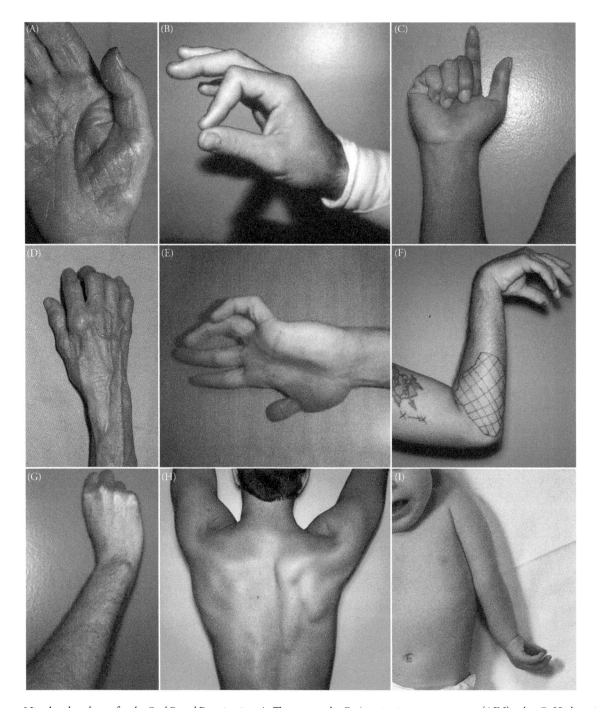

Figure 10.17 Nine hands to know for the Oral Board Examination. A: Thenar atrophy. B: Anterior interosseous nerve (AIN) palsy. C: High median nerve palsy. D: Wasting of first dorsal interosseous muscle. E: Ulnar Nerve Clawing at the metacarpophalangeal. F: Radial nerve palsy. G: Posterior interosseous nerve (PIN) palsy. H: Right suprascapular nerve palsy. I: Waiter's tip posture.

abductor pollicis brevis as well as sensory loss in the median nerve distribution.

D. Wasting of First Dorsal Interosseous Muscle

This photograph shows severe atrophy of ulnar-innervated hand muscles. This can be seen with a low or high ulnar nerve lesion. With ulnar nerve lesions, the patient would typically have sensory loss as well. If there is no sensory abnormality, you should consider a lesion affecting the deep branch (motor) of the ulnar nerve or ALS.

E. Ulnar Nerve Clawing

This patient has hyperextension at metacarpophalangeal joints of the little and ring fingers. The patient is trying to extend the fingers but is unable to because of imbalance and weakness in ulnar-innervated intrinsics.

F. Radial Nerve Palsy

This patient has wrist and finger drop. The triceps muscle has normal strength. Sensory loss would be present in the posterior forearm (shown) and dorsum of wrist. The lesion is in the mid or distal arm (in this case, "X" marks site of entrapment and percussion tenderness).

G. Posterior Interosseous Nerve Palsy

In this patient with PIN palsy, the wrist is in dorsiflexion and is strong, but radially deviated. It is unable to be dorsiflexed in neutral position. The patient has finger drop at the metacarpophalangeal joints. Cutaneous sensation is normal. The lesion is in the proximal forearm just below the elbow. Contrast with the patient who has radial nerve palsy in F.

H. Right Suprascapular Nerve Palsy

Atrophy of the supraspinatus and infraspinatus is seen. The right scapular spine is more prominent because of the associated muscle loss. Right-side shoulder abduction is mildly affected in this muscular patient because of compensation of the well-functioning deltoid muscle. External rotation would be weak, and there would not be any sensory abnormality.

I. Waiter's Tip Posture

This would be the expected appearance of an infant with a birth-related upper trunk (C5, C6) palsy. There is no shoulder abduction because of loss of C5 function (no deltoid or supraspinatus). There is no elbow flexion from C6. The arm is internally rotated because of overpull of the lower portion of the functioning pectoralis major muscle (C7-T1) and paralysis of the infraspinatus muscle (C5). Triceps is strong. Wrist and hand function is typically preserved.

11.

EPILEPSY, FUNCTIONAL, AND PAIN NEUROSURGERY

Nitin Tandon and Konstantin V. Slavin

Several aspects of the management of seizures and epilepsy are relevant to a general neurosurgical practice, which we cover in this chapter. First and foremost, all candidates should know how to manage a patient presenting with a new-onset seizure or in status epilepticus with a brain lesion or after a craniotomy. Second, candidates are expected to be able to explain how to perform fundamental epilepsy procedures such as a temporal lobectomy for hippocampal sclerosis or resection of an epileptogenic lesion—this may be combined with the need for intracranial recordings with implanted electrodes. Third, it is useful to have a clear process in place for mapping language and motor function for the resection of tumors located in the eloquent cortex. Lastly, the thought process behind developing an appropriate plan for the surgical management of movement disorders and the technical nuances of managing such cases will be discussed.

CASE 1

CLINICAL PRESENTATION

A 34-year-old right-handed chemical engineer, originally from Denmark, now living and working in the United States, had an episode of confusion and difficulty finding words to express himself while at work. This episode lasted about 10 minutes, during which his colleagues said that he could not speak fluently and only made unintelligible sounds. He was taken for an evaluation at a local emergency department for a presumed stroke, which included magnetic resonance imaging (MRI). The MRI revealed a brain mass, and he was referred to your office. He has had no further seizures and denies any other significant medical history. On your examination, he is neurologically intact—specifically, he has no dysfluency, no dysnomia, and no comprehension or speech production errors. He states that his native tongue is Danish and that he also speaks German and English.

DIAGNOSTIC TESTS

The patient has undergone MRI testing with and without contrast (Figure 11.1). This revealed a lesion in the mid-portion of the left temporal lobe that measures about 3.5 cm in diameter, has ill-defined boundaries, and is hypo-intense on T1-weighted imaging and hyper-intense on T2-weighted and fluid-attenuated inversion recovery (FLAIR) sequences. There is enhancement after contrast administration and mild mass effect from the mass on the temporal horn of the lateral ventricle.

ANALYSIS OF THE CASE

Likely Diagnosis

These imaging studies, coupled with the history of a single episode that is most consistent with a seizure in a young otherwise healthy male, who has since made a rapid and complete recovery, raise the possibility of a neoplasm as opposed to a vascular lesion in the temporal cortex. It is not uncommon for patients to have no symptoms with a gradually enlarging mass. The probability that this represents an inflammatory or ischemic lesion is very low, given the imaging findings and the clinical presentation.

Indications for Surgery

This non-contrast-enhancing lesion is most likely to be a low-grade glioma. Initial management options include biopsy or resection. Given that the lesion is superficial and the patient is young (which pushes the plan strongly in favor of a maximal resection), it is most reasonable to proceed with plans for a resection rather than an initial biopsy.

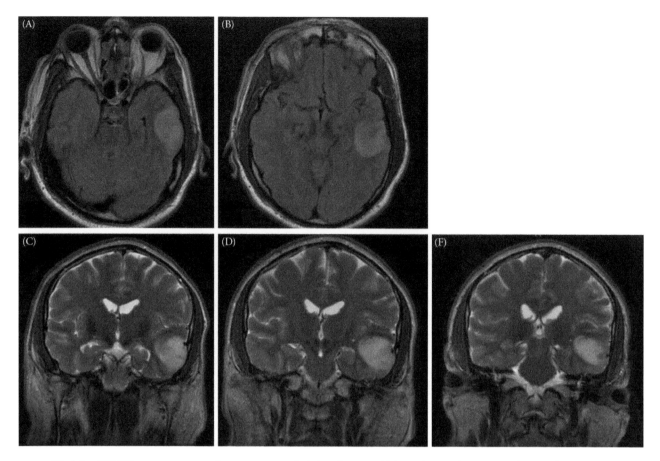

Figure 11.1 (Top) Axial FLAIR sequence images showing a mass in the left mid temporal lobe and coronal T2-weighted images (bottom row) showing the relationship to the superior temporal gyrus and the vein of Labbe.

Management Options

An important consideration is the relationship of the mass to the critical language cortex in the temporal lobe. The mass is located in the middle temporal lobe, and it is therefore likely that it abuts or involves language cortex. Given that the patient is right-handed, the likelihood is high that he is left-hemisphere dominant for language. He is also a polyglot, and Danish and English are of greatest importance to him. From various studies of polyglots, it is clear that primary and secondary languages occupy distinct, although usually adjacent, cortical substrates. Therefore, it is important to map at least the 2 languages most important to this patient. Most centers now use some type of noninvasive activation study (functional magnetic resonance imaging [fMRI] or magneto-encephalography [MEG]) to localize language in such cases, and these studies would be helpful in this case to lateralize language and to try to localize the relationship between language function and the lesion.

fMRI mapping of language function was carried out in this patient. Language was mapped with visual and auditory cues (Figure 11.2). Visual naming was performed in

both Danish and English. The patient had a difficult time understanding the auditory cues, and performance was low on that task but good on the others. The activation map clearly shows that the left hemisphere is dominant for language and that Broca's area is well localized. However, no activation is seen around the lesion. This raises an important issue—is the sensitivity of fMRI good enough that we can assume that the patient has no useful language function in the vicinity of the mass? The answer is no. In the best studies, the sensitivity and specificity of fMRI in detecting essential language sites localized by electrical cortical stimulation mapping (CSM) is about 80% to 85%. Therefore, fMRI should be used chiefly to lateralize language function and not to replace CSM to localize language sites. Given the proximity of language sites to the tumor in this case, the standard approach is to perform an awake craniotomy with language mapping to enable resection with minimal compromise of language.

There are certain prerequisites for an awake craniotomy and language mapping: The patient must be cooperative and not claustrophobic. There should be no history of anxiety attacks or panic disorder. The functions (e.g., naming or

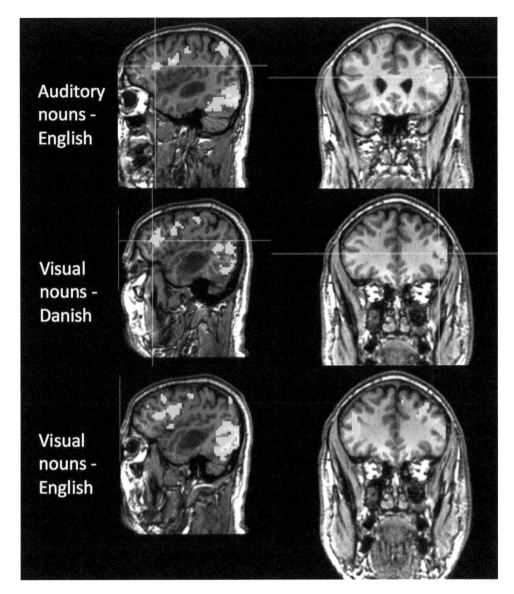

Figure 11.2 Sagittal (left column) and coronal (right column) views of a blood oxygen level dependent (BOLD) functional MRI sequence during auditory and visual cued object naming. Strongly left lateralized activity in the frontal lobe is seen. Activity is also seen just posterior to the lesion.

repetition) that the surgeon wishes to map should be nearly or completely intact (trying to map a significantly impaired function is often a futile process because patients generally wake up in the operating room a bit worse than they were in the clinic, given the lingering presence of even the short-acting anesthetic agents). The surgeon and the neuro-anesthesiologist should have a standing protocol in place for awake craniotomies. In general, the patient is not intubated, but a laryngeal mask airway is placed, and the anesthetic agents used are mostly, if not completely, intravenous agents. These include remifentanil or sufentanil for pain and dexmedetomidine and/or propofol for the anesthetic. Inhalational anesthetics are used minimally or not at all.

Given that electrical stimulation of the brain is likely to result in the production of seizures, a preoperative loading dose of anticonvulsants is helpful. It is best to do this a day or so before the procedure so that the patient is not sedated by the loading dose of the anticonvulsant during the awake portion of the operation. Phenytoin or fos-phenytoin (18 mg/kg load) is preferred for this purpose, although leveti-racetam (15 mg/kg) or lacosamide (3 mg/kg) can also be used in case of intolerance or allergy to phenytoin. Steroids (dexamethasone, 8–10 mg) should be given in each case, and mannitol can be used on an individual basis, based on the patient's age and the degree of mass effect.

Details of the Procedure

The patient is positioned lateral with a large shoulder roll and is held in place with tape and restraints. The head is immobilized with pins, which minimizes movements, particularly during micro-dissection, although positioning on a doughnut is also acceptable (in this case, a post is clamped to the skull after the craniotomy to ensure minimal head movements). The head is always in a lateral orientation, slightly extended, and should be such that the patient appears comfortable and the anesthesiologist has easy access to the airway.

A field block is created using a long-acting topical anesthetic such as 0.25% bupivacaine. After the craniotomy flap is elevated, the dura is also infiltrated with local anesthetic, the patient is awoken, and the laryngeal mask airway (if used) is removed. A neurophysiologist or a neuropsychologist well versed in language mapping then presents stimuli to the patient while the surgeon proceeds with electrical CSM. Stimulation is carried on after the patient is familiarized with the testing process, and a balanced Faradic current to avoid charge deposition in the brain is used. An Ojemann stimulator (Integra) or a Grass S88X stimulator is commonly used. A train of balanced square waves is delivered at 50 Hz. Each set of waves varies from 200 to 500 μs in duration (longer duration waves are useful for mapping in children), and these are delivered for 3 to 5 seconds during task performance. Stimulation currents range from 1 to 10 mA, and mapping is performed at 10 mA, or at 1mA below the potential that results in after-discharges or overt phenomenology, whichever is lower. Concurrent electrocorticography is essential to monitor for after-discharges and seizures. It also provides visible evidence of induced electrical artifacts in the recording that indicate that all the equipment is working and the electrical circuit is complete.

The tasks used for CSM vary across institutions, but the following are commonly used:

- *Object naming* using pictorial stimuli (e.g., Boston Naming Test)

- *Repetition* of spoken phrases

- *Spontaneous speech* (e.g., counting, reciting the alphabet, nursery rhymes); this is useful in localizing sites of speech arrest.

- *Auditory naming*—naming driven by a phrase or a sentence (e.g., question: "what a king wears on his head"; answer: " crown").

Stimulation sites where the task results in a delay, paraphrasia, anomia, or speech arrest are noted, as are those locations where stimulation produces overt sensori-motor phenomenology (Figure 11.3). CSM carries a small risk for producing seizures, and such seizures may severely limit the

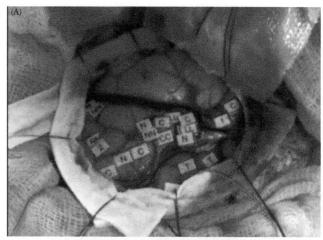

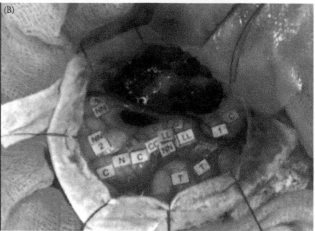

Figure 11.3 Intraoperative photographs showing the left temporal lobe (surgeon's orientation) and the results of the language mapping (*top*). Single alphabets are for the maps in English and double letters are for mapping in Danish. N = Auditory cued naming; C = Comprehension; L = N+C; T = tongue deviation. The Vein of Labbé is situated near the posterior boundary of the tumor. The post resection images (*bottom*) show preservation of the language sites as well as cortisectomy both anterior and posterior to the vein of Labbé, that skeletonize yet preserve the vein.

mapping process or lead to a postponement of the planned resection. Therefore, patients should receive therapeutic doses of anticonvulsants before mapping. Despite this, stimulation of peri-lesional cortex can result in seizure induction. This can be controlled by irrigation of the brain surface with ice-cold saline.

In the patient in this case, English and Danish were both mapped. This facilitated a resection of the tumor, part of which was located posterior to the vein of Labbé. The patient recovered from surgery well and was discharged home on postoperative day 2.

COMPLICATIONS

In addition to complications that are generic to any craniotomy, such as infections, cerebrospinal fluid (CSF) leak, hemorrhage, and stroke, particular complications related to this case are as follows:

1. Postoperative seizures: These are managed by maintaining high doses of anticonvulsants for 2 to 4 weeks after surgery in any patient who presented with a gliomas and a seizure.

2. Postoperative language deficit: This is minimized by the intraoperative mapping and monitoring of language function.

3. Delayed postoperative language deficit: This is not uncommon and could be related to edema or ischemia around the resection cavity. An MRI to rule out a stroke should be obtained (Figure 11.4) as should an electroencephalogram (EEG).

CASE 2

CLINICAL PRESENTATION

A 22-year-old right-handed woman is referred by her neurologist for definitive management of her epilepsy that is not well controlled with anticonvulsant medications. Her current seizures began at the age of 15 years. She has an aura of a rising sensation in her abdomen followed by a loss of awareness and inability to respond to questions, and she is told that she is confused for a few seconds after each event. She has 3 or 4 seizure events a month. Additionally, she has had a total of 5 grand mal seizures over the past 7 years. She has previously been on and has failed adequate drug treatment with oxcarbazepine, levetiracetam, and valproic acid. She is currently taking a combination therapy of lamotrigine and lacosamide. She is accompanied at the clinic visit by her mother, who states that the patient is a product of a full-term normal vaginal delivery and also that none of her siblings have ever had seizures. The patient did have febrile convulsions at 2 and 3 years of age. A total of 5 separate events occurred, all in the context of body temperatures greater than 102°F. The patient was placed on phenobarbital at that time, and this was stopped when she turned 6 years old. She was seizure free and off medications for 9 years, until her seizures recurred at age 15.

DIAGNOSTIC TESTS

The patient's video EEG reveals inter-ictal EEG spikes at F8-T4 and right hemispheric seizure onsets, maximum at

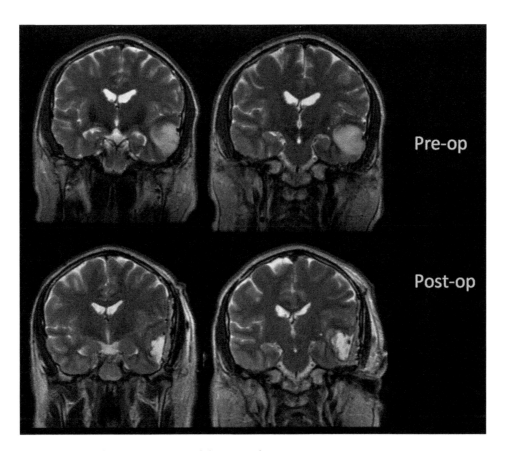

Figure 11.4 Coronal MRI views to show the resection cavity and the extent of resection.

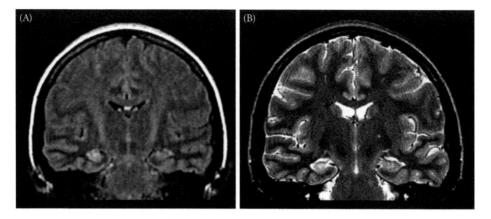

Figure 11.5 Coronal FLAIR (left) and T2 (right) images showing increased signal and volume loss in the right hippocampus.

the same electrodes. The video shows stereotypic seizure semiology for all recorded seizures with a sudden cessation of activity, loss of responsiveness, right-hand automatisms, and tonic posturing of the left hand. The seizure lasts about 2 minutes, and the patient is able to speak immediately thereafter and regains full awareness and orientation soon after the termination of the ictal rhythm on the scalp EEG recordings. The MRI reveals volume loss of the right hippocampus along with increased signal in the hippocampus on FLAIR sequences (Figure 11.5). No other abnormalities are detected in the brain. The patient's neuropsychological testing reveals a full-scale intelligence quotient (IQ) of 110, with a verbal IQ of 114 and a performance IQ of 104. The testing reveals deficiency in visuospatial memory, consistent with a right mesial temporal abnormality. Positron emission tomography reveals hypometabolism in the right mesial temporal lobe (Figure 11.6).

ANALYSIS OF THE CASE

Likely Diagnosis

This patient has a classical history of mesial temporal or hippocampal sclerosis causing medically intractable complex partial seizures. The history of febrile convulsions is typical, as is the latency between the seizures in early childhood and the onset of intractable epilepsy in the teenage years. The seizure semiology is characteristic for mesial temporal seizures, further evidenced by the EEG recordings. In summary, the patient has classical imaging and electrophysiologic features of right mesial temporal lobar epilepsy (MTLE).

Indications for Surgery

After failing adequate treatment with 3 anticonvulsants, the probability of an additional anticonvulsant leading to a durable cessation of seizures is less than 3%. This patient

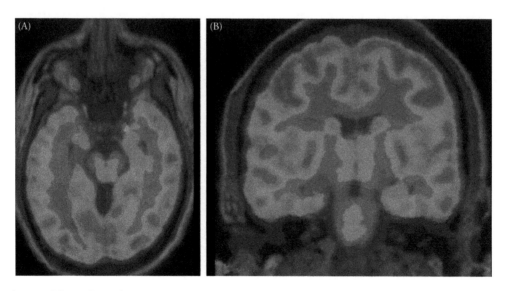

Figure 11.6 Axial and Coronal fluoro-deoxy glucose PET images showing hypo-metabolism in the right temporal lobe.

has failed treatment with 4 anticonvulsants; therefore, the probability of an additional trial with another anticonvulsant leading to seizure control is miniscule. Surgical treatment—anterior temporal lobectomy for MTLE—has been shown in a prospective randomized trial to be much more effective than treatment with anticonvulsants. Thus, some approach that targets the right mesial temporal lobe should be the management plan in this case.

Given that the patient is right-handed, the probability of meaningful or memory function being present in the right hemisphere is very small, and this is borne out by the neuropsychological tests that are concordant with this being a disease of the language-nondominant hemisphere. This may be confirmed by fMRI to lateralize language, but an invasive test such as an intra-carotid amytal injection (Wada test) is generally unnecessary in this case. Therefore, no additional testing is necessary before definitive surgical intervention for the epilepsy.

Management Options

Several approaches are described for a temporal lobe epilepsy. These include anterior temporal lobectomy (ATL) with amygdalo-hippocampectomy (AH), a selective amygdalo-hippocampectomy, or a laser interstitial thermal ablation (LITT) of the hippocampus. Here, we describe a classical ATL + AH and the LITT.

Details of the Procedure—ATL + AH

The patient is positioned with a shoulder roll under the right shoulder and with the head in a lateral orientation, right side uppermost. It is useful to tilt the vertex slightly toward the floor and to extend the neck. A small inverse question-mark incision is made to encompass most of the temporalis muscle, and a myo-cutaneous flap is elevated. A craniotomy flap is elevated extending as low in the middle cranial fossa as possible, the superior aspect of the mastoid air cells may need to be drilled down, and this region is then closed off with bone wax. The dura is then opened in a C-shaped fashion. Electrocorticography is then carried out in conjunction with the neurologists, and the diagnosis of antero-mesial temporal epilepsy is confirmed. The approximate distance from the tip of the temporal pole to a spot 5 cm from it along the middle temporal gyrus is marked as the posterior extent of the lateral resection.

A corticectomy is then made in the superior temporal gyrus (STG) (or in the middle temporal gyrus if on the left side) and taken forward to the temporal pole. The pia-arachnoid is coagulated and sharply divided. A subpial approach is then used to elevate the STG away from the sylvian fissure and then, more inferiorly, from the inferior limb of the circular sulcus of the insula (Figure 11.7). Next, a vertical corticectomy, extending downward from the posterior edge of the STG corticectomy and staying at or anterior to the 5-cm mark, is performed. The inferior edge of this is extended medially, and the basal cortex is aspirated in sub-pial fashion until the collateral sulcus is identified. The collateral sulcus is then exposed, with care taken to preserve the pia within it, and is traced superiorly until the white matter of the temporal lobe is exposed. Dissection is carried further superiorly along the line of the collateral sulcus until the temporal horn of the lateral ventricle is exposed. After the temporal horn is exposed, the cut in the STG and the superior circular sulcus of the insula is connected to this—by cutting across the temporal stem.

Last, a cut is made in the floor of the temporal horn, along a groove called the lateral ventricular sulcus, down

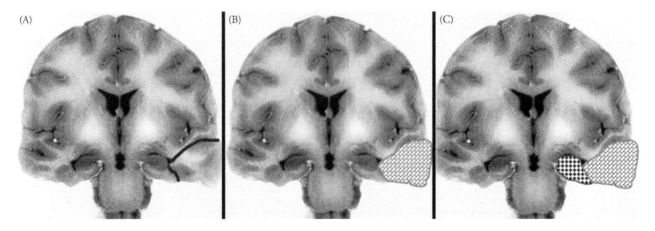

Figure 11.7 Coronal views showing the landmarks and the stages in a temporal lobectomy. Left: the superior temporal sulcus and the collateral sulcus are highlighted. Middle: The neocortical resection extends to the ventricle and stops at the collateral sulcus; Right: The medial temporal resection includes the amygdala and hippocampus.

to the basal pia. In this fashion, the temporal pole is removed en-bloc, and attention is directed to the hippocampus and amygdala. The choroid plexus is then identified, and the amygdala is resected below an imaginary line connecting the choroidal point—a pale-blue translucent portion of the choroidal fissure—to the genu of the middle cerebral artery. The subpial technique is used to resect the medial structures, preserving the contents of the ambient cistern—the posterior cerebral artery and the third nerve. Next, the hippocampus is retracted slightly laterally away from the choroidal point. Using microsurgical techniques, the fimbria of the hippocampus is aspirated to expose the vessels in the hippocampal hilus. The hilus is further exposed along its length, and the vessels are coagulated and cut as far distal as possible to prevent inadvertent damage to "en-passage" vessels supplying the brainstem. The hippocampus is rotated laterally, and the tail is then cut, after which the hippocampus is removed and submitted for subsequent histopathologic analysis. Remnants of the uncus and the tail of the hippocampus are aspirated using sub-pial resection techniques. The surgical bed is copiously irrigated, and the dura is closed in a watertight fashion.

The "selective" AH targets removal of the medial structures through either a trans-sylvian approach or a selective removal of the inferior or middle temporal gyri. Meta-analyses comparing the outcomes of these minimalist approaches with a traditional resection suggest similar or only slightly better neuropsychological outcomes combined with somewhat worse seizure-free outcomes. This paradox, of a smaller resection resulting in a similar neuropsychological outcome, can be explained as a consequence of the collateral damage to white matter pathways, associated with selective approaches.

Details of the Procedure—LITT

LITT is accomplished by controlled heating of brain tissue using a laser fiber that is stereotactically implanted inside a sheath through which local cooling is accomplished using either saline (Medtronic Visualase system) or air (Monteris). For hippocampal trajectories, a stereotactic frame (rather than a stereotactic arm, which may be less precise) is preferred to guide the implantation. An occipital entry point is used to target the long axis of the hippocampus, and the trajectory is optimized to ablate as much of the hippocampus and amygdala as possible (Figure 11.8). A stab incision is made in the scalp corresponding to the entry point and a twist drill hole with the drill guide precisely positioned using the stereotactic frame. After the dura is coagulated, the laser applicator sheath is placed to the target using a guide rod via an anchor bolt placed in the skull. The precise length of the probe, as well as confirmation of the positioning, is optimized using intraoperative imaging with fluoroscopic navigational guidance, computed tomography (CT) scanning or MRI. After placement of the laser applicator sheath, a laser fiber (400 µm core silica fiber-optic cable with a 10 mm cylindrical diffusing tip) is placed into the sheath. Precise placement of the laser probe is confirmed in the MRI scanner (patient is transported from the operating room to the MRI scanner under anesthetic if the procedure is not being performed in an interventional MRI environment) using a volumetric T1 acquisition reformatted in all 3 cardinal planes.

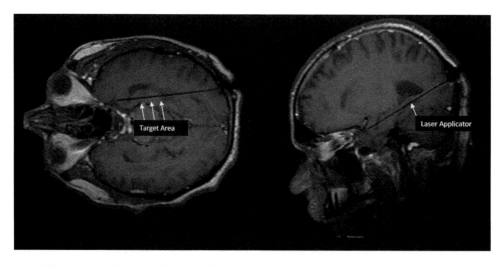

Figure 11.8 Two orthogonal plans showing placement of the laser fiber in the hippocampus for targeted ablation.

The ablation is monitored in the MRI scanner using 2 oblique views, each orthogonal to the other, chosen such that the full length of the probe is visible. Magnetic resonance (MR) thermal imaging is acquired continuously throughout the therapy, with a time resolution of 5 s. Thermal images are processed on a computer work station and color-coded temperature maps and thermal damage estimates overlaid on the structural MR images in near real time. Temperature control points are placed in the ventral thalamus to deactivate the laser if at any time during the treatment the estimated temperature exceeded 50°C. Additional control points are placed along the long axis of the fiber to deactivate the laser if the computed temperature exceeds a temperature of 90°C, to prevent steam formation or damage to the sheath. Low power test pulses are initially applied (3–4 W, 15–45 s) to verify locus of thermal delivery prior to ablation. Ablation is carried out at between 60% and 95% of the peak output of the 15W laser. Once ablation at a given site was judged as satisfactory (generally 1–3 minutes), based on real time monitoring of the damage map by the neurosurgeon in the MRI control room, the laser fiber is manually withdrawn in small increments to produce a cylindroidal thermal lesion along the trajectory. After ablation is complete, a postablation T1 contrast MRI is used to directly evaluate the extent of ablation and to derive confirmation of the targeting. Thereafter, the laser applicator is fully withdrawn, the anchor bolt removed, and the incision closed. Early studies suggest that the neuropsychological outcomes, particularly with regard to preventing naming deficits, are better with this approach than with traditional or selective resections, but the seizure-free rates are less than with a traditional temporal lobectomy.

In this case, the patient underwent an uneventful resection and had no discernible neuropsychological compromise at follow-up neuropsychological testing carried out 1 year later.

COMPLICATIONS

In addition to complications that are generic to any craniotomy, such as infections, CSF fistula, hemorrhage, and stroke, particular complications related to this case are as follows:

1. Anterior choroidal artery stroke (Figure 11.9) is the most common vascular injury that can occur and is usually related to excessive manipulation in the choroidal fissure or overzealous resection of the mesial structures. The patient will emerge from anesthesia hemiparetic or hemiplegic, with a contralateral hemianopsia. Speech is affected in the dominant hemisphere.

2. CSF rhinorrheas can be due to a leak through the dura into the mastoid air cells if these are not well sealed with bone wax.

3. Damage to visual pathways can occur by excessive retraction of the roof of the temporal horn where the optic tract is located. In the LITT procedure, this can occur due to thermal injury to these pathways.

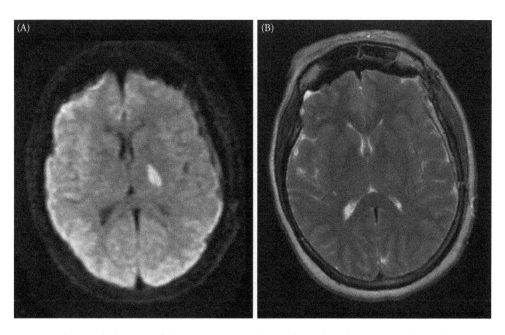

Figure 11.9 Fluoroscopic image showing the location of the Deep Brain Stimulation electrode in the cross hairs of the Leksell stereotactic arc.

4. Diplopia from damage to cranial nerve III can occur. The third nerve is located in the ambient cistern and is routinely visualized during resection of the uncus. If the subpial technique is not used, or excessive bipolar coagulation is used near the ambient cistern, injury to this nerve may occur. In the LITT procedure, this may occur if the fiber is too close to the cavernous sinus (more anteriorly situated than it needs to be).

PAIN

Historically, surgery for pain has been a large part of general neurosurgical practice. A variety of destructive and decompressive interventions have been developed over the years, and a number of comprehensive textbooks have summarized neurosurgical involvement with management of all kinds of medically refractory pain syndromes. Over the past 40 to 50 years, the field of pain surgery has expanded tremendously. Introduction of nondestructive options, primarily along the lines of electrical and chemical neuromodulation, has shifted the majority of care away from neurosurgeons and toward the continuously growing cohort of pain specialists, most of whom come from anesthesia, physiatry, and neurology backgrounds.

Nevertheless, surgical management of pain remains an important section of today's neurosurgery. It is included in the core neurosurgical education curriculum and is an integral part of neurosurgical knowledge that is tested during the Oral Board Examination. Not surprisingly, cases involving complex pain conditions that require neurosurgical interventions routinely show up during examinations, and it is expected that examinees are comfortable performing these interventions and are able to discuss indications, surgical details, outcomes, and complications.

CASE 3

CLINICAL PRESENTATION

A 49-year-old woman presents with complaints of sharp and shooting pain in the left side of her face. The pain started 4 years ago and has become progressively worse over time. It comes as a series of extremely painful attacks that last from a few seconds to about a minute, and, between the attacks, she is pain free. The neurological examination is intact; the areas that tend to trigger her pain are located in the upper lip and the gum of the upper jaw on the left side only; she is hesitant to brush her teeth, chew, and talk because each of these activities is associated with facial pain. She is currently being treated with oral gabapentin with only partial improvement of pain; previously, she tried oral carbamazepine, which was very effective in controlling her pain but produced severe hyponatremia that prompted the change in medication regimen.

DIAGNOSTIC WORKUP

The first question is, obviously, what is the diagnosis? There are a number of tests that would help in establishing it. A correct answer would be trigeminal neuralgia (TN), and, because it is a clinical diagnosis, the next steps in confirming it would be to obtain a detailed history and a standard imaging of the brain (preferably, MRI of the brain with and without contrast, with emphasis on cerebellopontine angles), mainly to rule out secondary TN due to demyelinating disease (e.g., multiple sclerosis) or mass lesions (e.g., tumors, vascular malformations).

TREATMENT OPTIONS

If the MRI does not show an underlying pathologic condition that would present with secondary TN, the classical clinical presentation and failure of medical management should be considered an indication for surgical treatment—and here the correct step would be to present the patient with all 3 main surgical options while discussing advantages and shortcomings of each. In a young and otherwise healthy person with classical TN, a procedure of choice would be microvascular decompression (MVD) of the trigeminal nerve through retromastoid craniectomy or craniotomy under general anesthesia. Patients who are not medically fit to undergo open cranial surgery under general anesthesia (age by itself is not a contraindication because there is a good amount of literature showing safety of MVD in elderly patients) may choose to proceed with percutaneous destructive surgery that may be done with radiofrequency (RF) thermocoagulation, glycerol gangliolysis, or balloon compression. Each of these is considered an appropriate intervention with consistently good results and expected partial sensory loss, with a general correlation between degree of sensory loss and duration of beneficial effects. RF retrogasserian thermocoagulation is considered the most selective intervention and is done with the patient awake because positioning of the electrode tip is determined by the patient's feedback. Glycerol gangliolysis may also be done in awake patients but requires much less patient participation. Balloon compression may be safely done under brief general anesthesia or deep sedation because no patient cooperation is needed. Finally, an option of stereotactic radiosurgery (SRS) has to be brought up because this modality is an accepted way to treat TN—although it is generally less effective compared with other surgical interventions, at least in terms of the probability of making the patient pain free without medications and in terms of immediacy of pain relief (The SRS effect may take between a few weeks to a few months to reach maximum, as opposed to open surgery and percutaneous destructions, which are expected to render the patient pain free by the end of surgery.) SRS appears to be most preferred by the patients because of its perceived lower invasiveness and minimal pain and discomfort experienced during the procedure.

In cases in which the MRI of the brain shows demyelination, the choice of surgical intervention would shift away from MVD and more toward the percutaneous destruction or radiosurgery. Conversely, if one detects a mass lesion in the vicinity of the trigeminal nerve root, the surgical treatment should be focused on eliminating the lesion (surgery or SRS) rather than proceeding with treatment of its symptom (TN). In radiosurgical treatment of tumors that present with TN, it is recommended to use standard tumor-related treatment protocols rather than a highly focused high-dose SRS, which is usually reserved for idiopathic TN or secondary TN due to multiple sclerosis.

Detailed knowledge of the surgical procedure is expected during the Oral Board Examination—particular attention is generally paid to choice of anesthesia, positioning, approach, use of physiologic monitoring, and certain procedural nuances that may avoid certain complications. Complications are expected to happen no matter what, and it is very important to know what to expect, what can be done to minimize the risk, and, most important, how to handle the complications when they occur.

MICROVASCULAR DECOMPRESSION

MVD is considered a procedure of choice for classic TN due to its nondestructive nature and based on its consistently shown best long-term success rate in terms of completeness of pain relief and incidence of recurrences. The procedure is done under general anesthesia; the patient is placed in a supine position with a shoulder roll or in a "park bench" lateral position with head turned horizontally so the sagittal plane is parallel to the floor. The incision is made behind the hairline—the goal of bone opening (with craniotomy or, more commonly, craniectomy) is to expose the junction of transverse and sigmoid sinuses and open the dura in such a way that the cerebellar hemisphere may be retracted medially and caudally to follow the superolateral corner of the posterior cranial fossa (the angle between the tentorium and petrous bone) to the arachnoid membrane of the cerebellopontine angle cistern.

Multiple nuances are expected to be mentioned. First, it is recommended to use intraoperative physiologic monitoring, usually with continuous recording of bilateral brainstem auditory evoked responses (BAERs) and the electromyographic activity of the ipsilateral muscles innervated by the trigeminal (masseter) and facial (frontal, periorbital, and perioral) nerves. Second, it is recommended to wax the mastoid air cells that are exposed or violated during the drilling process. As a matter of fact, it is recommended to wax them twice—first during the opening and then again just before the closure. The next issue is the use of the microscope. It is expected that the intradural part of the procedure will be done under surgical microscope. Use of the endoscope to provide better visualization of neurovascular conflict may also be mentioned, but not using it would not be considered a departure from standard care because endoscope-assisted MVD so far is not universally accepted. The same is true of the use of rigid retractor to expose the cerebellopontine angle: if the preoperative diuretics and spontaneous egress of CSF after opening the cerebellopontine angle cistern provide sufficient relaxation of the cerebellum, use of rigid retractor may be avoided. It is advisable to identify the cranial nerve VII-VIII complex that lies more inferiorly and more posteriorly to the cranial nerve V root in order to orient oneself. The greater petrosal vein of Dandy may be safely coagulated and cut; not doing this may result in hard-to-control venous bleeding if the uncut vein avulses from the tentorium in the middle of nerve root dissection (which is almost guaranteed to happen during the Oral Board Examination).

In most cases, the offending vascular loop conflict will be easily identified. There may be 1 or 2 arterial vessels that are compressing, indenting, and displacing the trigeminal nerve root a few millimeters away from the brainstem. Preoperative high-resolution imaging may help to visualize the vascular structure before the operation. The most common offending vessel is the superior cerebellar artery, which is encountered in approximately 67.5% of patients; the second most common is the anterior inferior cerebellar artery in 20% of cases; and in 25% of cases, a venous structure (such as an aberrant trigeminal vein) might be the cause of the conflict—this structure is visible on contrast-enhanced T1-weighted MRI and not on magnetic resonance angiography. After the vessel is dissected away from the nerve (not the other way around!), the decompression is completed by placing a nonabsorbable felt-like material between the nerve root and the vessel. The most commonly used material is shredded Teflon that is rolled into small patties or pledgets, which are inserted one after another to separate the vessel and nerve root. If the compression is venous (much less often), the vein is coagulated and cut. It is important to inspect the entire cisternal segment of the nerve—from its entry into the brainstem all the way to the porus trigeminus because missed vascular compression may result in incomplete pain relief or early pain recurrence. In rare cases in which there is no identifiable vascular compression, one may use so-called internal neurolysis, combing the nerve root between its fascicles with a blunt hook or gently compressing the nerve (as was suggested in the 1950s, before MVD was introduced), rather than rushing to open transection of the nerve root (trigeminal rhizotomy).

On completion of MVD, the dura is closed either primarily or with a dural patch, and the bone defect is closed with autologous bone or cement with or without a plate. It may be helpful to mention multiple other steps that are routinely used (e.g., preoperative antibiotic, surgical timeout, use of Mayfield or similar head holder), but the examiners' usually pay attention to more specific surgical details.

COMPLICATIONS

The patient may develop CSF leak (particularly if the dural closure was not watertight), hearing loss (which will be partial if one forgets to wax the air cells and the patient develops muffled hearing from CSF in the mastoid cells, or complete if one does not use BAER monitoring and inadvertently stretches cranial nerve VIII during retraction), facial numbness due to excessive manipulation of the trigeminal nerve root, or incomplete pain relief after the MVD. Each of these complications has to be properly addressed as soon as it is discovered. CSF leak may require reexploration for patching the dural defect. Hearing loss would necessitate a consultation with an ear, nose, and throat specialist but, just like facial numbness, is unlikely to require additional intervention. Incomplete—or absent—pain relief may indicate that the compression was missed or the pledgets have moved; this may necessitate reexploration and redecompression. However, if the pain returned more than 6 months after MVD, the risk of development of facial numbness from reexploration becomes so high that it may be prudent to consider other interventions rather than repeating MVD.

PERCUTANEOUS INTERVENTIONS

It would be great to be equally familiar with all 3 destructive interventions that are commonly used for TN, but it is mandatory to know at least 1 of them in minor detail. The choice between RF thermocoagulation, glycerol gangliolysis, and balloon compression is usually dictated by the surgeon's training and individual preferences, but in our practice we use the most selective intervention (RF thermocoagulation) whenever the patient is able to cooperate during the surgery and the pain involves either second, or third, or both second and third, branch distribution. In patients with first branch involvement and in those with dementia or cognitive impairment or any other issues (including language barrier) that would prevent them from clearly communicating during the surgery, we prefer using the balloon compression approach, which does not require the patient's cooperation and may be done under brief general anesthesia or deep sedation.

The entry point and direction for the cannula are chosen based on Härtel stereotactic technique of foramen ovale cannulation, with the skin entry placed 2 to 3 cm lateral to the corner of the mouth and 1 cm inferior to it. The cannula is aimed toward the ipsilateral medial epicanthus or slightly medial to the midpupillary line and to a point 1 to 3 cm in front of the tragus. The operator's finger is placed in the patient's mouth to prevent penetration of oral mucosa. We routinely use a submental-vertex view of the patient's skull through a standard C-arm fluoroscope. Some other centers use a C-arm direction that is parallel to the Härtel's approach tilting the C-arm until the foramen ovale is clearly visualized.

The process of cannula insertion during RF procedures usually requires brief sedation; the patient is awakened when the cannula is in place and the preganglionic nerve fibers are stimulated with low-voltage current to check the location of paresthesias and define the sensory threshold. When the electrode is in the correct place (we usually use a curved electrode designed by Tew), the RF lesion is created by heating the electrode to 65° to 70° C for 60 to 90 seconds and then testing the patient for the expected loss of sharp-dull discrimination and disappearance of trigger zones. The lesion is repeated in a different location if the painful regions are not covered by a single thermocoagulation. A straight electrode may be advanced deeper to reach fibers of different branches; the curved electrode may be repositioned by retracting it into the cannula, rotating the cannula and then redeploying the electrode in a different direction because an attempt to rotate the electrode itself would result in electrode fracture. When the loss of sharp-dull discrimination is confirmed, the electrode and the cannula are removed.

Balloon compression follows the same general approach—it may be worthwhile to move the entry point slightly higher, keeping it 2 to 3 cm lateral to the labial commissure to allow for more flat path for the balloon. The cannula is loaded with a sharp stylet to penetrate the skin; this sharp stylet is replaced with the blunt stylet when the cannula is 4 to 5 cm deep in the soft tissues. This is done to minimize risk for complications such as carotid artery puncture. After the stylet penetrates the dura of the foramen ovale, the cannula is lodged in the foramen and then the stylet is replaced with the balloon, which is then advanced into the Meckel's cave under direct radiographic control with the C-arm in lateral projection. The balloon with a stylet in it is advanced until it is completely outside of the cannula and inside Meckel's cave. When it is inflated with 1 mL of radiographic contrast (the contrast formulation should be safe for intrathecal application), the balloon would assume a typical pear-shape appearance that indicates its position under the dural fold of porus trigeminus (Figure 11.10). This is the site where actual compression takes place, and during the balloon inflation, it is not unusual to see a short period of bradycardia due to trigeminovagal reflex. The balloon is kept inflated for 90 seconds or so, although there are some published reports in which the balloon was inflated for a much longer time. The compression may be repeated if desired, and then the balloon and the cannula are removed. In case of balloon rupture, it may be replaced with another one; the contrast leaking into CSF as a result of such rupture is expected to be harmless.

COMPLICATIONS

Sensory loss after either of percutaneous destructive trigeminal surgeries is not considered a complication; it is an expected effect of nerve destruction. The extreme numbness that is perceived as pain is called anesthesia dolorosa (AD)—and this is indeed a rare and hard-to-treat complication. The best strategy to deal with AD is to avoid it, which is the rationale for not raising the temperature of the RF probe too high (above 85°C) or lesioning for too long (longer than 90 seconds), and for not keeping the balloon inflated for longer than 3 minutes or inflating it with more than 1 mL of contrast. However, if AD does occur, the treatments are quite limited and not always effective. One would usually start AD treatment with tricyclic antidepressants (e.g., amitriptyline, nortriptyline) and use surgical interventions only if medical treatment fails. Both destructive surgeries (trigeminal tractotomy and nucleotomy, either open or CT guided; Figure 11.11) and neuromodulation (motor cortex stimulation; Figure 11.12) have been tried for AD with varying degrees of success.

If the carotid artery is inadvertently penetrated during access to the foramen ovale, it is recommended to withdraw the cannula and abort the procedure. Because the carotid puncture is extracranial, the risk to the patient remains low, but it would be prudent to wait 1 or 2 weeks before attempting repeat trigeminal intervention.

STEREOTACTIC RADIOSURGERY

Despite its relatively low effectiveness, SRS is an established modality for treatment of TN. Just like with everything else during the Oral Board Examination, it is advisable to avoid using the brand names, particularly because all currently available SRS devices (Gamma Knife, frame-based and frameless linear accelerators, including CyberKnife) have been reported to be used for TN treatment. The target of SRS is the cisternal segment of the trigeminal nerve root (Figure 11.13)—it is best visualized with special MRI sequences

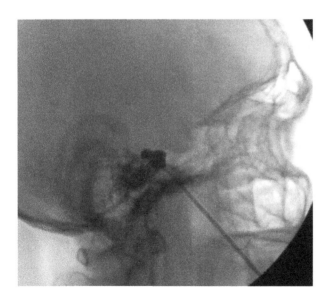

Figure 11.10 Intraoperative fluoroscopic image during trigeminal balloon compression procedure. Note the typical "pear-shape" appearance of the balloon indicating correct position of the balloon inside the Meckel's cave.

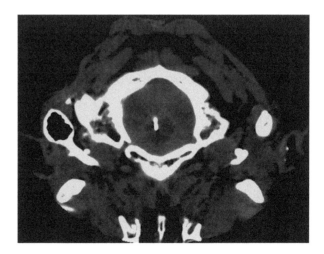

Figure 11.11 CT-guided trigeminal tractotomy/nucleotomy: the contour of the uppermost spinal cord is delineated with intrathecal contrast; the needle is reaching the surface of the cord; and the electrode is in the posterolateral quadrant of the cord (the patient is positioned prone in CT scanner).

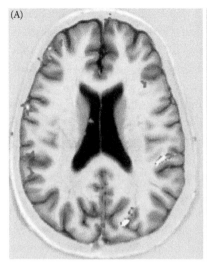
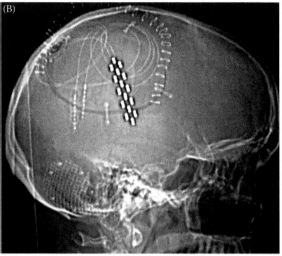

Figure 11.12 A. The functional MRI indicates location of the hand/face motor activation in planning of motor cortex stimulation for deafferentation facial pain. B. An epidural paddle type electrode is placed over the mapped representation of the face in the contralateral motor cortex, in addition to fMRI guided navigation, we use intraoperative recording of cortical activity for physiological localization of the motor cortex. Note the mesh in retromastoid area from previous intradural trigeminal rhizotomy procedure.

(e.g., FIESTA, CISS). If the patient cannot undergo MRI because of an implanted pacemaker or defibrillator, CT cisternography may be used for SRS targeting. The usual dose for the first time SRS for TN would be 80 Gy, this number varies from center to center. As mentioned earlier, it takes some time for the SRS effect to reach maximum,

which makes it different from other surgical interventions that work immediately. The results of SRS for TN are also less impressive than those of other approaches but are well received by the patients.

CONTINGENCY PLANS

If the surgical procedures do not work, or if the pain recurs, the surgery may be repeated. It is not uncommon for TN patients to require more than 1 surgery, and there are no data to suggest that either SRS or percutaneous interventions make subsequent MVD less effective or vice versa. The challenge usually is to differentiate TN from trigeminal neuropathic pain (TNP) that is associated with constant pain and sensory deficit; even though TNP resembles a less typical presentation of TN (so-called TN type 2, in which constant pain dominates clinical picture but triggerable shooting pains are also present). Recurrent TN, even in presence of neurological deficits, is an indication for surgery, but TNP is not expected to improve with either MVD or destructive interventions. Instead, TNP would be expected to respond to neuromodulation approaches such as peripheral nerve stimulation (PNS).

CASE 4

CLINICAL PRESENTATION

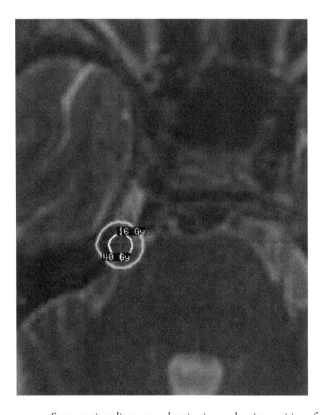

Figure 11.13 Stereotactic radiosurgery planning image showing position of the isocenter over the cisternal segment of the trigeminal nerve root.

A 68-year-old woman presents with severe pain in her hip, pelvis, and leg on the right side. The patient was diagnosed with metastatic cervical cancer that invaded her lumbar plexus on the right side. The tumor was deemed unresectable, and the patient underwent a course of radiation treatment and continues to receive systemic chemotherapy. Since the pain has become refractory to systemic opioid therapy, a neurosurgical service is being consulted for consideration of pain-relieving surgical interventions. The patient's neurological examination is consistent with right lumbar plexopathy. She has a working colostomy and suffers from chronic urinary incontinence, most likely due to focal invasion of pelvic structures. Her spine imaging does not show any neoplastic involvement of the vertebral column; there is no abnormal enhancement to suggest metastatic tumors on her brain imaging. She does, however, have metastases in her liver and lungs.

SURGICAL DECISION-MAKING

In this clinical situation, the main question that should be asked by the surgeon is what is the patient's life expectancy, because this will determine the choice of surgical intervention. As with most chronic pain conditions that require surgical intervention, there are 2 general approaches that are commonly used—neurodestruction and neuromodulation. The destruction is often irreversible, not testable with certainty, and not adjustable. Moreover, the results of destructive interventions are relatively short-lasting because pain would frequently recur in 6 to 12 months, possibly due to inherent plasticity of the nervous system. Nevertheless, it remains attractive due to its immediate onset of action and lower costs because an expensive implant is not needed for modulation.

This choice between destruction and modulation comes up frequently when dealing with cancer-related pain because destructive interventions, such as cordotomy and myelotomy, may be done in a minimally invasive fashion, and the short duration of the pain relief may be sufficient for many patients in terminal stages of malignancy. Electrical stimulation of the spinal cord and peripheral nerves may not be as effective because of the nature of the cancer pain: both SCS and PNS seem to work best for neuropathic pain conditions, and cancer pain has a major nociceptive component due to actual injury of the tissues. Two alternatives for high-dose systemic opioids are intrathecal drug delivery (opioids, calcium-channel blockers, various adjuvants including local anesthetics and adrenergic agents) and surgical interruption of pain-transmitting pathways—and for the patient presented here, the unilateral nature of the pain would make her a good candidate for a cordotomy procedure.

If the patient's life expectancy is longer than 6 months, the preference is given to intrathecal drug delivery, the modality that includes implantation of a programmable pump, commonly referred to as "morphine pump." If, on the other hand, her life expectancy were 3 months or less, a cordotomy would be a more reasonable surgical choice.

INTRATHECAL MORPHINE PUMP

The main rationale for intrathecal drug infusion is the ability to obtain good pain relief with significantly lower dose of the drug (so-called equianalgesic ratio) because the effect of 1 mg of intrathecal morphine is roughly equivalent to 100 mg of intravenous morphine. Such significant reduction of the medication dose translates into a better safety and satisfaction profile and allows one to avoid oversedation, constipation, and other dose-related opioid side effects. Intrathecal delivery also allows better compliance, more steady effect without dosing-related fluctuations, and, with most recent pump models, an option of on-demand boluses, similar to the familiar approach of patient-controlled analgesia, in addition to the continuous intrathecal infusion at a steady rate.

CHOICE OF INTRATHECAL MEDICATION

The only 2 pain-relieving medications that are approved for use in intrathecal pumps are morphine sulfate and ziconotide. Although morphine sulfate is a well-known medication that is familiar to both physicians and patients, ziconotide is a unique calcium channel antagonist that is a synthetic form of the conotoxin peptide, an analgesic substance derived from a cone snail, Conus magus. The side-effect profile of ziconotide is very different from that of opioids, and the best way to avoid development of psychiatric symptoms is to start with a low dose of medication and increase it slowly until desired pain relief occurs.

Many other medications are suggested for intrathecal use despite lack of regulatory approval. These off-label medications include hydromorphone, bupivacaine, clonidine, fentanyl, and others. The recommendations on choice of intrathecal medications are updated every several years with published guidelines that summarize consensus of an expert panel on polyanalgesic use. The most recent guidelines list three first-line choices for neuropathic pain (morphine, ziconotide, and morphine + bupivacaine) and 4 first-line choices for nociceptive pain (morphine, hydromorphone, ziconotide, and fentanyl). Other medications and their combinations are listed as second through fifth lines in step-like algorithms.

So how does one decide whether the patient is a candidate for intrathecal drug delivery? It is considered a standard operating procedure to perform a trial of intrathecal morphine before implanting the intrathecal pump. Although many different approaches for trialing exist (single bolus, multiple boluses, implanted catheter for either continuous infusion or periodic administration of escalating dose, epidural or intrathecal, medication only or placebo controlled), but none is superior to the others. The simplest approach is to give a single intrathecal injection of a test dose of medication (usually 1 mg of preservative-free morphine sulfate) through a regular lumbar puncture and then monitor the patient for 6 to 8 hours for degree of pain relief and development of any side effects. Usually, a more than 50% reduction in the pain intensity is considered a positive result that would justify proceeding with implantation of the pump. Less than 50% reduction in pain and no side effects may be an indication for repeating the trial with a higher dose of morphine, and good pain relief but development of side effects may be a reason to repeat the trial with a lower dose of medication.

IMPLANTATION OF THE PUMP

Surgery for implantation of the pump is done under general anesthesia—the patient is placed in a lateral position, and the incisions are planned over the midlumbar area to insert the catheter and over the abdominal wall to place the pump. Choice of the side depends on the presence of colostomy, nephrostomy, or surgical scars. Although in principle there are many different kinds of pumps, the usual choice is to use programmable pumps that allow one to change the daily dose of medication by simple reprogramming rather than by replacing the medication with a different drug concentration.

To reduce the risk for catheter fracture or migration, it is recommended to use oblique paramedian approach. It is also recommended to use fluoroscopic guidance and to enter the thecal sac below the level of L2—to reduce the risk of inadvertent injury of the conus. Special kink-resistant catheters are loaded with a flexible guidewire; they are inserted in cephalad direction through a Tuohy-type needle. The catheter is usually advanced to a mid-thoracic level, and its location is controlled with fluoroscopy. After the guidewire is removed, the spontaneous flow of CSF from the catheter indicates patency of the tubing and subarachnoid position of the catheter tip. It is important to anchor the catheter to the fascia—most often; an injectable anchor from the catheter kit is deployed over the catheter and sutured to

the fascia with nonabsorbable suture. After that, the catheter is advanced to the pump pocket in the abdominal wall through a catheter passer. A standard shunt passer may be used for this purpose.

The pump is filled with medication before it is attached to the catheter. After the catheter and pump are connected, the pump is placed in its abdominal wall pocket, the catheter is coiled under the pump, and then the pump is secured to the underlying abdominal fascia with nonabsorbable sutures. Care is taken to avoid making the pump pocket too large because the pump may flip or migrate or too small in order to avoid excessive tension of the tissues. After the closure, the pump is programmed to start continuous infusion of the intrathecal medication, and an initial bolus is administered to clear the internal pump tubing and the entire catheter and then to fill them with the medication.

COMPLICATIONS

Despite being a very straightforward surgical procedure, implantation of an intrathecal drug delivery system is associated with all kinds of complications, including surgical issues (e.g., hematoma, cord or nerve root injury from needle insertion, CSF leak, seroma formation, wound infection), hardware-related issues (e.g., disconnection, catheter migration, catheter fracture [Figure 11.14], pump

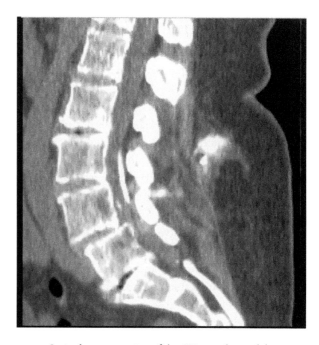

Figure 11.14 Sagittal reconstruction of the CT scan obtained during a "pumpogram" for suspected fracture/disconnection of the intrathecal catheter indicates contrast extravasation in extraspinal location. The catheter enters intrathecal space but the medication does not reach the spinal canal due to a leak at the anchoring site, presumably due to needle penetration of the catheter at the time of its original implantation.

stall), and therapy-related issues (e.g., overdose resulting in respiratory depression, underdose resulting in withdrawal symptoms, itching and leg swelling from morphine administration, psychosis from ziconitide).

INTRATHECAL CATHETER-TIP INFLAMMATORY MASS (GRANULOMA)

A separate concern is a possibility of development of an intrathecal catheter-tip granuloma (Figure 11.15). This is an inflammatory mass that is not associated with any kind of infection; it forms inside the intrathecal space, interfering with medication release and distribution, and becomes attached to the spinal cord and nerve roots, sometimes to a point of causing neurological deficits due to cord compression.

Most catheter-tip granulomas occur with high concentrations of morphine sulfate, with use of morphine citrate, or

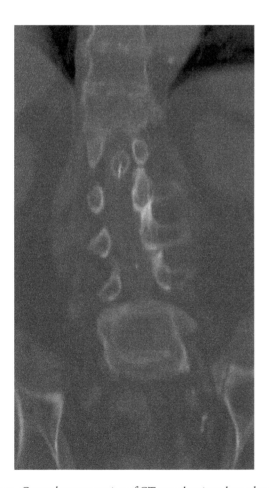

Figure 11.15 Coronal reconstruction of CT scan showing a hyperdense intrathecal lesion that formed around the tip of intrathecal catheter. Such intrathecal inflammatory mass may present with nerve compression symptoms or be an incidental finding during routine imaging study.

with high doses of medications, but they are also described with other medications, including hydromorphone and fentanyl. Most granulomas remain asymptomatic and present as an incidental finding on follow-up imaging, but in some patients they manifest with gradual loss of efficacy (because the drug stays inside the granuloma and gets absorbed into the bloodstream instead of circulating in CSF) or neurological deficits due to direct compression of the underlying spinal cord. The pumps that are being implanted today are considered MRI conditional and should not prevent the patient from undergoing a MRI scan if clinically warranted. It is recommended to interrogate the pump after MRI to make sure the motor restarted after exposure to the strong magnetic field; some pump models require medication withdrawal and reservoir refill after MRI.

Asymptomatic granulomas do not require surgical intervention—if desired, the medication dose, concentration, infusion rate, or medication itself may be changed to stop granuloma progression. Minimally symptomatic granulomas would usually require stopping the pump and not restarting it until granuloma disappears, but if the patient is overtly symptomatic and presents with cord compression, it is recommended to decompress the cord with laminectomy and duraplasty. Aggressive removal of granuloma, which was advocated in the past due to concerns about a possible infectious nature of the inflammatory mass, is no longer recommended—partly because it is now confirmed that granulomas are sterile and partly because inflammatory reaction around the mass results in significant risk for neurological injury from granuloma resection.

OVERDOSE AND UNDERDOSE

Because the pump has to be refilled on a regular basis, there is a possibility of human error with missing the pump port (so-called pocket refill) or injecting the drug into a wrong port, or hitting the catheter with the needle and accidentally injecting 3 to 6 months' worth of medication directly into the spinal fluid. There may also be an error in using the wrong concentration of the drug or with programming a wrong infusion rate. The end result of this complication will be either a dramatic overdose of the patient with all signs of opioid toxicity (e.g., respiratory depression, somnolence, or coma) or development of withdrawal symptoms if the lower drug concentration was used, the pump was improperly programmed, or the catheter became obstructed or disconnected.

Treatment of overdose includes initiating supportive measures such as intubation and respiratory support in the intensive care setting, administering proper medications (e.g., naloxone), stopping the pump, and emptying the pump reservoir. Withdrawal symptoms, if recognized on time, are best treated with administration of opioids orally or parenterally. Incomplete pain relief may indicate catheter obstruction; the other possible explanations would include development of tolerance and disease progression.

CORDOTOMY

But what if the patient's life expectancy is shorter than 6 months? Implantation of an intrathecal pump in such a situation would not be appropriate for logistical and cost-effectiveness reasons. Instead, one would consider using a destructive option, which in this case of unilateral treatment-resistant pain from known malignancy would be a contralateral cordotomy. The target for intervention is the lateral spinothalamic tract that transmits pain information from the contralateral side of the body toward the brain. This tract is located in the anterior (ventral) half of the lateral columns and projects anteriorly to the dentate ligament. Fibers of spinothalamic tract are somatotopically organized, and the cervical fibers project more medially within the tract than the thoracic, lumbar, and sacral fibers.

Classical cordotomy consisted of a mechanical transection of the anterolateral quadrant of the spinal cord with a dedicated right-angle instrument (the cordotome). Most often, open cordotomy was done at the upper thoracic level, and the surgical approach would include hemilaminectomy on the side of surgery contralateral to the side of pain. A less invasive alternative is CT-guided cordotomy in which the RF electrode is inserted through a special needle at the C1-C2 level and then a lesion is made in the location chosen based on the patient's feedback in response to electrical stimulation. CT-guided cordotomy may be done on an outpatient basis; the entire procedure takes place in the CT scanner suite.

For a CT-guided approach, we start the procedure with an injection of myelographic dye to define the borders of the spinal cord and to clearly visualize the cord on axial CT images. The infraauricular area is sterilely prepared, the needle insertion point is infiltrated with local anesthetic, and then the lateral upper cervical puncture is performed using standard landmarks. With the patient lying supine, the entry point is chosen 1 cm below the tip of mastoid process, and the needle is aimed slightly caudal and parallel to the floor. If needed, a series of images is obtained during the insertion process to confirm the needle direction. The needle used for cordotomy is a standard cut-tip needle, large enough to accommodate the special RF electrode (Kanpolat CT cordotomy kit [KCTE]); curved and closed-tip needles that are usually used for lumbar punctures (Touhy- and Whitaker-type needles) would not be appropriate. After the intrathecal space is entered, the stylet of the needle is replaced with the electrode and the spinal cord entry is confirmed by the change in electrical impedance. The electrode is aimed anterior to the dentate ligament; its position is checked with axial CT images (Figure 11.16). To confirm the correct position of the electrode tip, the electrical stimulation is used to elicit paresthesias. The curved tip of the electrode allows one to insert it in different directions in order to reach the correct location inside the spinothalamic tract. For the patient described here, we would target the left (contralateral to the side of pain) lateral spinothalamic tract and look for paresthesia coverage in the hip, pelvis, and right leg. After the paresthesias cover the painful region, a thermal RF lesion is created, usually with 70° to 72°C for 60 seconds. As a result of the lesion, the patient develops partial numbness in the area of the pain as well as significant and immediate improvement of pain. After this is achieved, the electrode and the needle are withdrawn, and the insertion point is covered with a bandage.

COMPLICATIONS

In general, unilateral cordotomy is a very safe intervention. Development of neurological deficits is rare and may be detected early because the patient stays awake during the procedure and is asked to move the ipsilateral extremities

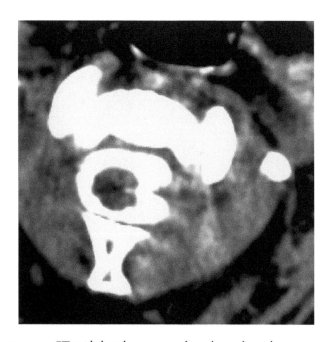

Figure 11.16 CT-guided cordotomy procedure: the myelographic contrast facilitates visualization of the spinal cord at the upper cervical level with a needle reaching the surface of the spinal cord and the electrode entering the ventrolateral quadrant of the spinal cord.

every few minutes during each step of the procedure. Sensory deficits are usually well tolerated; motor deficits occur rarely and are unlikely to be severe or permanent. Theoretically, it is possible to injure the vertebral artery or the upper cervical nerve root during the approach, but very small caliber of the needle and CT guidance are intended to minimize these risks. A serious problem may arise from a loss of ability to breathe when asleep (so-called Ondine's curse), which is a feared complication of bilateral high cervical cordotomy. This is the main reason the cervical cordotomy is reserved for unilateral pain; bilateral pain is better treated with midline myelotomy, and if the patient with unilateral pain later develops pain on the opposite side (ipsilateral to cordotomy), then the second cordotomy may be done on the upper thoracic level so the risk for central hypoventilation is minimized.

CASE 5

CLINICAL PRESENTATION

A 52-year-old man presents with severe pain in his right foot for the last 20 months. The pain started almost immediately after a trivial injury of the foot when a shopping cart rolled over it. At that time, the patient was diagnosed with a hairline fracture of his metatarsal bone and did not require any surgery. His foot was immobilized with a splint for few weeks, but despite apparent healing of the fracture, the patient continued to have pain. In addition to this, he developed severe sensitivity to any kind of touch, pressure, or manipulation of his foot and after a year or so started exhibiting muscle atrophy, hair loss, toenail fragility, coldness, and pale discoloration of the distal part of the right leg from midcalf down to his toes. The pain improved only temporarily with various interventional treatments in the pain clinic. Currently, he is referred for neurosurgical evaluation by his pain specialist in hopes of qualifying for some kind of pain-relieving surgery.

DIAGNOSTIC IMPRESSION

Making the diagnosis in such a case of peripheral pain may be challenging because the pain frequently does not follow the clear anatomic border of a dermatome or sensory distribution of a specific peripheral nerve. In the past, the pain described here would be referred to as *reflex sympathetic dystrophy*; use of this descriptive term is related to frequently encountered sympathetic features (e.g., coldness, discoloration, impaired perspiration) and development of "dystrophy" or gradual atrophy of the soft tissues. Currently, this

term is abandoned—instead, the correct diagnosis is *complex regional pain syndrome* (CRPS) type 1.

The distinction between CRPS type 1 and type 2 is in involvement of a named nerve. Existence of such an involved nerve would be referred to as *causalgia*, or what is currently called CRPS type 2. Both types 1 and 2 may be sympathetically maintained or sympathetically independent; presence or absence of autonomic features does not change the diagnosis or treatment.

There is no particular tool to diagnose CRPS. Structural imaging is expected to be normal; in advanced cases, the imaging would confirm the presence of tissue atrophy on the symptomatic side. Thermography was proposed as a diagnostic test for CRPS because most patients would have a pronounced asymmetry in tissue temperature between the normal and affected sides.

TREATMENT

The best treatment for CRPS is mobilization of the affected extremity. CRPS symptoms do indeed resemble findings observed in so-called disuse syndrome, as one would develop, for example, after prolonged wearing of a cast. However, it is difficult to participate in therapy while suffering from uncontrollable pain. Therefore, it is recommended to proceed with aggressive pain management before therapy is initiated. The surgery referral would be appropriate if the patient fails to improve in response to standard medical treatment with anticonvulsants and antidepressants. Usually, the patient would receive local anesthetic or sympatholytic blocks from a pain specialist before being referred for surgical treatment.

Current surgical treatment of pain in CRPS is straightforward. Although there is a destructive option of sympathectomy, it is rarely, if ever, used now for anything other than hyperhidrosis. Over the last several decades, electrical neuromodulation, particularly spinal cord stimulation (SCS), has become an accepted surgical treatment of CRPS pain, and a published randomized prospective study supported its efficacy. In fact, SCS is the most common surgical procedure done specifically for the treatment of pain, and CRPS is one of its most established indications.

SPINAL CORD STIMULATION

Several criteria qualify a patient for a SCS procedure. These include presence of chronic (>6 months), severe (numeric rating scale of 6 or higher), disabling (affecting one's functionality) pain; established medical diagnosis; favorable psychological evaluation results; the patient's ability and willingness to operate the implanted device; preserved sensation in the painful region; and finally—and perhaps most important—successful trial of stimulation. Most prerequisites can be checked during initial evaluation; psychological evaluation requires separate referral; the patient education prepares him- or herself for the surgical interventions. Finally, the trial of SCS allows one to determine its efficacy and the severity of side effects, if any, related to the stimulation.

In cases of documented CRPS, it may make sense to intervene before the usual 6 months of conventional treatment are over. Early physical therapy is the key to success, but, as mentioned earlier, it is hardly possible for patients to participate in therapy as long as they are in severe pain.

The target for SCS is the dorsal column. Despite many discussions and arguments, the gate control theory of pain that postulates an ability to suppress the pain by delivering nonpainful information to the interneurons of the spinal cord is still the most likely explanation, at least for paresthesia-based SCS. The craniocaudal location of the SCS target is determined by the location of pain—those with pain in the lower back and legs would usually achieve best results with stimulation of the lower thoracic region (between T7 and T10), pain in feet and perineal area would require stimulation below T10, and the pain in arms and hands would respond to SCS at the mid and low cervical levels.

There are many types of SCS systems—percutaneous and paddle-type leads (Figure 11.17), rechargeable and non-rechargeable devices, constant current and constant voltage-based systems, but most of them use implantable pulse generators and not RF receivers, which have become obsolete over the years. Choice of device (percutaneous vs. paddle) is determined by several practical nuances—patients with lack of true epidural space due to previous laminectomy, those with tight stenosis at the level of stimulation, and those with history of multiple device migrations would do better with a paddle-type electrode that is implanted through a small laminectomy or laminotomy. Other patients probably would do just as well with percutaneous electrodes that are much less invasive and may be advanced over multiple spinal levels through a simple epidural entry with a Tuohy-type needle. However, relative unfamiliarity of neurosurgeons with percutaneous implantation technique may be another reason that most electrode leads implanted today by neurosurgeons are of the paddle type.

SPINAL CORD STIMULATION TRIAL

The usual approach to SCS is to do a trial with percutaneous electrodes (unless the patient has one of the issues listed earlier that requires paddle electrode), and then, during the

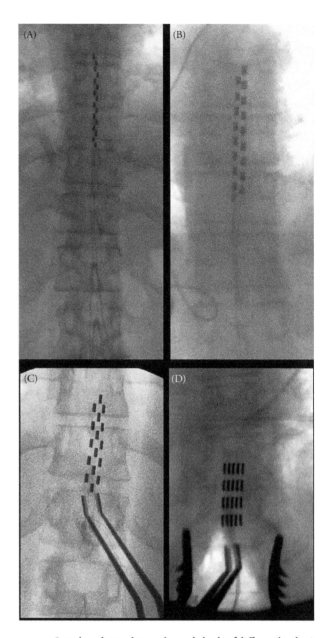

Figure 11.17 Spinal cord stimulation electrode leads of different kinds: A. Percutaneous 8-contact cylindrical electrodes; B. Percutaneously insertable narrow paddle electrodes; C. Three-column paddle-type electrode; D. Five-column paddle-type electrode. The bayonet-shaped insertion tool is intended to advance and steer the paddle type electrode while avoiding putting direct pressure on the thecal sac.

5 to 7 days of the trial, to determine the patient's response. The electrodes are placed with the patient awake in prone position under fluoroscopic guidance, and the intraoperative testing helps to determine paresthesia coverage with the goal of covering all painful areas with stimulation-induced paresthesias in a concordant fashion. If the electrodes are intended to be temporary, they are simply sutured or taped to the skin for the duration of the trial; these electrodes are removed at the end of the trial, and the permanent implantation includes placement of a new electrode that is then

connected to the generator. Another option is to keep the same electrodes that were used for the trial—in this case, they should be anchored to the fascia and connected to a set of extensions that is then tunneled under the skin to a distant exit site. At the end of this "tunneled trial," the incision is reopened, the extension cables are cut and discarded, and the electrodes are tunneled to the generator pocket. The main advantage of the tunneled trial is that the electrodes that were tested during the trial remain in use for long-term stimulation. The disadvantages of this approach are that the patient requires electrode placement in the operating room, as opposed to the doctor's office or the procedure room, and that another trip to the operating room is required even if the trial fails because the anchored electrodes need to be taken out by reopening the original incision.

IMPLANTATION OF PERMANENT DEVICE

This stage of surgery is usually done under general anesthesia in a prone or lateral position depending on the chosen location for the generator. We prefer placing the generator into the abdominal wall, where it is easier to program and charge—this requires lateral positioning of the patient; others use the flank or buttock for generator placement and this may be done in prone position. The electrode is connected to the generator after it is tunneled to the generator pocket.

The pocket depth is dictated by the need for recharging: nonrechargeable devices may be placed up to 4 cm deep under the skin, but rechargeable devices should be no more than 1.5 to 2 cm under the skin surface. The size of the generator pocket should match the size of the generator. Making the pocket too large may result in device rotation and possible seroma formation. Making the pocket too small would produce significant tension of the tissues and elicit pocket-site pain after the implantation. Most companies making devices also make plastic templates that may help in sizing the pocket before the generator insertion.

POSTOPERATIVE CARE:

Current SCS devices allow for multiple programs to be used based on the patient's preference. These programs include different combinations of stimulating contacts, different frequencies and pulse widths of stimulation, and different amplitude ranges within which the patient can vary the intensity of stimulation. Nevertheless, it is common for SCS patients to undergo reprogramming sessions in the postoperative period, usually once every 1 to 3 weeks, to optimize the coverage and achieve reliable pain relief.

Currently, there are at least half a dozen SCS devices that may be used for most indications. Most of them have unique features, such as adaptable stimulation that changes based on the patient's position, ability to deliver burst or very high-frequency stimulation, special programming approaches that allow for independent current delivery to multiple contacts, different paddle configurations with 2 to 5 columns, and smaller paddle electrodes that may be implanted through a percutaneous approach.

Most devices implanted today have limitations in terms of MRI compatibility. None is MRI safe, but some have conditional approval for use in 1.5T or 3T scanners for certain parts of the body or even for whole-body scanning as long as certain conditions are met. There are now MRI-conditionally approved paddle electrodes from every big SCS device manufacturer, but the conditions of approval vary from one paddle to another, and it is recommended to check the latest approval status before allowing the patients with these paddles in place to undergo MRI examination.

The actual treatment of CRPS starts after SCS implantation. The pain relief allows the patient to start intensive physical therapy that may reverse trophic changes and muscle atrophy associated with this condition. Eventually, if the pain subsides, the stimulation may be stopped. Subsequently, the device may be safely removed if it has not been used for 6 months or longer.

COMPLICATIONS

Use of SCS devices is associated with several types of complications and side effects. Some of them are procedure related and include hematoma, infection, damage to the nervous tissue (spinal cord or nerve roots), and internal or external CSF leak that may occur if the underlying dura was inadvertently violated during electrode insertion. Others may be related to the hardware and surgical technique; these include device migration, fracture, and disconnection. Finally, there is a group of therapy-related effects, including loss of stimulation benefits, development of unpleasant paresthesias, pain from stimulation, and discomfort during recharging.

Most of these complications are easy to recognize and treat. Loss of stimulation may be remedied by reprogramming; this may also be used to eliminate unpleasant paresthesias or stimulation-induced discomfort. Sometimes changing electrode polarity will suffice, but in other cases, the entire stimulation paradigms have to be changed to either higher frequency, bursting mode, or wider pulse widths. Pocket hematoma or seroma may have to be drained. Migrated electrodes have to be revised and repositioned; repeated migration of percutaneous leads may be a reason to switch to a paddle-type electrode, but one has to keep in mind that paddle leads are not immune to migration either.

Infection should be treated cautiously, and superficial infection of soft tissues may be resolved with a short course of antibiotics. Deep infections and those involving the back incision usually indicate that the hardware is involved. In situations like this, it is recommended to remove the entire system and replace it with a new one a few months later after the infection has cleared.

Hematoma is of particular concern when it occurs in the epidural space. Development of cord compression symptoms after electrode implantation should prompt urgent surgical decompression (Figure 11.18). Sometimes, the symptoms are caused by the paddle, which itself behaves as a mass lesion and therefore has to be removed during the decompressive intervention. However, it is also possible that the cord was damaged during the insertion procedure, and the deficits may be a result of the cord edema. To minimize this risk, it is recommended to use intraoperative neurophysiologic monitoring during asleep implantation cases. It is also advisable to avoid aggressive epidural manipulation, to start with adequate exposure in longitudinal and transverse directions, and to obtain preoperative imaging of the operated area (in this case—thoracic spine) to avoid any surprises such as herniated disks or stenosis.

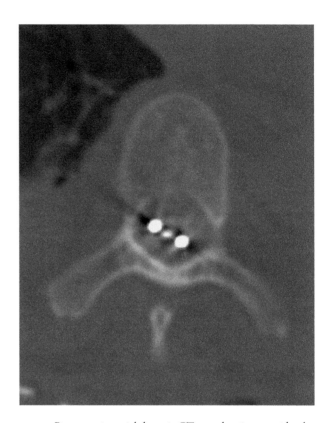

Figure 11.18 Postoperative axial thoracic CT scan showing an epidural hematoma that is pushing the electrode against the thecal sac in a patient with newly developed neurological deficit several hours after uneventful insertion of the spinal cord stimulation electrode.

CONTINGENCY PLANS

If conventional SCS does not provide expected pain relief, one may explore alternative options. In addition to new stimulation paradigms (e.g., high frequency, high density, burst stimulation), there is an option of intrathecal drug delivery, similar to what was discussed earlier. There is anecdotal evidence that addition of local anesthetic, such as bupivacaine, to the opioid medication may be more effective in pain control in CRPS cases.

Anecdotal reports have been made of destructive surgery and central neuromodulation procedures, such as deep brain stimulation, used for CRPS treatment. The results, however, have been somewhat discouraging, particularly in advanced and more chronic cases.

12.

PEDIATRIC NEUROSURGERY

Jodi L. Smith

HISTORY AND PHYSICAL EXAMINATION

You are covering for your pediatric neurosurgery partner, who is on a well-deserved 2-week vacation, when you are called by the neonatal intensive care unit (NICU) to evaluate and treat a 1-hour-old male infant with spina bifida (SB) born by caesarean delivery at 37+6 weeks estimated gestational age with a birth weight of 4.95 kg. At birth, he received stimulation and brief blow-by oxygen for cyanosis. At the time of your examination, he is awake, alert, and in no acute distress. He is on room air. He has severe macrocephaly, frontal bossing, scalp vein distension, and cranial suture diastasis. His anterior fontanelle is convex and tense. His head circumference (occipital frontal circumference [OFC]) is 50 cm. He moves his extremities and withdraws to tickle in all 4 extremities. He flexes and extends his hips and knees bilaterally but has weak ankle dorsiflexion and no plantar flexion bilaterally. His back reveals an open neural tube or myelomeningocele (MMC) defect (Figures 12.1 and 12.2).

IMAGING STUDIES

Imaging studies reveal extreme hydrocephalus with severe dilatation of the lateral ventricles and complete effacement of the sulci. The cerebral cortex is extremely thinned and is compressed against the inner table of the calvarium (Figure 12.3).

ANALYSIS OF CASE AND SURGICAL PLAN

MMC defects result from incomplete development of the primary neural tube. This, in turn, results in protrusion of malformed neural tissue and meninges through an opening in the vertebral arches, muscle, fascia, and skin with associated loss of motor and sensory function below the level of the defect. In addition, most neonates have associated malformations, including hydrocephalus, Chiari II malformation, orthopedic deformities of their lower extremities, and urogenital anomalies from involvement of sacral nerve roots.

PREOPERATIVE EVALUATION

Neonates with SB present with a sac-like protrusion containing a neural placode and cerebrospinal fluid (CSF) ventral to the placode. Examination should include measurement of the OFC as well as assessment of general vigor (especially cry and suck); upper and lower extremity motor and sensory function; anal sphincter function; site, level, and size of the MMC defect; and orthopedic deformities, such as club feet and kyphosis and/scoliosis. One should also look for signs and symptoms of hydrocephalus and Chiari II malformation. The neonate in this case has at least 2 major problems that must be treated: myelomeningocele defect and extreme hydrocephalus.

MMC closure in a newborn is relatively straightforward. Key aims of this procedure include the preservation of neurological function, detection of associated anomalies, and prevention of postoperative complications, with early closure representing an important component of initial management. Closure may be delayed up to 72 hours without an increase in complications.

Preoperatively, the patient should be maintained in a prone position to prevent rupture of the MMC sac and trauma to the neural placode. The defect should be covered with a sterile, saline-soaked gauze to prevent desiccation of the exposed neural tissue. To prevent rapid evaporation of the saline, the dressing is covered with a plastic wrap and sterile saline is trickled onto the gauze at a rate of 3 ml/hr.

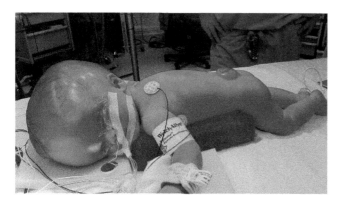

Figure 12.1 One-hour-old male infant born at 37+6 weeks with a lumbosacral myelomeningocele defect and severe hydrocephalus with associated macrocephaly.

Intravenous fluids are started and systemic antibiotics (e.g., ampicillin and gentamicin) are given. A head ultrasound is obtained to evaluate for hydrocephalus.

The goal of surgery is anatomic reconstruction of the defect, closing the neural placode into a neural tube to establish a microenvironment conducive to neuronal function. The exposed neural tissue is functional and should be preserved. This requires preservation of the vascular supply to the placode which passes through the laterally reflected dura to supply the MMC.

PROCEDURE: MYELOMENINGOCELE CLOSURE

Closure of the MMC defect involves the following steps: (1) separation of the neural placode from the skin by first making an incision at the junction of the normal and abnormal thin skin around the entire circumference of the MMC; (2) separation of the placode from the abnormal thin skin to prevent formation; (3) pial-to-pial closure of the placode into a tube using interrupted 7-0 nylon sutures

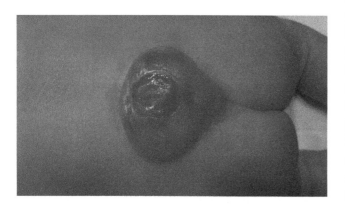

Figure 12.2 Lumbosacral myelomeningocele defect in a 1-hour-old male infant born at 37+6 weeks.

(Figure 12.4); (4) disconnection of the dura at its most lateral extent where it is attached to the underside of the skin lateral to the open skin edge, leaving a small rim of dura attached to the skin edge which will strengthen the skin edge and aid in skin closure; (5) watertight closure of the dura around the newly created neural tube, without constricting the underlying neural tissue or interfering with its vascular supply, using a running 6-0 silk suture (Figure 12.5); (6) mobilization and midline approximation of lateral paraspinous muscles and fascia if possible; (7) surgical correction of any significant kyphotic deformity if present (Figure 12.6); (8) mobilization of the skin, including the subcutaneous layer; and (9) tension-free closure of the skin in the midline with interrupted or running 5-0 nylon sutures (Figure 12.7).

The timing of CSF diversion is controversial and depends on the severity of the hydrocephalus. More than 85% of infants with SB develop hydrocephalus. Identifying impending hydrocephalus can help achieve optimal neurological function. The goal is to maintain appropriate ventricular system pressure and CSF volume. The patient in this case has obvious severe hydrocephalus (Figures 12.1 and 12.3) and would benefit from shunt placement at the time of MMC repair to reduce the risks for CSF drainage and/or wound breakdown postoperatively.

PROCEDURE: SHUNT PLACEMENT

After informed consent is obtained and a time-out performed, intravenous access is achieved, cardiopulmonary monitoring is established, the patient is intubated, and general anesthesia is induced. In an infant with extreme hydrocephalus requiring shunt placement, one could use a fixed medium or high pressure or a programmable type of shunt valve and either a frontal or an occipital approach. If a right occipital approach is chosen, the infant is positioned supine with the head turned to the left, a gel donut placed under the head, and a gel roll placed under the shoulders bilaterally posteriorly. All pressure points are carefully padded. Two linear incision sites are marked—one in the right occipital region 3 cm lateral to the midline and 1 cm superior to the lambdoid suture and the other one in the abdominal midline 2 fingerbreadths inferior to the xiphoid process. The entire area between and including the two incision sites is prepared thoroughly with a solution of 2% chlorhexidine gluconate and 70% isopropyl alcohol and, after allowing the prepared area to dry for at least 3 minutes, the drapes are applied in a sterile fashion. Before opening the incisions, a prophylactic antibiotic is administered (e.g., cefazolin [Kefzol] 25mg/kg). The incisions are infiltrated

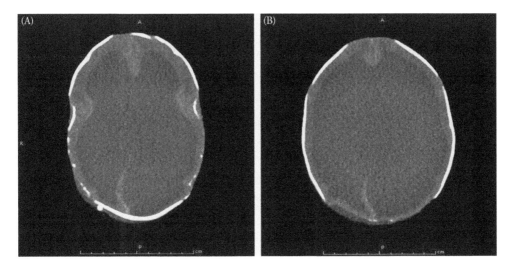

Figures 12.3A, B. Head CT axial images showing extreme hydrocephalus with severe dilatation of the lateral ventricles and a thin rim of cortical mantle in a 1-hour-old male infant born at 37+6 weeks with a myelomeningocele defect.

with 0.25% bupivacaine (Marcaine) with 1:200,000 units of epinephrine and then opened with a No. 15 scalpel blade.

The midline abdominal incision is carried down through the subcutaneous tissue to the rectus fascia using bovie electrocautery. The fascia is opened in the midline to expose the pre-peritoneal space. The peritoneum is identified, grasped with forceps or a hemostat, and opened with scissors. Entrance into the peritoneal cavity is confirmed with a No. 4 Penfield and the peritoneum is retracted with micro-hemostats.

Next, the cranial incision is opened and the pericranium is stripped. A small burr hole is made by hand with a drill bit and enlarged slightly with a 2-mm Kerrison rongeur. A tunneling device is then used to create a subcutaneous tunnel between the cranial and abdominal incision sites and a pediatric integral shunt system with reservoir is brought onto the field, assembled, and primed. The shunt is passed within the tunnel and both ends of the shunt are covered with bacitracin-soaked sponges.

Next, the dura is cauterized and opened, and an antibiotic-impregnated ventricular catheter is passed into the occipital horn of the right lateral ventricle. The length of the catheter is determined before placing the catheter by measuring the patient's head from the entry site in the right occipital region to just past the right coronal suture. This will place the tip of the ventricular catheter within the frontal horn of the lateral ventricle. CSF is sent for routine studies including cell count, differential, culture and sensitivity, Gram stain, glucose, and protein. The ventricular catheter is secured to the shunt reservoir with a 3-0 silk tie. The distal shunt tubing is examined for CSF flow and the tubing is passed into the peritoneal cavity. Intrathecal antibiotics are

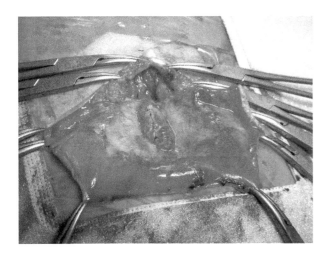

Figure 12.4 Anatomical reconstruction of the placode into a tube using interrupted 7-0 nylon sutures.

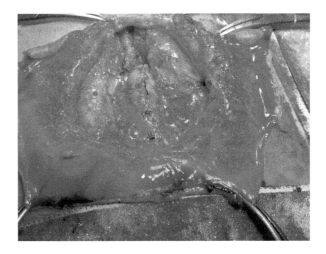

Figure 12.5 Closure of the dura around the newly created neural tube using a running 6-0 silk suture.

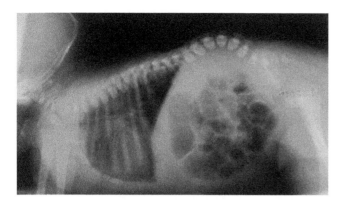

Figure 12.6 Significant kyphotic deformity in a newborn infant with a myelomeningocele defect.

injected through the reservoir into the ventricle, including 10 mg of intrathecal vancomycin in 1 mL of preservative-free normal saline and 4 mg of intrathecal gentamicin in 2 ml of preservative-free normal saline.

Finally, the incisions are irrigated with bacitracin solution and then closed with antibiotic-impregnated sutures as follows. The peritoneum is closed in a purse string fashion using a 4-0 Vicryl suture. The abdominal fascia is closed with simple interrupted 3-0 Vicryl sutures and the subcutaneous and subcuticular layers are closed with buried interrupted 3-0 and 4-0 Vicryl sutures, respectively. The skin is closed with a running 5-0 Monocryl suture and/or a topical skin adhesive. Regarding the cranial incision, the galea is closed with buried interrupted 4-0 Vicryl sutures, and the skin is closed with a running 5-0 Monocryl suture and/or a topical skin adhesive. Sterile dressings are then applied.

Of note, more recently, fetal surgery has been advocated as a means of improving neurologic outcome based on the results of the Management of Myelomeningocele Study (MOMS) trial. This study compared the outcomes of in utero MMC repair with standard postnatal repair. In this trial, prenatal surgery for MMC reduced the need for shunting and improved motor outcomes at 30 months. However, this procedure was associated with both maternal and fetal risks (e.g., increased risk for preterm delivery and uterine dehiscence at delivery). Moreover, the risk for recurrent tethered spinal cord in children who have undergone this method of MMC closure is currently unknown.

Infants with SB may also present with a symptomatic Chiari type II malformation. Chiari II malformations can cause deterioration of respiration, swallowing, and overall neurological functioning. This can be an important cause of death for patients with SB. Chiari II malformations consist of a spectrum of abnormalities, including lacunar skull (i.e., thinning and scalloping of the calvarium producing a "copper-beaten" appearance), small posterior fossa, low-lying transverse sinus and torcular Herophili, fenestrated falx, heart-shaped tentorial incisura with upward herniation of the cerebellum, medullary kinking, beaking of the tectal plate, prominence of the massa intermedia, enlargement of the suprapineal recess, elongation of the fourth ventricle, syringohydromyelia, and downward displacement of the cerebellar vermis, fourth ventricle, medulla, and pons through the foramen magnum (Figure 12.8). Neonates with symptomatic Chiari II malformation present with inspiratory stridor, apnea, dysphagia or nasal regurgitation, aspiration, weak or absent cry, weakness and/or spasticity in the upper or lower extremities, and opisthotonic posturing. Older children and adolescents have a more insidious

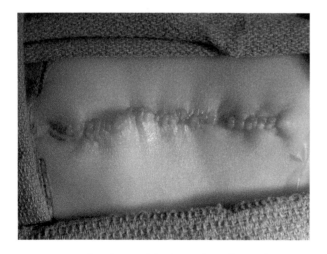

Figure 12.7 Tension-free closure of the skin in the midline with interrupted or running 5-0 nylon sutures.

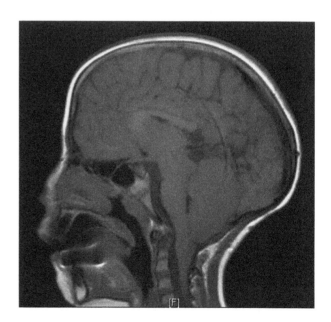

Figure 12.8 Sagittal brain MRI image in a child with spina bifida showing findings of a Chiari II malformation.

presentation with syncopal episodes, nystagmus, oscillopsia, lower cranial nerve palsies, hyperreflexia, and spastic quadriparesis. Treatment consists of surgically decompressing the posterior fossa and upper cervical spinal canal (typically a bony decompression only because of the low-lying torcular region) after making certain that the patient's shunt is functioning appropriately. Symptomatic Chiari II malformations need prompt neurosurgical intervention.

COMPLICATIONS

Two potential complications of MMC repair are CSF drainage and postoperative wound breakdown. CSF drainage most often results from untreated hydrocephalus and requires CSF diversion by means of ventricular shunt placement. Wound breakdown frequently results from a tight skin closure leading to compromise of the vascular supply. Wound dehiscence is managed most effectively with wet-to-dry dressing changes, which facilitate wound healing by secondary intention. Several complications can occur with shunting and these are discussed in Case 3.

CASE 2

HISTORY AND PHYSICAL EXAMINATION

After finishing with the MMC repair and shunt placement in the baby with SB discussed previously, you are called by the craniofacial clinic to see another baby. The patient is a 4-month-old male who was born at 40 weeks estimated gestational age by cesarean section, weighting 8 lbs, 6 oz. There were no problems with pregnancy, labor, or delivery. He has been meeting developmental milestones appropriately. His past medical history is otherwise unremarkable, he is on no medications, and he has no known drug allergies. His family and social histories are noncontributory.

In the clinic, his neurological examination is normal for his age. However, he has a severely abnormal head shape with palpable and visible ridging along the entire metopic suture creating a beak-shaped forehead with a midline frontal keel, posterior retrusion of the lateral aspects of the supraorbital ridges bilaterally, and hypotelorbitism. In addition, his bifrontal cranial dimension is abnormally narrowed, and there is compensatory widening of the biparietal diameter.

IMAGING STUDIES

The patient has metopic craniosynostosis resulting in trigonocephaly. The diagnosis is made clinically. Although unnecessary and relatively undesirable due to potential harmful effects of radiation exposure, the diagnosis can also be established radiographically with a plain film of the skull or head computed tomography (CT) with or without 3-dimensional reconstructions (Figures 12.9 and 12.10).

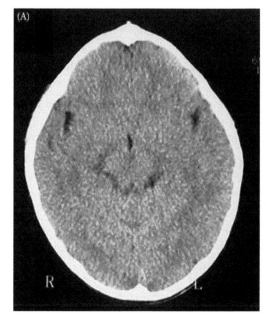 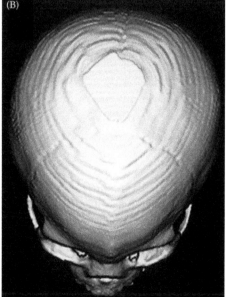

Figures 12.9A, B. Axial (A) and 3D vertex (B) head CT views in a male infant with premature closure of the metopic suture and associated trigonocephaly.

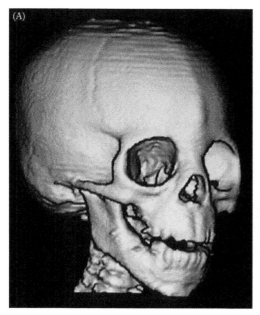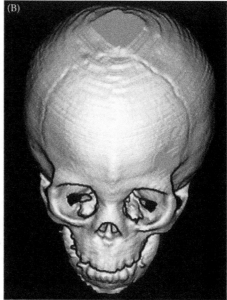

Figures 12.10A, B. Anterolateral (A) and frontal (B) 3D head CT views in male infant with trigonocephaly owing to premature fusion of the metopic suture.

ANALYSIS OF CASE AND SURGICAL PLAN

The cranium consists of several plates of bone separated by sutures—fibrous joints that function by depositing bone at their margins in response to brain expansion. The skull grows to accommodate brain growth, especially during the first 2 years of life when brain volume can increase up to 3 times its size at birth. The cranial sutures must remain open for the skull to grow and achieve its characteristic normocephalic shape. When 1 or more cranial sutures close too early, the skull ceases to grow in the direction perpendicular to the closed suture but continues to grow parallel to the closed suture. Craniosynostosis is the term used to describe this condition, and the shape of the skull is altered in a predictable way with recognizable patterns that depend on which suture is fused. The correct treatment of any craniosynostosis requires that the correct diagnosis is made.

There are two primary goals of treatment of craniosynostosis: (a) to release the fused suture(s) to allow the brain to grow and expand normally and prevent problems associated with increased intracranial pressure and (b) to establish the normal contour of the skull and thereby minimize psychosocial effects. One way to accomplish these goals is to perform a bifrontal craniotomy and remove the supraorbital bar. The supraorbital bar is then split down the midline where the metopic suture is fused, and a bone graft is positioned and fixed in between the bones to widen the bar. Finally, the reconstructed forehead is reshaped and secured to the widened supraorbital bar, and together they are rigidly fixed in position to the nose and lateral orbits.

Premature closure of the *metopic* suture as seen in the child presented here results in trigonocephaly. Morphologic findings in metopic synostosis are due to restricted growth of the frontal bones in the plane perpendicular to the fused metopic suture and compensatory skull growth parallel to the fused suture at the unfused sagittal, coronal, and lambdoid sutures. This leads to a triangular-shaped head, with varying degrees of bifrontal narrowing and biparietal expansion.

There are at least 4 key principles of surgery. First, if untreated, metopic synostosis will lead to severe deformity of the forehead and orbits that worsens with head growth. Second, treatment is surgical and is best carried out by a pediatric neurosurgeon and craniofacial surgeon, with a pediatric anesthesiologist administering the anesthesia. Third, surgery is usually performed between 4 and 8 months of age since the calvarial bone has developed sufficient thickness to enable fixation and provide structural stability, the bone is malleable making remodeling easier, rapid brain growth helps bone remodeling, bony defects heal more quickly, and early correction prevents further compensatory deformities. Finally, overcorrection can diminish the need for reoperation.

Special equipment used in the surgical correction of metopic synostosis include at least 2 large-bore peripheral intravenous catheters, an arterial line, a Foley catheter, a precordial Doppler and end-tidal CO_2 monitor to detect air embolism, corneal protectors, resorbable craniofacial plate-and-screw fixation hardware, a sterile hot water bath to facilitate bending of the plates, bone benders, and high-speed drill and saw systems. In addition, the infant should be typed and crossed for at least 1 unit of packed red blood cells.

PROCEDURE

Surgical correction of metopic craniosynostosis can be performed open or endoscopically. Surgical technique is tailored to the severity of the calvarial vault and skull base deformity created by the metopic synostosis. Resection of the affected suture alone will not correct the associated compensatory skull shape changes and fronto-orbital abnormalities that accompany premature fusion of the metopic suture. The best surgical results are achieved with extensive reconstruction and active reshaping of the fronto-orbital deformity by widening and advancement of the supraorbital rim and reshaping of the frontal bone. A description of the open technique follows.

The patient is taken to the operating room (OR) and placed on the operating table in a supine position. A time-out is performed per institutional protocol. After adequate intravenous access and cardiopulmonary monitoring are established, the patient is intubated, and general anesthesia is induced. A Foley catheter, arterial line, and precordial Doppler are placed. The head is positioned supine on a well-padded horseshoe head holder, a gel roll is placed behind the shoulders, and all pressure points are carefully padded (Figure 12.11). Corneal protectors are placed bilaterally

in a sterile fashion. The hair is clipped along the proposed incision line (or completely if the parents desire). A 2-0 silk suture is pressed against the scalp just posterior to the coronal suture to create a line extending from ear to ear. This is used as a reference line to mark a scalloped-patterned bicoronal incision, taking care to stay well behind the hairline (Figure 12.11B). The incision is thoroughly prepared with a solution of 2% chlorhexidine gluconate and 70% isopropyl alcohol.

Prior to opening the incision, a prophylactic antibiotic is administered (e.g., Kefzol 25mg/kg). The incision is infiltrated with 0.25% Marcaine with 1:200,000 units of epinephrine and then opened with a No. 15 scalpel blade beveled in the direction of the hair follicles to avoid cutting across their shafts and to minimize visibility of scarring. The anterior and posterior scalp flaps are elevated in the subgaleal/supraperiosteal plane using bovie electrocautery to maximize hemostasis. The posterior scalp flap is reflected posteriorly to the mid-parietal region; the anterior scalp flap is reflected to approximately 1 cm above the orbital rims (Figures 12.12 and 12.13A).

The pericranium is incised parallel to the rim and periorbital dissection proceeds in a subperiosteal plane using periosteal elevators to preserve the periorbital fascia. An osteotome is used to free the supraorbital nerve from its bony encasement. Periorbital dissection, bilaterally along the superior and lateral aspects the orbits, mobilizes the globes and exposes the frontozygomatic sutures bilaterally, the nasofrontal suture in the midline, and the entire supraorbital rim (Figure 12.13B). The temporalis muscles and fasciae are opened, and the anterior aspect of muscle and

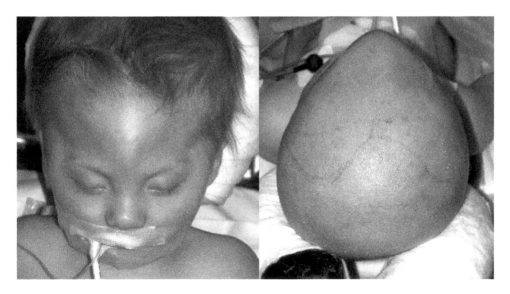

Figures 12.11A, B. Frontal (A) and vertex (B) views of a trigonocephalic 4-month-old male infant positioned supine on a horseshoe head holder for surgery and showing a scalloped-patterned bicoronal incision.

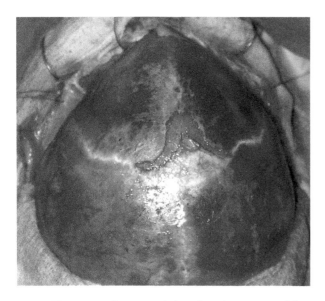

Figure 12.12 Vertex view of trigonocephalic infant after exposure of the calvarium anterior and posterior to the coronal suture. The posterior scalp flap is reflected posteriorly to the mid-parietal region; the anterior scalp flap is reflected to approximately 1 cm above the orbital rims.

fascia are reflected anteriorly out of the infratemporal fossa with the anterior scalp flap (Figure 12.14). Next, the craniofacial surgeon marks (a) a bifrontal craniotomy encompassing the fused metopic suture and (b) the supraorbital bar, including an extension behind the sphenoid wing on both sides (Figure 12.13).

The bifrontal craniotomy is performed by the neurosurgeon, with the posterior extent of the bone flap extending posterior to the coronal sutures bilaterally and the anterior boundary extending to 1 cm above the supraorbital rims (Figure 12.13). A high-speed craniotome is used to place burr holes in strategic locations to prevent weakening of the supraorbital bar and facilitate subsequent elevation of the bone flap. The dura is carefully stripped along the anterior cranial fossae to the level of the crista galli in the midline

as well as along the lateral aspects of the greater sphenoid wings and temporal fossae bilaterally using periosteal elevators. The temporal extensions of the supraorbital bar are freed up by making osteotomies with the drill.

Together, the neurosurgeon and craniofacial surgeon remove the supraorbital bar, which serves as the foundation of the reconstruction. To do this, osteotomies are carried out across each orbital roof, taking care to protect the brain and contents of the orbit with malleable brain retractors, but not retracting excessively, as the cuts are made. The orbital osteotomies extend medially just anterior to the cribriform plate and laterally to the frontozygomatic sutures. Osteotomies are also made through the lateral orbital walls beginning at the frontozygomatic sutures and extending back to join the osteotomies of the temporal extensions.

An osteotome is used to make vertical osteotomies through the pterional regions, taking care to prevent injury to the temporal and frontal lobes. A reciprocating saw is used to create an osteotomy at the nasion at the level of the nasofrontal suture. The supraorbital bar is then removed intact and placed on the back table in a saline-soaked sponge. The bone edges are waxed for hemostasis, and the dura is inspected for rents, which, if observed, are repaired primarily with 4-0 nonabsorbable, braided nylon suture.

At this point, the craniofacial surgeon commences with reconstruction of the bone. A series of curves are cut on the endocranial surface of the supraorbital bar as needed to allow in-folding of the temporal extensions, and the supraorbital bar is widened using an autograft of bone harvested from the parietal region and placed in between the 2 halves of bone created by cutting the bar in the region of the metopic suture (Figure 12.15). A resorbable plate is placed obliquely at the midline, and additional triangular plates are placed at the junction of the supraorbital bar with the lateral temporal extensions to allow for in-folding of

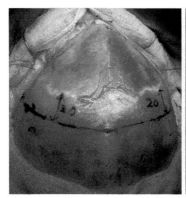
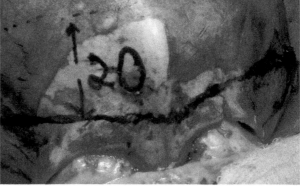

Figures 12.13A, B. Vertex (A) and frontal (B) views in trigonocephalic infant after periorbital dissection, bilaterally along the superior and lateral aspects the orbits to mobilize the globes and expose the frontozygomatic sutures bilaterally, the nasofrontal suture in the midline, and the entire supraorbital rim.

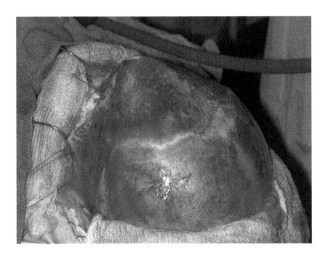

Figure 12.14 Lateral view of trigonocephalic infant after the temporalis muscles and fasciae are opened, and the anterior aspect of muscle and fascia are reflected anteriorly out of the infratemporal fossa with the anterior scalp flap.

the extensions. The plates are heated in a sterile water bath and then secured to the bar using 4-mm resorbable screws (Figures 12.15 and 12.16). The frontal bone is reshaped using bone benders, inner and outer cortex burring, and barrel-stave osteotomies. After remodeling, the frontal bone is anchored to the supraorbital bar in its new position by securing it to the previously placed plates using 4-mm screws (Figure 12.15).

At the end of the procedure, the wound is extensively irrigated with antibiotic solution and 0-Prolene sutures are placed to reapproximate the scalp flaps. The galea is then closed using buried interrupted 3-0 Vicryl sutures. The scalp is closed using a running, noninterlocking 5-0 Monocryl suture, and a sterile dressing is applied. The corneal protectors are removed prior to extubation.

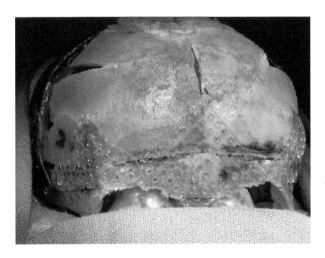

Figure 12.15 Frontal view of trigonocephalic infant after remodeling and anchoring the frontal bone to the supraorbital bar in its new position by securing it to resorbable plates using 4-mm screws.

COMPLICATIONS

Serious complications can occur during surgical correction of metopic synostosis. Detection of possible air emboli warrants immediate flooding of the field with irrigation, lowering the head of the bed, and waxing of all bone edges. It is essential to know the amount of blood that is lost during the procedure and to monitor the coagulation status and platelet count. Give blood products when indicated and promptly replace fluid losses to maintain hemodynamic stability. When possible, dissect in a supraperiosteal plane to minimize blood loss from the bone, and wax all bone edges when cut.

Dural lacerations must also be repaired to prevent persistent CSF leak. Additional risks include increased blood loss and the need for blood transfusion intraoperatively, postoperative wound infection with the potential for operative management, injury to the brain, and persistent asymmetry and/or bony defects requiring further surgery.

CASE 3

HISTORY AND PHYSICAL EXAMINATION

A 7-year-old boy presents to your emergency department (ED) with persistent headaches and vomiting after sustaining a concussion. He reportedly collided with another child on the playground 5 days prior to his arrival in the ED. On examination, he is awake, alert, and oriented but has mental slowness. He has bilateral papilledema but no evidence of Parinaud's syndrome. He has right upper extremity dysmetria on finger-nose-finger testing and is hypersensitive to noise and light. Otherwise, he is neurologically intact. His imaging studies are presented.

IMAGING STUDIES

A head CT scan is obtained. The scout reveals splaying of the coronal suture and multiple craniolacunae (Figure 12.17). The axial cuts on the CT scan show massive enlargement of his lateral and third ventricles, transependymal CSF absorption, and a small aqueduct with calcification in the tectum consistent with a tectal plate glioma (Figure 12.18). A brain magnetic resonance imaging (MRI) scan was subsequently obtained which revealed hydrocephalus secondary to obstruction of the aqueduct resulting from a small tectal plate glioma (Figure 12.19). Like the head CT, the brain MRI also reveals severe transependymal CSF absorption.

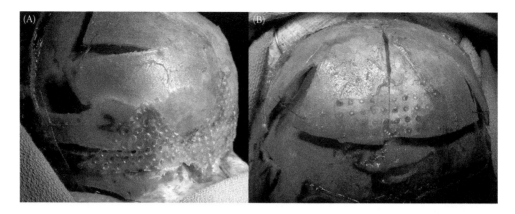

Figures 12.16A, B. Additional views of the reconstructed and expanded skull in a trigonocephalic infant after remodeling and anchoring the frontal bone to the supraorbital bar using resorbable plates and screws.

ANALYSIS OF CASE AND SURGICAL PLAN

The patient has hydrocephalus diagnosed 5 days after sustaining a concussion. With bilateral papilledema, his symptoms are most likely the result of hydrocephalus and not post-concussive. In the case of a child presenting with acute hydrocephalus later in like this child, always consider the possibility of tumor or occult infection as the cause.

Treatment of hydrocephalus from obstruction of the aqueduct in an older child (2 years of age or older) can include placement of a shunt or performing an endoscopic third ventriculostomy (ETV). ETV involves the use of a rigid endoscope to create an opening in the floor of the

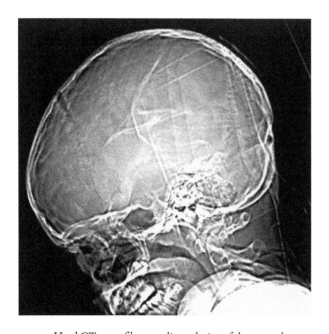

Figure 12.17 Head CT scout film revealing splaying of the coronal suture and multiple craniolacunae in a 7-year-old boy with newly diagnosed, symptomatic, obstructive hydrocephalus.

third ventricle just in front of the mammillary bodies. This is done through a frontal burr hole approach. The opening in the floor of the 3rd ventricle is widened with a Fogarty balloon catheter. CSF can flow through this opening into the basilar cisterns and bypass the area of aqueductal stenosis. ETV eliminates the need for a shunt but has failure rates comparable to a shunt.

Risks and benefits for each procedure should be explained to the patient's parents and a decision made as to which surgical procedure is the right procedure for the patient. The child in this case underwent placement of a right parieto-occipital programmable shunt with a siphon guard (Figure 12.20). His opening pressure at the time of catheter placement in the OR was >56 cm H20. The shunt was initially set at 130 mm Hg, and the setting was confirmed with a lateral skull film. The tectal plate glioma was managed conservatively.

He did very well initially with good ventricular decompression and resolution of his preoperative symptoms. However, about 6 months later he presented with recurrence of his headaches, vomiting, and lethargy. The ED calls you to see this child after a head CT showed an interval increase in ventricular size (Figure 12.21).

Children with shunt-dependent hydrocephalus require life-long follow-up to make sure that the shunt is functioning adequately. Two key points to remember when taking care of children with shunted hydrocephalus: (a) it is always the shunt, and (b) the parents are always right. In a child with shunted hydrocephalus who presents with signs and symptoms of hydrocephalus, a shunt malfunction must be considered. A head CT or fast spin MRI is obtained and must be compared to a similar study from a time when the patient was doing well in order to evaluate for ventricular enlargement (Figure 12.21). A shunt series is also obtained to look for kinking or discontinuity of the shunt system

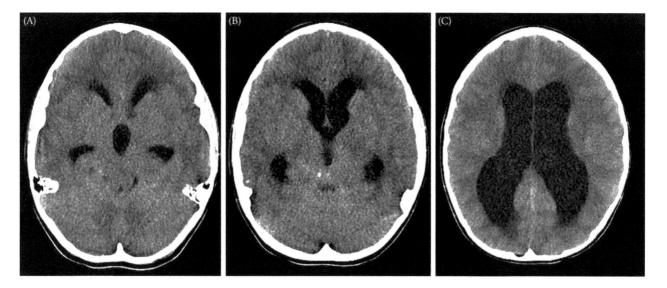

Figure 12.18 Head CT axial images from a 7-year-old boy with newly diagnosed, symptomatic, obstructive hydrocephalus showing massive enlargement of his lateral and third ventricles, transependymal CSF absorption, and a small aqueduct with calcification in the tectum consistent with a tectal plate glioma.

(Figure 12.22), catheter malposition, inadequate length of the distal shunt tubing, or a CSF pseudocyst. Remember—if you order a study, look at it—do not depend on the radiologist's interpretation. In the face of ventricular enlargement and symptoms of elevated intracranial pressure (ICP), a shunt malfunction is presumed, and the patient is taken for shunt exploration and revision.

A proximal shunt malfunction is typically associated with precipitous development of elevated ICP so that the shunt should be revised shortly after patient arrives at the hospital. In contrast, most distal shunt malfunctions not associated with a short catheter are due to infection, which

can be determined by tapping the shunt and looking for a CSF pseudocyst on the shunt series or abdominal ultrasound/CT (Figure 12.23). Hence, in the face of a distal shunt malfunction, one should look carefully at the CSF prior to performing a shunt revision to make sure an infection is not present.

A child with an abdominal pseudocyst will present with abdominal distension and headaches. The head CT typically shows ventricular enlargement consistent with a shunt malfunction related to decreased abdominal CSF absorption. If a CSF pseudocyst is found, consider the shunt infected until proven otherwise.

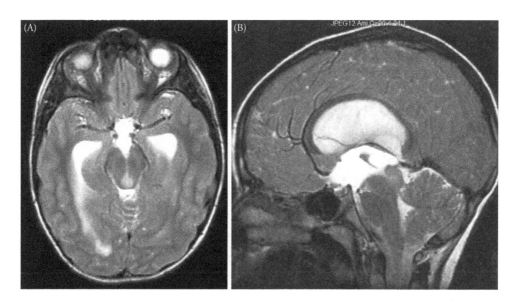

Figure 12.19 Brain MR axial (left) and sagittal (right) images showing obstruction of the aqueduct resulting from a small tectal plate glioma.

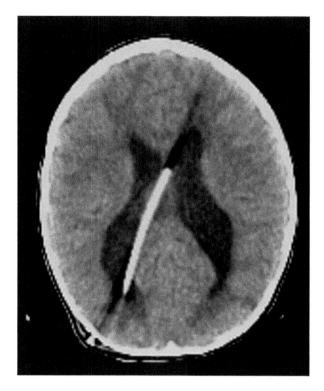

Figure 12.20 Head CT axial image after placement of a right parieto-occipital programmable shunt with a siphon guard.

In 70% of patients with a shunt malfunction, there are overt signs of elevated ICP such as headaches, vomiting, and lethargy. Patients will progress to stupor, coma, and death if the shunt is not promptly revised. In the other 30%, there are subtle signs of deterioration as the ventricles enlarge over time, which include changes in behavior, chronic daily headaches, and a decline in school performance.

Electively lengthen a shunt if the child is known to be shunt dependent from prior shunt malfunctions or if the head CT scan shows slit ventricles (Figure 12.23) and/or a thick calvarium, since both features have been shown to be associated with shunt dependency. Never place a connector at the abdominal end of the incision because this will limit the ability of the distal shunt tubing to elongate with continued growth of the child and will frequently result in separation of the shunt tubing at the site of the connector. If a child has not had any shunt problems previously and is completely asymptomatic with a short shunt, continued observation is recommended, and the shunt is not lengthened electively. However, close follow-up is crucial since the child may develop subtle signs of decompensated hydrocephalus.

COMPLICATIONS

Several complications can occur with shunting. Shunt tubing is made of silicone elastomers, and it can calcify and break over time, especially in the neck above the clavicle where there is increased motion (Figure 12.22). Distal shunt tubing can also erode into abdominal viscera and be seen protruding from the anus. Intraventricular hemorrhage can occur at the time of a proximal shunt revision as the obstructed catheter is removed. Oftentimes, choroid plexus is stuck to the fenestrated end of the ventricular catheter and can cause bleeding as the catheter is removed (Figure 12.24). In this situation, the shunt operation may need to be aborted and an external ventricular drain (EVD) placed until the blood clears from the CSF.

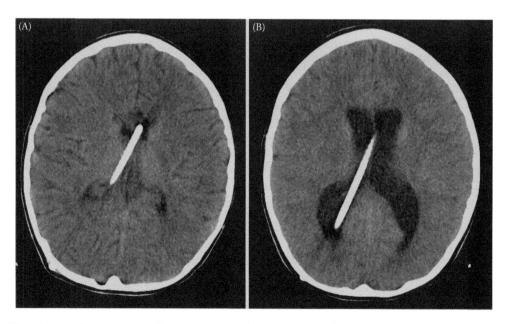

Figure 12.21 Head CT axial images showing an interval increase in ventricular size concerning for shunt malfunction.

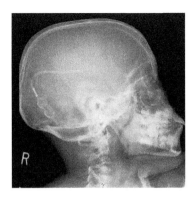

Figure 12.22 Lateral skull view of shunt series showing discontinuity of the shunt system.

Over shunting or over drainage can lead to the formation of subdural hematoma(s), craniosynostosis with craniocerebral disproportion, and/or slit ventricle syndrome. A child suffering from slit ventricle syndrome (Figure 12.25) typically complains of headaches, nausea, and dizziness, especially when upright and most often later in the day.

Shunt infection is another possible complication of shunting. Shunt infection increases the mortality rate and risk of seizures and results in decreased IQ. There is a 2% to 8% incidence of infection with each shunt operation, and 5% to 15% of shunts become infected over the life of the shunt. Shunt infections typically occur within the first 6 months after a shunt is placed. Specifically, 70% of shunt infections are diagnosed within the first month after surgery, and 90% within 6 months after surgery. Shunt infection is rare after 6 months. Risk factors for shunt infection include young age, poor skin condition, length of the operation, CSF leak from the incision, number of shunt revisions, and concomitant infection.

A child with a shunt infection typically presents with increasing irritability, persistent low-grade fever, decreased appetite, and abdominal pain within 2 weeks after shunt placement/revision. The ventricles may be stable on a head CT, whereas a CSF pseudocyst may be seen on the shunt series. Fever in the early postoperative period (i.e., <6 months) is concerning for a shunt infection and should be considered as such until proven otherwise. If a shunt infection is suspected, a shunt tap is performed with a 25 gauge butterfly needle using sterile technique, and CSF is sent for routine studies including protein, glucose, cell count and differential, gram stain, and culture and sensitivities. A complete blood count, erythrocyte sedimentation rate, and C-reactive protein are also sent. Once CSF has been obtained, broad spectrum intravenous antibiotics are started such as vancomycin and cefotaxime. The most common organism causing shunt infection is staphylococcus.

If the white blood cell count is elevated in the CSF and/or CSF cultures/S gram stain are positive, the child is taken to the OR for complete shunt removal and placement of an EVD and a temporary central venous line. The antibiotics are tapered based on the results of the culture and sensitivity studies. CSF is sent until cultures are negative. The child remains externalized on intravenous antibiotics for up to 14 days after the first negative CSF culture. Once the infection has been adequately treated, the EVD is removed and a new shunt is placed.

CASE 4

HISTORY AND PHYSICAL

A 16-year-old young man presents to your ED with progressively worsening headaches for 10 days and vomiting for 2 days. He has a history of sinusitis, treated with oral antibiotics. On examination, he is neurologically intact except for very mild bilateral upper extremity dysmetria on finger-nose-finger testing. Imaging studies are presented.

IMAGING STUDIES

The imaging studies (Figures 12.26) demonstrate a 4.3 × 3.4 × 3.9 cm mass likely arising from the posterior and inferior aspect of the fourth ventricle or cerebellar tonsils. The differential diagnosis includes ependymoma, medulloblastoma, and pilocytic astrocytoma. There is moderate hydrocephalus and compression of the brainstem at the level of the foramen magnum secondary to the mass.

ANALYSIS OF CASE AND SURGICAL PLAN

Posterior fossa tumors are common in children. Some of the more common posterior fossa tumors include (a) cystic cerebellar astrocytoma (juvenile pilocytic astrocytoma), typically located medially in the vermis or laterally in the cerebellar hemisphere or peduncle (Figure 12.27); (b) medulloblastoma (cerebellar primitive neuroectodermal tumor), typically arising from the superior medullary velum and growing to fill the fourth ventricle (Figure 12.28); (c) ependymoma, typically arising from the floor of the fourth ventricle and extending out the foramina of Luschka into the cerebellopontine angle (Figure 12.29); and (d) hemangioblastoma, a cystic tumor with mural nodule found most commonly in children with von Hippel Lindau syndrome (Figure 12.30A).

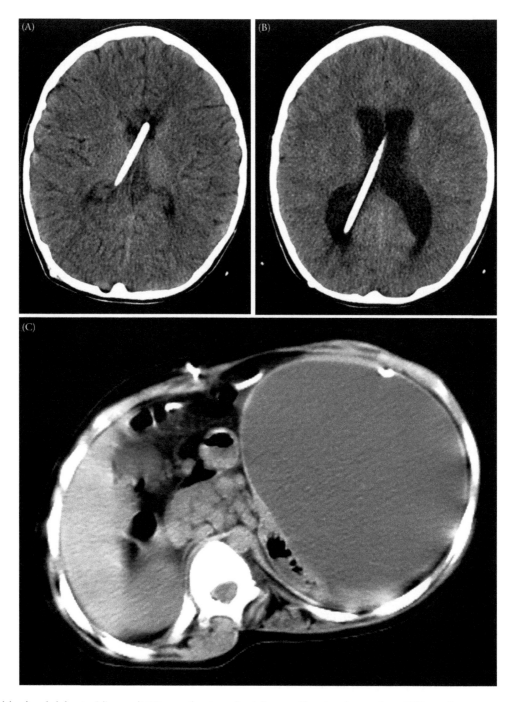

Figure 12.23 Head (top) and abdominal (bottom) CT scans showing a distal shunt malfunction due to a large CSF pseudocyst.

PREOPERATIVE/
OPERATIVE MANAGEMENT

When a child presents with a posterior fossa tumor, it is crucial to obtain a brain *and* full spine MRI (Figures 12.30 B, C) with and without contrast and typically under general anesthesia. These studies enable the neurosurgeon to determine whether the tumor arises from the cerebellar hemispheres, vermis, or fourth ventricle and whether the tentorial notch, brainstem, or lateral recesses of the fourth

ventricle are involved—information that is key to understanding potential for harm to surrounding tissues and to making appropriate judgments regarding the extent of tumor removal at the time of surgery. These studies also reveal whether the patient has hydrocephalus and whether there are drop metastases present.

In the face of symptomatic obstructive hydrocephalus, the patient often requires emergent CSF diversion which is accomplished by placement of a frontal EVD according to external anatomic landmarks and sterile technique and

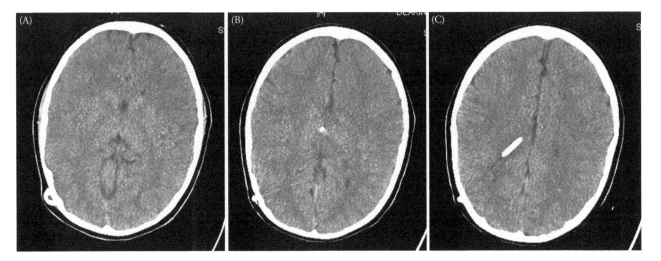

Figure 12.24 Head CT scan axial views showing IVH in a patient who presented with a proximal shunt malfunction due to ventricular catheter obstruction. Choroid plexus was stuck to the fenestrated end of the catheter, and removal of the catheter resulted in significant IVH requiring EVD placement.

tunneled to and secured at a distant exit site. In the past, placement of a ventriculoperitoneal shunt was advocated as a means of treating symptomatic hydrocephalus in these patients; however, shunts have fallen out of favor recently because they take away the patient's chance to be shunt independent and expose the patient to potential perils of upward herniation and shunt dependency. If the patient is only mildly symptomatic and surgery is imminent, acetazolamide (Diamox) may be used (25 mg/kg/day divided 3 times daily). At the time of admission, the patient is started on dexamethasone (Decadron; up to 4 mg every 6 hours) along with an histamine-2 blocker. The patient is typed and cross-matched for 1 to 2 units of packed red blood cells.

A surgical consent is obtained. Frequently, parents will ask about prognosis. Prognosis with medulloblastoma depends on age at time of diagnosis (<2 years old with worse prognosis), amount of resection (best prognosis if able to resection all but 1.5 cm²), and presence of drop metastases. All patients require adjuvant chemotherapy (and craniospinal radiotherapy if >3–4 years of age). Recent genomic studies have identified 4 distinct, nonoverlapping molecular variants of medulloblastoma: WNT, SHH, group C, and group D, each with distinct demographics, clinical presentation, transcriptional profiles, genetic abnormalities, and clinical outcome. Prognosis with ependymoma depends on the extent of resection; radiotherapy is sometimes used to treat residual tumor

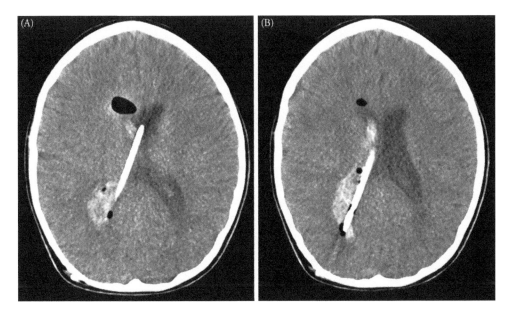

Figure 12.25 Head CT scan axial views in a patient with shunt-dependent hydrocephalus showing slit ventricles.

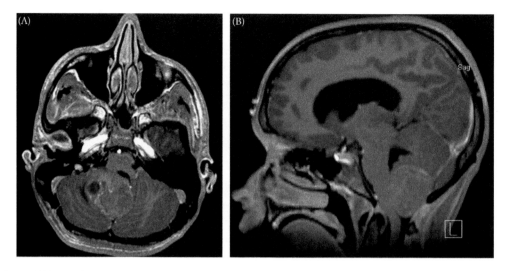

Figures 12.26A, B. 16-year old boy with a 4.3 × 3.4 × 3.9 cm contrast-enhancing posterior fossa mass and associated obstructive hydrocephalus: sagittal (A) and axial (B) views.

in children more than 3 to 4 years of age. With cerebellar astrocytoma, gross total removal of the tumor is typically curative, and no adjuvant therapy is required.

The timing of surgery depends on the patient's presenting signs and symptoms. Typically, the operation is performed the next operating day after imaging studies have been performed. The operation can be performed either in the prone or sitting position. The prone position minimizes the risk for air embolus. If the sitting position is used, a central venous line should be placed, and a precordial Doppler

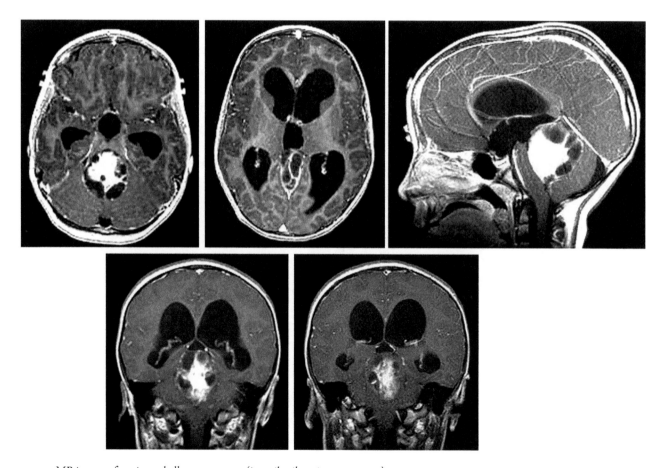

Figure 12.27 MR images of cystic cerebellar astrocytoma (juvenile pilocytic astrocytoma).

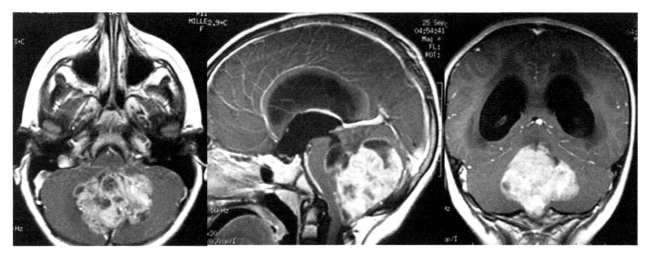

Figure 12.28 MR images of medulloblastoma (cerebellar primitive neuroectodermal tumor).

and end-tidal CO_2 monitor should be used to detect air embolism during the operation.

With pediatric patients, the type of head fixation device depends on age and skull thickness. Typically, a 3-pin skull clamp is used with pediatric pins if the patient is 3 to 7 years of age or adult pins if older than 7 years (Figure 12.31). A well-padded horseshoe head holder is used for patients who are younger than 3 years, and special care is taken to prevent pressure on the globes. When positioning the patient prone, the neck may be gently flexed to provide better access to the posterior fossa, but one should leave roughly 2 to 3 fingerbreadths between the chin and

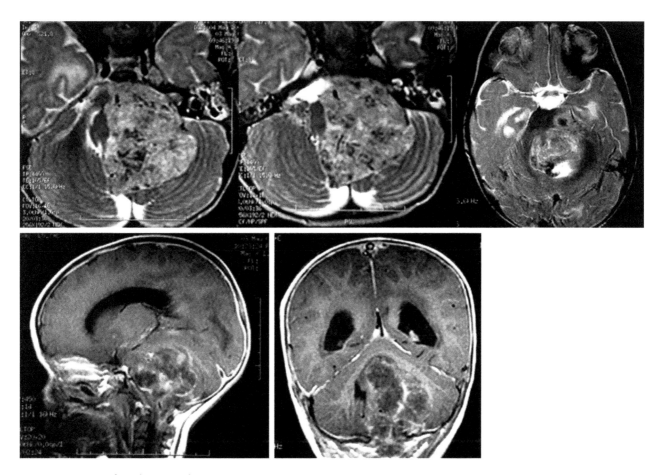

Figure 12.29 MR images of anaplastic ependymoma.

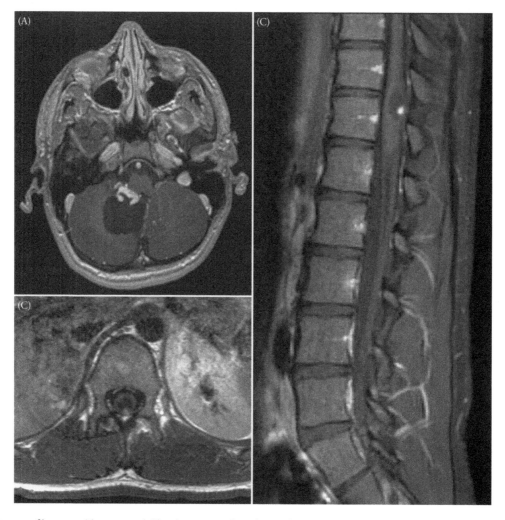

Figures 12.30 MR images of hemangioblastoma in child with von Hippel Lindau syndrome: brain, axial (A); spine, sagittal (B); and spine, transverse (C).

the sternal notch or neck to prevent compromise of venous return. Cranial nerve monitoring may be helpful especially if the tumor extends out the cerebellopontine angle. An intravenous antibiotic (usually a cephalosporin if the patient is not allergic) is given just before the time of EVD insertion if placed intraoperatively or within 1 hour of making the incision.

If an EVD is not inserted preoperatively or in the OR before positioning, it is important to prepare for an occipital burr hole (i.e., 6–7 cm superior to the inion and 3 cm lateral to midline) and make sure there is an EVD catheter on the operating field. A midline suboccipital skin incision is made from the external occipital protuberance to the C2 level and extended down to bone in the midline fascial plane. The ligaments attaching the dura to the undersurface of the foramen magnum are stripped with an up-angled curette, and a craniotomy bone flap is turned, using a high-speed drill with footplate attachment and extending from below the transverse sinus superiorly to the foramen

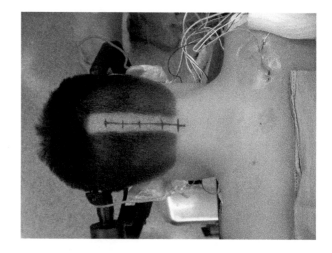

Figure 12.31 Sixteen-year-old boy with a posterior fossa tumor positioned prone in 3-point skull fixation with electrodes in place for intraoperative monitoring of cranial nerves 7–12 on the right.

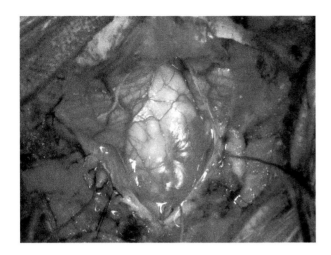

Figure 12.32 View of a posterior fossa hemangioblastoma after opening the dura.

magnum inferiorly, after placing burr holes along the superior aspect of the flap. The lateral extent of the craniotomy depends on the size and location of the tumor. Posterior cervical laminectomies are also performed based on the caudal extent of the tumor.

The dura is opened in a Y-shaped fashion and tacked up to the adjacent muscle or/fascia, and the arachnoid is also opened and tacked up to the dura (Figure 12.32). Opening the arachnoid over the cisterna magna enables CSF to drain and provides relaxation of cerebellum. The tumor is removed taking care to avoid injuring the floor of the fourth ventricle, the deep cerebellar nuclei, and the middle cerebellar peduncles but with the goal of achieving a complete resection if safely possible. To get to midline tumors, one can open the vermis vertically in the midline, open it transversely, or use a tela choroidea approach whereby the cerebellar hemispheres are retracted laterally and the vermis is elevated to expose the tela choroidea (i.e., the arachnoid and blood vessels going to choroid plexus). The dura is then closed in a watertight fashion with a patch graft consisting of harvested pericranium or a dural substitute and the bone flap is replaced with titanium microplates and screws. The incision is closed in multiple layers.

Complete excision is the goal for nearly all focal low-grade astrocytomas or non-infiltrating posterior fossa tumors (Figure 12.33). The initial objective in most cases is brainstem decompression and reduction of tumor bulk. Attachments of tumor to brainstem, cerebellar peduncles, or cranial nerves are usually taken down last using the operating microscope. Care must be taken to avoid injury to the deep cerebellar

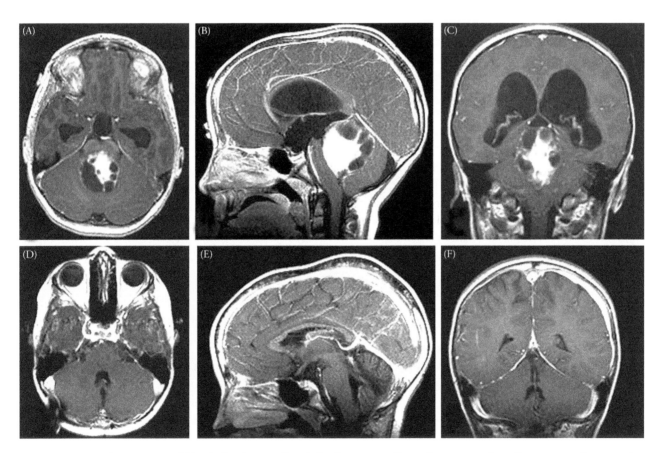

Figure 12.33 MR images from an 8-year-old boy before (top panel) and after (bottom panel) complete excision of a midline posterior fossa juvenile pilocytic astrocytoma.

nuclei, cerebellar peduncles, and floor of the fourth ventricle. All radiographically enhancing tissue should be removed completely—including the cyst wall if it enhances.

COMPLICATIONS

Several complications can occur with posterior fossa tumor resections. During the opening of the dura, the surgeon must be ready for possible torrential bleeding from intradural venous lakes /or the circular sinus. Such bleeding is typically controlled with cotton patties containing Gelfoam powder soaked in thrombin, hemostatic clips, or over sewing of the dural edge to stop the bleeding. It is essential to know the amount of blood that is lost during the procedure and to monitor the coagulation status and platelet count. Give blood products when indicated and promptly replace fluid losses to maintain hemodynamic stability.

Another possible complication that the surgeon must always be ready for is venous air embolism. A precordial Doppler and end-tidal CO_2 monitor help to detect air embolism during the operation. If suspected and a central venous line is present, the anesthesiologist can try to aspirate air through the central venous line. At the same time, the surgeon inspects the field to determine the source of the venous air embolus. Common sites include the diploic space of bone, veins located laterally along the craniocervical junction and between C1 and C2, and the cut edge of muscle. Detection of possible air emboli warrants immediate flooding of the field with irrigation, lowering the head of the bed, and waxing of all bone edges. Jugular venous compression can be performed to decrease venous return and facilitate identification of an air leak by causing bleeding from the site that is the source of entry of air into the systemic circulation. If the end-expired CO_2 continues to decrease, the end-expired nitrogen continues to increase, or the mean arterial pressure begins to decrease, the wound should be closed rapidly and the patient transported intubated to the intensive care unit for further management.

Cerebellar mutism or posterior fossa syndrome is a rare complication of removal of midline cerebellar tumors. The exact mechanism of this syndrome is poorly understood. It involves an array of signs and symptoms, including decreased or absent speech, dysphagia, cranial nerve palsies, decreased motor movement with inability to coordinate voluntary movements, ataxia, and emotional lability. Patients are usually very whiny, irritable, and unable to speak for a finite period after surgery. It can occur immediately or appear in a delayed fashion. It is not uncommon for a child to speak a few words after surgery and then be mute the following day. Cerebellar mutism may be present for up to 3 to 6 months but is usually more short-lived. There are no reported cases in which a child with cerebellar mutism did not recover functional speech.

CASE 5

HISTORY AND PHYSICAL EXAMINATION

A 10-year-old girl presents to your ED because of sudden onset of left face, arm, and leg weakness. She was recently diagnosed by her pediatrician with Grave's disease and associated hyperthyroidism. Other past medical history was unremarkable except for seasonal allergies treated with an antihistamine. General physical exam did not reveal any rashes, birthmarks, cardiac abnormalities, or hepatosplenomegaly. Neurological exam was notable for mild flattening of the left nasolabial fold, mild left hemiparesis, with 4+/5 strength in all muscle groups of the left upper extremity, slower sequential finger taps on the left, and an upgoing toe on left Babinski testing.

IMAGING STUDIES

MRI demonstrated acute infarction in the right posterior frontal and anterior parietal lobes and a small infarct in the left frontal lobe (Figures 12.34 and 12.35). Magnetic resonance angiography (MRA) demonstrated narrowing of both middle cerebral arteries (MCA), right greater than left (Figure 12.36). Conventional angiography demonstrated distal narrowing of the right internal carotid artery (ICA) with non-visualization of the right MCA and prominent lenticulostriate branches. She also had relative narrowing of the distal left ICA with non-visualization of the proximal segment of the left anterior cerebral artery (ACA) and severe stenosis of the proximal segment of the left MCA branches. Posterior and external carotid circulations were normal. A comprehensive stroke workup was otherwise normal.

ANALYSIS OF CASE AND SURGICAL PLAN

This patient has moyamoya syndrome associated with Grave's disease. Moyamoya disease, a known cause of pediatric stroke, is a cerebrovascular occlusive disorder that can lead to devastating, permanent neurologic disability if left untreated. It is characterized by progressive stenosis of the intracranial internal carotid arteries and the proximal segments of their distal branches along with the nearly

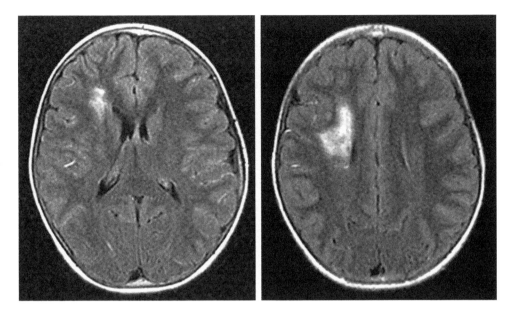

Figure 12.34 Axial MR FLAIR images from 10-year-old girl with sudden onset of left face, arm, and leg weakness showing acute infarction in the right posterior frontal and anterior parietal lobes.

simultaneous appearance of basal arterial collateral vessels which vascularize hypoperfused brain distal to the occluded vessels. Moyamoya disease may be idiopathic or may occur in association with other syndromes. *Moyamoya disease* typically refers to the idiopathic form of the arteriopathy, whereas *moyamoya syndrome* signifies cases in which the characteristic angiographic findings occur in association with other pathologic processes such as neurofibromatosis, sickle cell anemia, Down syndrome, and Grave's disease. Most children with moyamoya disease present with recurrent transient ischemic attacks or strokes. There is no definitive medical treatment. Numerous direct and indirect

revascularization procedures have been utilized to improve the compromised cerebral circulation, with outcomes varying according to procedure type. Such techniques improve the long-term outcome of patients with both idiopathic and syndrome-associated moyamoya vasculopathy.

PREOPERATIVE EVALUATION/ MANAGEMENT

Although it is a relatively uncommon clinical entity, moyamoya disease must be considered in the differential diagnosis of any child who presents with symptoms of

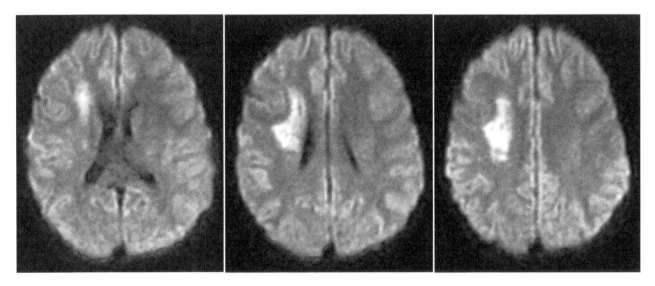

Figure 12.35 Axial MR DWI from 10-year-old girl with sudden onset of left face, arm, and leg weakness showing acute infarction in the right posterior frontal and anterior parietal lobes.

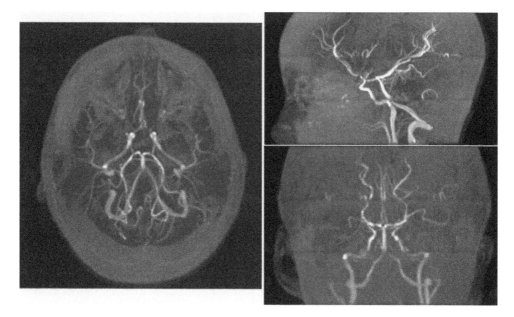

Figure 12.36 MRA from 10-year-old girl with sudden onset of left face, arm, and leg weakness showing narrowing of both MCAs, right greater than left.

cerebral ischemia (e.g., a transient ischemic attack manifesting as episodes of hemiparesis, speech disturbance, sensory impairment, involuntary movement, and/or visual disturbance), especially if the symptoms are precipitated by physical exertion, hyperventilation, or crying. Radiologic imaging plays a key role in the diagnostic evaluation of these patients. A head CT is typically the first study obtained when patients present with symptoms of cerebral ischemia. In patients with moyamoya disease, the head CT frequently demonstrates areas of hypodensity consistent with infarction in cortical watershed zones, basal ganglia, deep white matter, and/or periventricular regions.

Brain MRI/MRA (Figure 12.36) and CTA typically reveal diminished flow voids in the supraclinoid ICA, proximal MCA, and proximal ACA vessels and prominent flow voids in the basal ganglia and thalamus resulting from dilated moyamoya vessels that traverse these regions to supply hypoperfused brain distal to the occluded vessels (Figure 12.37). Such flow voids are virtually diagnostic of moyamoya disease. MRI may also demonstrate multiple, small, asymptomatic areas of cerebral infarction, which are typically found in watershed regions between the cortical areas vascularized by anterior and middle cerebral arteries. Moreover, diffusion-weighted, perfusion echo-planar, and gradient-echo MRI techniques are useful for evaluating cerebral ischemia (Figure 12.35), with diffusion-weighted imaging leading to significantly earlier detection of ischemic lesions in patients with moyamoya disease.

The smaller moyamoya collateral vessels clearly are visualized better with conventional cerebral angiography, which is still the gold standard for diagnosing moyamoya disease (Figure 12.38). Bilateral selective external and internal carotid artery injections and a vertebrobasilar artery injection are essential to define the extent of preexisting collaterals from the extracranial circulation, to document areas of cerebral hypoperfusion, and to identify any coexisting

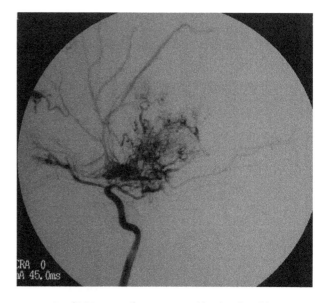

Figure 12.37 Axial MR images from 10-year-old girl with sudden onset of left face, arm, and leg weakness showing diminished flow voids in the supraclinoid ICA, proximal MCA, and proximal ACA vessels and prominent flow voids in the basal ganglia and thalamus resulting from dilated moyamoya vessels that traverse these regions to supply hypoperfused brain distal to the occluded vessels.

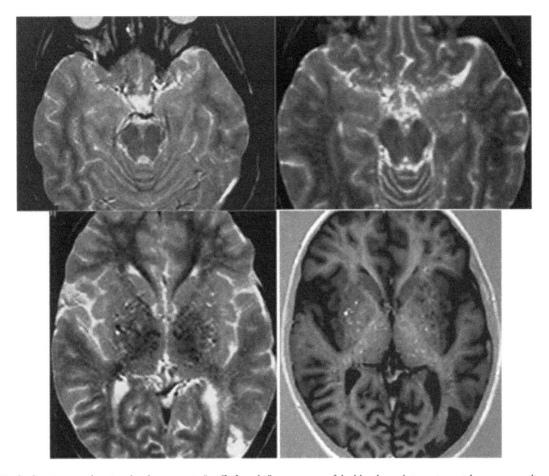

Figure 12.38 Cerebral angiogram showing the characteristic "puff of smoke" appearance of the blood vessels in patient with moyamoya disease.

aneurysms or AVMs. SPECT +/− diamox (vasodilatory stimulus) can also be used to detect regional perfusion instability (cerebrovascular reserve) and predict likelihood of further disease progression.

Children with moyamoya disease present with headaches, seizures, transient ischemic attacks (TIAs), and/or strokes. Once the diagnosis is made, it is unwise to wait for clinical symptoms before recommending surgery. Children who present with TIAs, even if accompanied by severe arteriographic disease, frequently have excellent outcomes if surgical revascularization is performed before infarction occurs. Patients are considered surgical candidates if diagnosis is established by angiographic criteria. These include stenosis or occlusion of the distal portion of the intracranial ICA and the proximal portions of the ACA and MCA and an abnormal vascular network seen during the arterial phase near the stenosed or occluded vessels that creates the characteristic "puff of smoke" appearance of the blood vessels in patients with moyamoya disease (Figure 12.38).

Currently, there is no known medical treatment capable of reversing, halting, or stabilizing the relentless progression of the arteriopathic process in moyamoya disease.

Nevertheless, aspirin plays a role in the treatment of this disorder. Aspirin is taken daily to avoid ischemic symptoms due to possible emboli from microthrombus formation at sites of arterial stenoses. If less than 6 years old, a patient receives 80 mg/day and the dose is gradually increased up to 300 mg/day in adolescents. Patients are monitored for side effects, such as easy bruising, bleeding, and gastrointestinal irritation, and the aspirin dose is adjusted as needed.

Although there are no prospective randomized controlled clinical trials to determine the efficacy of surgical revascularization in the treatment of moyamoya disease, there are numerous studies that provide strong support for surgical management. Revascularization surgery is generally recommended for the treatment of patients with recurrent or progressive cerebral ischemic events and associated reduced cerebral perfusion reserve. Numerous operative techniques have been described. At the present time, there is no standardized surgical approach for the treatment of moyamoya disease in children and numerous surgical procedures have been used in a variety of combinations. Such techniques aim to prevent further ischemic injury by increasing collateral blood flow to hypoperfused areas of cortex, with most using the external carotid circulation as a donor supply. Revascularization procedures can be divided into three main groups: (a) indirect (non-anastomotic) bypass techniques, (b) direct (anastomotic) bypass techniques, and (c) indirect and/or direct bypass techniques combined, which have the advantages (and disadvantages) of both direct and indirect revascularization procedures.

Numerous studies have reported on the technical aspects, indications, pitfalls, and efficacy of both direct and indirect revascularization techniques for the prevention of ischemic symptoms in patients with moyamoya disease. In general, these studies have documented good to excellent angiographic and clinical results with various surgical revascularization techniques, including good collateralization of the MCA territory, reduction in the size of the basal collateral vessels, improved cerebral blood flow, and partial or complete resolution of ischemic symptoms. Evidence suggests that essentially any surgically induced pathway that traverses the skull, dura, and arachnoid will permit the formation of cortical collaterals.

PROCEDURE

An indirect bypass technique that works very well in the treatment of children with moyamoya disease is pial synangiosis. Pial synangiosis involves the dissection of a scalp donor artery (most commonly the posterior/parietal branch of the superficial temporal artery [STA]) with a cuff of galea (Figure 12.39); opening the temporalis muscle and fascia in 4 quadrants and tacking up each quadrant with 3-0 vicryl suture; turning a frontotemporal craniotomy bone flap in the region

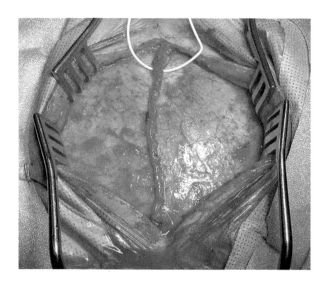

Figure 12.39 Parietal branch of the STA mobilized with its cuff of galea as part of a pial synangiosis indirect revascularization procedure in a child with moyamoya disease.

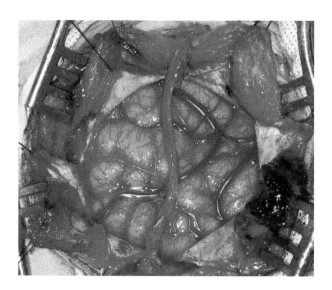

Figure 12.40 Opening of the temporalis muscle and fascia in 4 quadrants.

subjacent to the artery to expose the underlying dura; opening the dura in a stellate fashion, making at least 6 incisions without disrupting potential meningeal collateral vessels, in order to increase the surface area of dura exposed to the pial surface and thereby enhance formation of collateral vessels from the dural vascular supply (Figure 12.40); opening the arachnoid widely over the cortical surface exposed by the dural opening; and then suturing the intact donor artery by its galeal cuff directly to the pial surface using several interrupted 10-0 nylon sutures. The bone flap is then replaced using microplates and screws, and the scalp is closed by reapproximating the temporalis muscle and fascia except near the STA where it enters and exits the skull and then closing the galea with buried interrupted 3-0 vicryl sutures and the skin with a running non-interlocking 4-0 or 5-0 monocryl suture.

A cerebral angiogram and/or brain MRI/MRA is obtained 1 year following pial synangiosis. This typically shows excellent MCA collateralization from the donor superficial temporal artery as well as from other meningeal and scalp arteries near the craniotomy site. Patients undergoing pial synangiosis demonstrate an excellent neurological outcome with complete resolution or a significant reduction in the frequency and severity of TIAs during the first postoperative year, as well as an extremely low incidence of new strokes.

COMPLICATIONS

Risks of surgery are more often related to neurologic instability of the patient at the time of surgery and to the risks of anesthesia rather than to actual surgical manipulations. For example, patients with moyamoya disease not infrequently may develop their first stroke or ischemic symptoms following the administration of a general anesthetic. The increased risks of anesthesia result in large part from moyamoya vessels being extremely sensitive to changes in blood pressure, blood volume, and $PaCO_2$. To reduce the risk of intraoperative and perioperative neurologic morbidity, adequate cerebral blood flow must be maintained. To accomplish this, there must be meticulous management of blood pressure, fluid balance, temperature, and blood gases with strict avoidance of hypotension, hypovolemia, hyperthermia, and hypocarbia both intraoperatively and perioperatively. Intraoperative EEG monitoring with a full array of scalp electrodes can be helpful in the neurologic assessment of patients under general anesthesia. To help prevent hypovolemia during surgery, patients are admitted the evening prior to surgery for intravenous hydration at 1.5 times maintenance. Potential complications associated with surgical treatment of moyamoya disease include postoperative stroke, subdural hematoma, following both trauma and spontaneous, intracerebral hemorrhage, wound infection, and CSF leak.

REFERENCES

Adzick NS, Thom EA, Spong CY, et al. A randomized trial of prenatal versus postnatal repair of myelomeningocele. *N Engl J Med.* 2011;364 (11):993–1004.

Albright AL, Pollack IF, Adelson PD. *Operative techniques in pediatric neurosurgery.* New York, NY: Thieme; 2001.

Cheek WR, ed. *Atlas of pediatric neurosurgery.* Philadelphia, PA: W. B. Saunders Company; 1996.

Cohen AR. *Pediatric neurosurgery—tricks of the trade.* New York, NY: Thieme; 2015.

Goodrich JT. *Pediatric neurosurgery* (Neurosurgical Operative Atlas). 2nd ed. New York, NY: Thieme; 2008.

Northcott PA, Korshunov A, Witt H, et al. Medulloblastoma comprises four distinct molecular variants. *J. Clin Oncology.* 2011;29(11):1408–1414.

Scott RM, Smith JL, Robertson RL, et al. Long-term outcome in children with moyamoya syndrome following cranial revascularization by pial synangiosis. *J. Neurosurgery Peds.* 2004;100:142–149.

Smith JL. Understanding and treating moyamoya disease in children. *Neurosurg Focus.* 2009;26(4):E4.

13.

NEUROLOGY

Kristine O'Phelan

CASE 1

An 88-year-old African American woman presents to the emergency department complaining of abdominal pain and palpitations. She is found to have atrial fibrillation with rapid ventricular response. Her history is also notable for hypertension and hyperlipidemia, and she has been on dual antiplatelet medications. After admission to the hospital, she suddenly develops altered mental status and decreased movement in her limbs. When you arrive to examine her, she is able to open her eyes to pain, she does not track or answer questions, her pupils are reactive, and her corneal reflexes are diminished bilaterally. She has a weak cough/gag and extends her upper extremities to stimulation. Given her low Glasgow Coma Scale score she is intubated for airway protection.

A noncontrast computed tomography (CT) scan of the brain is performed (Figure 13.1).

The noncontrast CT of the brain does not demonstrate any acute hemorrhage; there is age-appropriate atrophy and evidence of prior ischemic events in the left cerebellar hemisphere and left thalamus.

WHAT IS THE DIFFERENTIAL DIAGNOSIS?

Given the acute onset of symptoms in a patient with vascular risk factors and imaging negative for a structural lesion, acute ischemic stroke is likely. Complicated migraine headache and seizures are possibilities when there are acute focal symptoms with negative imaging. However, this presentation would be atypical for those disorders.

WHAT FURTHER HISTORY DO YOU NEED?

You should determine the last time the patient was seen, know the duration of symptoms, and decide eligibility for thrombolytic treatment. In this case, the patient was last seen well 30 minutes ago. Serum glucose should be measured as hypoglycemia can produce focal neurological deficits. In this case, the serum glucose was 160 mg/dL. You should ask about medications the patient is taking to determine potential contraindications for thrombolysis, specifically anticoagulants. Recent trauma, surgery, or prior history of bleeding, particularly intracranial hemorrhage, are important to consider when deciding the best course of treatment.

WHAT FURTHER WORKUP AND TREATMENT IS INDICATED?

The patient should receive intravenous (IV) thrombolysis as she does not have any contraindications to this and is highly likely to have an acute ischemic stroke. Alteplase (Activase®)—a tissue plasminogen activator—is Food and Drug Administration approved in the United States for acute thrombolysis in ischemic stroke. The dose is 0.9 mg/kg up to a total dose of 90 mg with the first 10% given as an IV bolus and the remainder to run over 1-hour infusion.

Once that is started, a CT angiography of the head and neck are performed to evaluate the arterial vasculature for evidence of a large vessel occlusion (LVO) that may benefit from mechanical thrombectomy. Mechanical thrombectomy is indicated if there is an occlusion of the proximal middle cerebral artery (MCA), internal carotid artery (ICA), vertebral artery, or basilar artery within 6 hours of last known "well" time. Several clinical trials in 2015 have shown marked clinical improvement in patients with LVO who are treated with mechanical thrombectomy.[1] More recent studies are demonstrating benefit of mechanical thrombectomy in more distal MCA segments (M2, M3)[1] and even with later treatments—up to 24 hours post onset of stroke.[2–5]

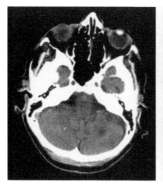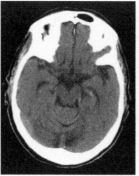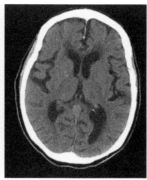

Figure 13.1 Noncontrast CT of the brain.

CT angiography and subsequently digital subtraction angiography revealed occlusion of the distal basilar artery (Figure 13.2).

Mechanical thrombectomy is attempted; however, no recanalization is achieved. The patient is brought back to the intensive care unit (ICU) and another noncontrast CT of the brain is performed.

The CT demonstrates acute infarcts of the pons and left cerebellum as well as extensive subarachnoid hemorrhage in the basal cisterns and Sylvian fissure, as well as parenchymal hemorrhage in the midbrain (Figure 13.3).

WHAT DO YOU DO NEXT?

This patient has an acute intracranial hemorrhage after IV thrombolysis. You should reverse the thrombolytic with the following: cryoprecipitate 10 units IV, Tranexemic acid 1 gm IV over 10 minutes, platelets 6–8 units. Send prothrombin time (PT), partial thromboplastin time (PTT), and fibrinogen to determine the need for further treatment, but do not wait for results to give reversal agents. This patient has suffered a devastating stroke complicated by intracranial hemorrhage with poor neurological outcome expected. You should have a discussion with her family regarding her wishes for further aggressive treatments including their risks and benefits and determine her goals of care.

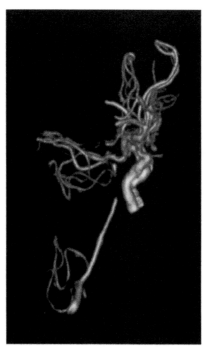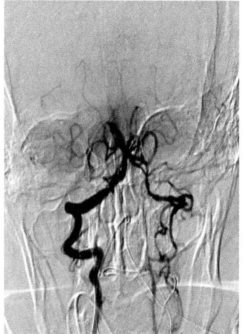

Figure 13.2 CT angiography (left); digital subtraction angiography (right).

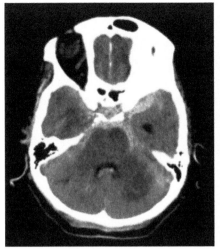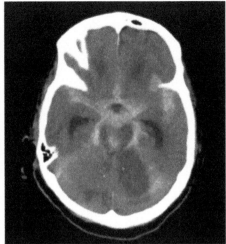

Figure 13.3 Noncontrast CT of the brain.

CASE 2

A 68-year-old man with a history of hypertension, hyperlipidemia, and obstructive sleep apnea is sent to your office for evaluation of leg weakness. He reports that he has been dragging his right foot for at least 6 months. He was initially evaluated by his primary physician and found to have an elevated creatine phosphokinase (CPK) level. This was thought to be due to his statin medication. However, the CPK elevation persisted after discontinuation of the drug and his weakness worsened. He reports no swallowing or chewing difficulty, no back pain, and no sensory complaints. An magnetic resonance imaging (MRI) of the spine was performed and he was referred to you.

MRI of the cervical and lumbar spine demonstrate canal stenosis and disc bulges at C4-5, C5-6, and L3-4 and canal narrowing at L4-5 (Figure 13.4).

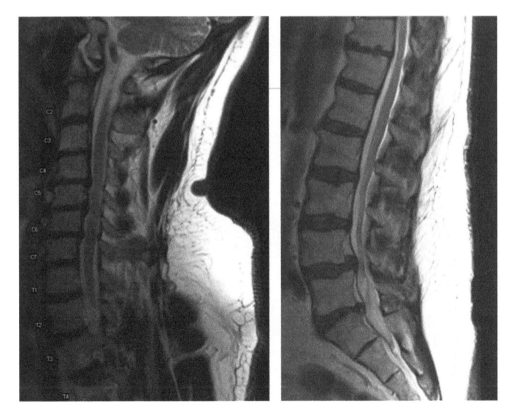

Figure 13.4 Sagittal MRI of the cervical (left) and lumbar (right) spine.

On exam, the patient is awake and alert and his cranial nerves are normal. Motor strength in the deltoids bilaterally are 4/5 without atrophy. There is spasticity of the lower extremities bilaterally, and he has difficulty standing on his right heel with atrophy of the tibialis anterior muscle on the right. Deep tendon reflexes are 2+ in biceps bilaterally and 3+ at the patella bilaterally with extensor plantar responses bilaterally.

DO THE FINDINGS EXPLAIN THE EXAM?

The patient's chronic weakness of tibialis anterior is not explained by the mild degree of canal narrowing seen on imaging. Additionally, the patient would not be expected to have increased deep tendon reflexes consistent with cervical myelopathy without more significant stenosis or spinal cord involvement on cervical MRI.

WHAT FURTHER WORKUP DO YOU ORDER?

An electromyography (EMG) and nerve conduction study was performed. It demonstrates denervation of the thoracic paraspinal muscles bilaterally without h reflex or f wave changes and no sensory abnormalities.

WHAT IS THE DIFFERENTIAL DIAGNOSIS?

The most likely diagnosis in this case is amyotrophic lateral sclerosis (ALS), also known as Lou Gehrig's disease with chronic onset, no sensory involvement, and evidence of upper and lower motor neuron abnormality. A predominantly motor polyneuropathy with cervical myelopathy would be less likely.

WHAT IS THE WORKUP?

An EMG and nerve conduction study will demonstrate selective involvement of motor roots consistent with motor neuron disease.

WHAT IS THE TREATMENT?

Treatment for ALS at this time is predominantly supportive. Disease modifying therapies are limited. Riluzole has been shown to slow the progression of the disease but does not change its outcome.

CASE 3

A 28-year-old man with a history of severe traumatic brain injury 4 years ago complicated by severe spasticity and baclofen pump placement for intrathecal baclofen therapy. He is brought to the emergency department after his family found him with an altered mental status.

On examination his temperature is 39° C, heart rate is 130 beats per minute (sinus tachycardia), and blood pressure is 95/50.

He is able to open his eyes to stimulation, pupils are reactive bilaterally, and corneal and cough reflex are intact. He is able to state his name and follow simple directions. He is not speaking in sentences and appears confused and agitated with diaphoresis. He is able to localize pain and has increased tone throughout with extensor plantar response bilaterally. A CT scan of the brain and kidney, ureter and bladder x-ray (KUB) are performed.

Noncontrast CT of the brain demonstrates right temporal encephalomalacia consistent with prior traumatic brain injury (Figure 13.5).

Figure 13.6 shows plain film of the abdomen showing normal bowel gas pattern and implanted baclofen pump in the right lower quadrant.

WHAT IS THE DIFFERENTIAL DIAGNOSIS?

Sepsis and metabolic encephalopathy must be considered in this patient with fever, tachycardia, hypotension, and altered mental status. However, acute withdrawal from intrathecal baclofen can also cause these symptoms, and in light of this patient's increased muscle tone and history of intrathecal baclofen therapy, this is the likely diagnosis. Serotonin syndrome and other withdrawal syndromes including withdrawal from gamma-hydroxybuteric acid should be considered.

WHAT IS THE WORKUP?

Blood cultures should be sent and other sources of infection investigated. Initiation of broad-spectrum antibiotics is prudent after cultures are collected until results exclude infection. Plain films of the abdomen can demonstrate evidence of a dislodged or fractured catheter, which may have disrupted baclofen delivery from the pump. The pump itself should be interrogated and the chamber should be checked.

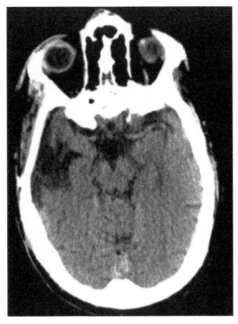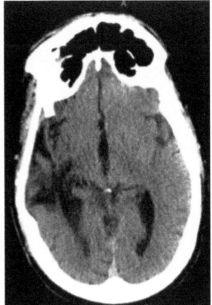

Figure 13.5 Noncontrast CT of the brain.

WHAT IS THE TREATMENT?

Acute withdrawal from intrathecal baclofen can be life threatening and manifests with altered mental status with confusion and hallucinations, which may worsen to stupor, seizures, and coma. Fever and muscle rigidity with resulting rhabdomyolysis are seen in severe cases. There is some

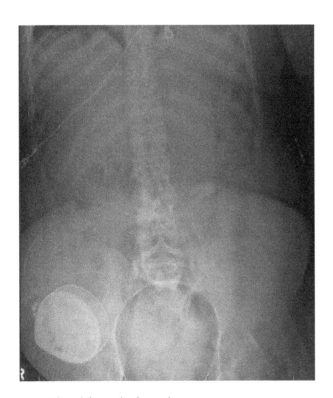

Figure 13.6 Plain abdominal radiograph.

degree of direct cardiac depression which when coupled with vasodilation from hyperthermia causes tachycardia and hypotension. The best treatment is restoration of intrathecal baclofen, either by resolution of pump malfunction or delivery of intrathecal baclofen via lumbar drain or lumbar puncture. If this is not feasible, oral baclofen can be given to mitigate symptoms of withdrawal. Oral baclofen alone is not expected to reverse withdrawal symptoms. The degree of response to oral baclofen is unpredictable; doses usually range between 10 to 20 mg every 6 hours via nasogastric tube. Benzodiazepines are useful to manage seizures, agitation, and muscle rigidity related to acute loss of GABA receptor activation by baclofen. Hyperthermia should be aggressively treated, and Cyproheptadine can be used as well; however, this is an "off label" use.[6]

CASE 4

A 58-year-old African American man presents to the emergency department complaining of 2 days of difficulty walking. He was treated for an upper respiratory infection 2 weeks prior to presentation. He describes dragging his foot first with a subsequent feeling of heaviness in his legs and now has difficulty holding objects in his hand. He describes pain in his back over the past day.

On examination, the patient is awake, alert, and fully oriented; his speech is mildly dysarthric and you notice his nasolabial folds are diminished bilaterally. He has full extraocular movements. Motor examination reveals 4/5 strength in

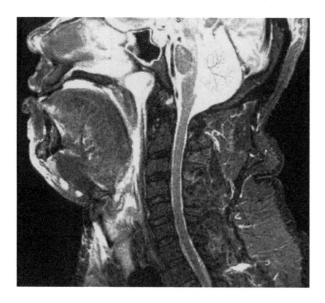

Figure 13.7 Sagittal MRI of the cervical spine.

albuminocytologic dissociation where the cerebrospinal fluid (CSF) protein is elevated without an increased number of cells. Serum markers can be sent for a number of variants of AIDP. These include GQ1b (Fisher variant), IgG to GM1, GM1b, GD1a, and Gal-NacGD (acute motor axonal neuropathy).

WHAT IS THE TREATMENT?

Immune modulation with either IV immune globulin or plasma exchange therapy are the treatments for Guillian Barré syndrome. Both have been shown to be equally effective in clinical trials. Intensive care unit admission for hemodynamic and respiratory monitoring is often warranted. Respiratory parameters with vital capacity and negative inspiratory force measured every 4 hours is standard. No steroids should be given; they are *not indicated* for Guillian Barré syndrome.

deltoids with 3/5 in handgrip; iliopsoas strength is 4/5 bilaterally with weakness distally as he is only able to wiggle his toes. Reflexes are absent throughout and toes do not move with plantar stimulation. MRI of the cervical spine is performed.

The MRI of the cervical spine does not demonstrate an acute process or cord compression (Figure 13.7).

WHAT IS THE DIFFERENTIAL DIAGNOSIS?

There are several processes that can cause weakness in this distribution. At the level of the brainstem, a demyelinating process or tumor could cause weakness; however, areflexia would not be expected. At the level of the peripheral nerves, Guillain-Barré syndrome or acute inflammatory demyelinating polyradiculoneuropathy (AIDP) is most consistent with the rapidly progressing weakness starting in a distal and progressing to a proximal distribution accompanied by areflexia. A preceding upper respiratory tract infection, diarrheal illness, or vaccination is commonly found. Diphtheria, porphyria, tick paralysis, West Nile infection, Lyme disease, and polio should be considered but are less common. At the level of the neuromuscular junction, myasthenia gravis and botulism can cause rapidly progressive weakness; however; the history and distribution of weakness are not typical in this case.

WHAT IS THE WORKUP?

Imaging of the brain and cervical spine should be obtained to exclude a structural lesion although the history and exam are not typical for this. A lumbar puncture should be performed to exclude infective processes. AIDP often causes an

CASE 5

A 64-year-old woman with poorly controlled hypertension suffers a spontaneous intracranial hemorrhage in the right posterior frontal lobe. She has been taken for a decompressive craniectomy due to acute symptoms of herniation with pupillary dilation and posturing. Postoperatively she is admitted to the ICU. The patient is able to open her eyes spontaneously, following directions on the right side, and has reactive pupils and a left hemiplegia.

On postoperative day 2, her neurological examination is worse. She is not opening her eyes, her pupils are reactive bilaterally, her gaze is persistently turned to the left side, and she can localize pain on the right side but does not follow directions. A noncontrast CT of the brain is performed.

This noncontrast CT of the brain demonstrates evidence of prior right craniectomy with a stable lobar hemorrhage. No worsening edema or shift of midline is noted and basal cisterns are open (Figure 13.8).

WHAT IS THE DIFFERENTIAL DIAGNOSIS?

The patient's worsening examination could be caused by multiple factors. The brain imaging excludes new hemorrhage or worsening edema and brainstem compression. Severe metabolic encephalopathy can cause neurological worsening postoperatively, and the patient should be evaluated for sepsis, hypernatremia, or organ failure. In this case, the patient's eye deviation is not explained by a metabolic encephalopathy. Subclinical seizures or nonconvulsive status epilepticus is highly likely given the eye deviation.

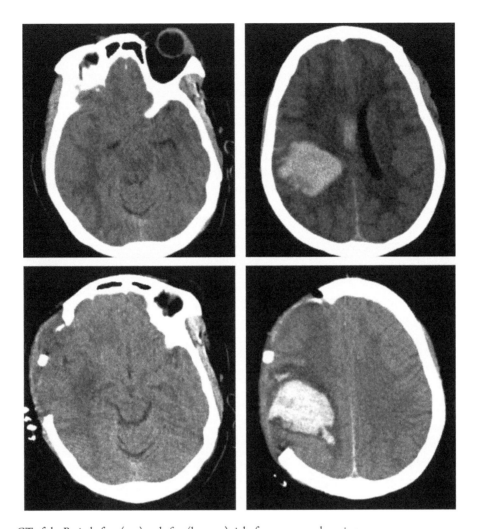

Figure 13.8 Noncontrast CT of the Brain before (top) and after (bottom) right frontotemporal craniectomy.

WHAT WORKUP AND TREATMENT ARE NEEDED?

In this case, treatment and workup should proceed simultaneously since delayed treatment of status epilepticus has been shown to lead to worse outcomes.

Lorazepam should be given up to a dose of 0.1 mg/kg in 4 mg doses. This patient is already intubated so her airway is secure. In unintubated patients, lorazepam should still be given with attention to the airway and preparation for intubation if needed. A dose of IV anticonvulsant should be given. This patient was already on Levetiracetam 750 mg twice a day. An additional 750 mg IV can be given with the standing dose increased to 1500 mg twice a day. Continuous electroencephalogram (EEG) monitoring should be obtained. If the patient continues to have either clinical or electrographic seizures, a second anticonvulsant can be added via IV with preparations to add a continuous infusion anticonvulsant if needed. IV anticonvulsants typically used for status epilepticus are phenytoin, levetiracetam, phenobarbital, and valproic acid (not used in this case due to acute hemorrhage and potential antiplatelet effect of this medication).

In this case, the continuous EEG shows spike and wave activity over the right hemisphere with occasional spread to the contralateral hemisphere consistent with ongoing seizure activity.

IV midazolam infusion was started to suppress seizure activity. The dose can be increased to 3 mg/kg/hr if needed. Other medications used for continuous seizure suppression are propofol and pentobarbital. All will cause some degree of hypotension, and vasopressors should be readily available to avoid hypotension and secondary brain insults.

CASE 6

A 42-year-old woman without a past history is referred to your office due to an abnormal MRI scan. She describes unsteadiness in her gait for the past month and now has noticed weakness of her left leg over the past week. She denies headache or fever. There is no history of trauma. She does report having a few days of decreased vision in her left eye 6 months ago, but it improved on its own and she did not seek medical attention.

Her examination reveals a temperature of 37°C, blood pressure 110/60, and heart rate 82 in normal sinus rhythm. She is in no acute distress, awake, alert, and oriented. Her pupils are reactive and show an afferent pupillary defect on the left. Visual fields to confrontation are full. Motor strength is full in the upper extremities and right lower extremity. The left iliopsoas is 4/5 and foot dorsiflexion is 3/5. Deep tendon reflexes are 3+ throughout with 5 beats of clonus bilaterally and extensor plantar responses. An MRI of the brain with contrast was performed.

MRI of the brain with contrast demonstrates many areas of white matter abnormality periventricularly without significant contrast enhancement. (Figure 13.9).

WHAT IS THE DIFFERENTIAL DIAGNOSIS?

Demyelinating disease is a likely diagnosis given the patient's age, history of prior deficit with remission, and imaging with predominantly white matter abnormality. The afferent pupillary defect is likely related to a prior episode of optic neuritis making multiple sclerosis more likely than an acute fulminating demyelinating process such as acute disseminated encephalomyelitis (ADEM). Small vessel vascular disease can sometimes cause periventricular white matter abnormalities but, considering the patient's age and lack of vascular risk factors, this is unlikely. Infectious processes are also less likely with a subacute onset and no headache or fever.

WHAT IS THE WORKUP?

A lumbar puncture should be performed and CSF sent for cell count, glucose, protein and bacterial culture. CSF polymerase chain reaction test (PCR) for Herpes Simplex Virus (HSV), Varicella Zoster Virus (VZV), Epstein Barr Virus (EBV), and Cytomegalovirus (CMV) should be sent to exclude a viral encephalitis. CSF oligoclonal bands, myelin basic protein, and immunoglobulin index should be sent. Serum neuromyelitis optica and Myelin oligodendrocyte glycoprotein (MOG) antibodies are also helpful if positive.

WHAT IS THE TREATMENT?

IV steroid therapy should be started with methylprednisolone 1000 mg IV daily for 5 days. Further evaluation for longer-term disease modifying therapies to reduce relapses, and new MRI lesion activity should be performed after CSF results are received.[7]

CASE 7

A 52-year-old woman is seen for intermittent sharp sensation of "electric shock" over her left cheek and temple for a year. She denies any other head pain, prior trauma, and tinnitus. She does notice that the pain is sometimes associated with chewing, talking, or washing her face. Her dental exam is normal and her neurologic exam is completely normal.

The MRI of the brain with contrast does not show any mass lesion, hemorrhage, ischemic area, or vascular abnormality (Figure 13.10).

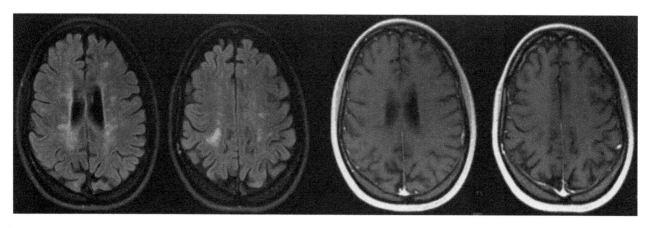

Figure 13.9 Axial MRI of the brain. FLAIR sequence (left) and contrast enhanced T1 sequence (right).

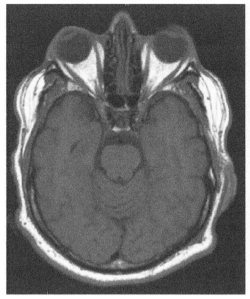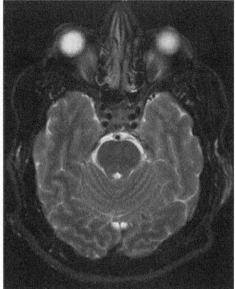

Figure 13.10 Axial MRI of the brain. T1 sequence (left) and T2 sequence (right).

WHAT IS THE DIFFERENTIAL DIAGNOSIS?

The patient's history is typical for trigeminal neuralgia (TN) or tic douloureux. Compressive lesions such as meningioma, cholesteatoma, acoustic neuroma, demyelinating processes, and vascular abnormalities in the region of the trigeminal nerve entry into the pons must be excluded. TN typically affects women more often than men; the incidence is 13 per 100,000 population. The incidence increases with age, and most idiopathic cases have onset after 50 years of age. Many are caused by compression of the trigeminal nerve root near its entry into the pons. Cases are divided into 3 types. Classical TN is caused by compression of the nerve by a vein or artery. Secondary TN is related to an underlying disease such as multiple sclerosis. The third type is idiopathic TN.

WHAT ARE THE AVAILABLE TREATMENTS?

Medical treatment should be started with carbamazepine (Tegretrol). Carbamazapine can produce dose-related side effects including drowsiness, unsteadiness, and dry mouth. Typical dosage for TN is in the 400–800 mg range. Baclofen and lamotrigine are possibly effective. In atypical TN, gabapentin and antidepressants may be efficacious.[8] Surgical treatment with microvascular decompression can have long-lasting benefit in classic TN with favorable long-term outcomes in the 70% to 80% range.[9] Surgical ablative procedures include needle-based approaches such

as radiofrequency thermocoagulation, glycerol injection, and balloon compression. Stereotactic radiosurgery such as gamma knife ablation of the ganglion has also been used.

REFERENCES

1. Powers WJ, Rabinstein AA, Ackerson T, et al. 2018 Guidelines for the Early Management of Patients With Acute Ischemic Stroke: a guideline for healthcare professionals from the American Heart Association/American Stroke Association. *Stroke.* 2018;49(3):e46–e110.
2. Altenbernd J, Kuhnt O, Hennigs S, Hilker R, Loehr C. Frontline ADAPT therapy to treat patients with symptomatic M2 and M3 occlusions in acute ischemic stroke: initial experience with the Penumbra ACE and 3MAX reperfusion system. *J Neurointerv Surg.* 2018;10(5):434–439.
3. Chen CJ, Wang C, Buell TJ, et al. Endovascular mechanical thrombectomy for acute middle cerebral artery M2 segment occlusion: a systematic review. *World Neurosurg.* 2017;107:684–691.
4. Grossberg JA, Rebello LC, Haussen DC, et al. Beyond large vessel occlusion strokes: distal occlusion thrombectomy. *Stroke.* 2018;49(7):1662–1668.
5. Nogueira RG, Jadhav AP, Haussen DC, et al. Thrombectomy 6 to 24 hours after stroke with a mismatch between deficit and infarct. *N Engl J Med.* 2018;378(1):11–21.
6. Albers GW, Marks MP, Kemp S, et al. Thrombectomy for stroke at 6 to 16 hours with selection by perfusion imaging. *N Engl J Med.* 2018;378(8):708–718.
7. Saulino M, Anderson DJ, Doble J, et al. Best practices for intrathecal baclofen therapy: troubleshooting. *Neuromodulation.* 2016;19(6):632–641.
8. Di Stefano G, Truini A, Cruccu G. Current and innovative pharmacological options to treat typical and atypical trigeminal neuralgia. *Drugs.* 2018;78(14):1433–1442.
9. Oesman C, Mooij JJ. Long-term follow-up of microvascular decompression for trigeminal neuralgia. *Skull Base.* 2011;21(5):313–322.

14.

COMPLICATIONS

Allan D. Levi and Roberto C. Heros

Complications form a very significant element of the Oral Board Examination. In fact, the scoring system gives a grade for "the handling of complications relevant to the neurosurgical treatment of your cases" (see Chapter 1 of this volume). The good news is that there really is a limited number of complications in neurosurgery, and if up front you have an answer for most complications, you will be ahead of the game. Again, we would emphasize that complications are expected on the Oral Board Examination, and when you get them, it does not mean that you are handling the case poorly.

When complications ensue, and they will, be ready to jump into the fire. Come in and see the patient, lay hands on, express your concern. Do not send your resident or nurse practitioner or delay the visit until Monday if the problems are occurring on the weekend.

To assist with board preparation, we have compiled some of the more common complications seen in neurosurgery, so that you can make a well-defined plan when hearing them on your examination. This way, you can easily respond without generating too much stress.

1. Postoperative neuropathic pain

2. Postoperative wound infection

3. Cerebrospinal fluid (CSF) leak

4. C5 nerve palsy

5. Postoperative cranial or spinal hematoma

6. Hyponatremia

7. Vasospasm

8. Intraoperative aneurysm rupture—open or endovascular

9. Major arterial injuries with cranial and spinal surgery

10. Uncontrolled intracranial pressure

11. Brain swelling during operative exposure

12. Esophageal injury

POSTOPERATIVE NEUROPATHIC PAIN

Postoperative neuropathic pain is associated with injury or irritation typically to a peripheral nerve. Such injuries can give rise to paresthesias, numbness, tingling, or electrical sensation. The pain associated with these nerve injuries is often unrelenting. It is typically described as burning.

Neuropathic pain is typically not responsive to anti-inflammatory agents or steroids and is poorly responsive to opioids.

Managing a neuropathic patient after cervical, lumbar, or peripheral nerve surgery is a very important component of the Oral Board Examination. It is clear that the primary line agents are antiepileptics, such as gabapentin (Neurontin) and pregabalin (Lyrica). Start with a low dose of gabapentin, such as 300 mg given orally 3 times daily, raising the dose until the patient achieves pain relief or cannot tolerate side effects; common side effects include drowsiness and peripheral extremity edema. Conversely, removing either of these medications requires a weaning process—particularly if the patient has been on the medication long term. Ruling out a surgical etiology for neuropathic pain such as a residual disk or constriction of the nerve by a band or hematoma is always important in the workup.

Occasionally, when all conservative treatments fail, consideration is given to a spinal cord stimulator or a peripheral nerve stimulator.

POSTOPERATIVE WOUND INFECTIONS

How to manage postoperative wound infections is a common question on the Oral Board Examination. Infections can occur after either cranial or spinal procedures. An aggressive stance is usually needed. The typical presentation is that of drainage, fever, pain, and wound redness. The differential diagnosis is often CSF leak. Ancillary testing, such as laboratory data, to look at the white blood cell count, erythrocyte sedimentation rate, and C-reactive protein, is always helpful.

With possible spine infections, it is important to distinguish between a superficial infection, or stitch granuloma in which there is typically no systemic symptoms, and a deep infection that often presents with fever, pain, and malaise. Deep infections require irrigation and debridement supplemented by intravenous (IV) antibiotics.[1] Typically, a minimum of a 2-week course of IV antibiotics for a deep infection is required, although there are many subtle factors involved in the final decision of how long to administer the antibiotics. In the presence of spinal instrumentation with an acute infection, the hardware can be left in, but the wound will require irrigation and debridement and removal of all necrotic material, placement of drains, and typically 6 weeks of IV antibiotics. If the patient presents with a chronic wound infection, and particularly if there is an associated osteomyelitis, the instrumentation frequently needs to be removed.

For cranial wound infections, the bone flap frequently needs to be removed, particularly if there is pus under the bone flap or any erosion of the bone suggestive of osteomyelitis. This is followed by irrigation and debridement, evacuation of an epidural abscess, and removal of devitalized wound edges. Drains form an important part of the treatment to prevent reaccumulation of infected fluids leading to a potential recurrent abscess. The patient will need the infection completely eradicated before reconsideration of cranioplasty, because obviously the previously infected bone flap cannot be used and should have been discarded. A minimum waiting time of 3 months, but preferably 6 months, before performing cranioplasty is necessary.

Postoperative meningitis is another important consideration for any cranial or spinal intradural procedure, or in cases in which CSF drains are used. It is critical to sample CSF if meningitis is suspected, to look for an elevated white blood cell count with elevated percentage of neutrophils, a reduction in glucose below 50% of serum value, and elevated protein.

Whenever a wound infection, whether cranial or spinal, is suspected, it is important *not* to start the patient on antibiotics and to let the situation define itself. If a "real" wound infection exists, it will declare itself with obvious signs such as swelling, redness, drainage, or systemic symptoms related to a deep wound infection. Antibiotics should not be started until cultures are obtained at surgery. Starting antibiotics empirically, before open surgical treatment of the infection, can result in a partially treated infection that becomes a chronic problem with possible development of a deeper infection, such as meningitis or osteomyelitis. In addition, if the patient has been taking antibiotics before the wound is opened and cultured, frequently the causative organism cannot be recovered at culture, and the patient needs to be unnecessarily treated empirically with broad-spectrum antibiotics, which is not satisfactory.

CEREBROSPINAL FLUID LEAK

CSF leak again is a very common complication presented on the Oral Board Examination. CSF leaks may present with positional headache or simply as an obvious clear liquid escaping from the wound or possibly a pseudomeningocele with a bulging wound (Figure 14.1). Postoperative imaging, including magnetic resonance imaging (MRI), can help define the borders of the spinal fluid leak, and very rarely a myelogram is required to determine the area where the leakage is emanating from. The incidence of CSF leaks after spinal surgery is in the range of about 3%.[2] It is certainly more common after revision surgeries. Minimally invasive surgeries have a similar incidence, but the likelihood that they will present with symptoms is less because the spinal fluid leak is contained by the muscles, which are still firmly attached to the spine, and there is no potential space in which the CSF can collect. The management is often multitiered; one can consider a blood patch, especially if it is a post–lumbar puncture headache. This works less frequently for a postoperative CSF leak. Often, what is required is to reexplore the wound and consider direct repair with sutures. Occasionally, indirect repair with glue needs to be done, often to supplement the repair with a lumbar or cervical CSF drainage, to help offset the pressure with the repair. Thoracic CSF leaks are certainly more difficult to treat, because the negative intrathoracic pressure encourages CSF to leak into the chest cavity; these leaks often require the adjunct of a cervical CSF drain.[3]

With postoperative cranial CSF leaks, one must always consider the issues of CSF drainage into air cells, such as the mastoid air cells after posterior fossa craniotomy or the frontal sinus air cells after an anterior fossa craniotomy. In these cases, one may encounter CSF from the wound,

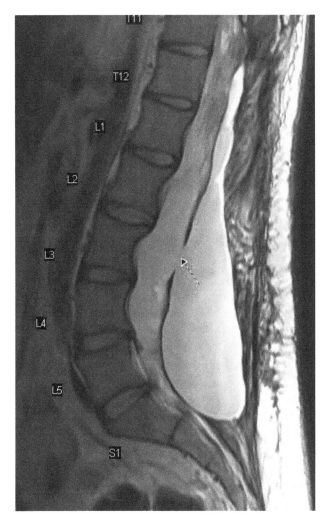

Figure 14.1 A large dorsal pseudomeningocele is seen after resection of a large lumbosacral schwannoma. The arrow points to the dural defect.

low-pressure headaches, or leakage of spinal fluid from the nose. Direct dural repair is often required in complex anterior skull base cases, and the use of a vascularized galeal flap may be required. Again, supplementation with a lumbar CSF drain may be important, particularly if there is no focal tumor mass effect, or raised intracranial pressure. Chronic problems with CSF leakage may be related to increased intracranial pressure and may require the placement of a ventriculoperitonal shunt.

C5 NERVE PALSY

C5 nerve palsy is another complication that can occur after cervical spinal surgery. It can happen either with anterior approaches, including anterior cervical discectomy, corpectomy, or posterior approaches, including a cervical laminectomy, cervical laminoplasty, or cervical laminectomy and fusion.

The important issue is to obtain a correct diagnosis. Typically, the weakness involves the deltoid supraspinatus and infraspinatus muscles and results in the inability to adduct the arm, and often weakness in the biceps muscles, which are also innervated by the C5 nerve root. The other important issue has to do with the onset of the symptoms; usually, if the onset is immediately after surgery, and particularly if it is complete, the prognosis is less certain and less favorable. Typical onset is in a delayed fashion, and this occurs in between 3% and 8% of posterior cervical procedures. The prognosis for delayed palsy is certainly better, and often the recovery is complete. It is important in the diagnostic workup to rule out structural causes such as a hematoma or a disk fragment, and if there are none, the treatment is conservative with physical therapy when appropriate.

If there is a severe injury and no hope for recovery through regeneration, one can consider a nerve transfer. This may involve a spinal accessory-to-suprascapular nerve transfer to reanimate the supraspinatus and infraspinatus muscles and using a branch of the radial nerve to the long head of the triceps to the axillary nerve to reinnervate the deltoid.

POSTOPERATIVE CRANIAL OR SPINAL HEMATOMA

Postoperative hematomas can occur after cranial neurosurgery in any number of locations: intralesional, intracerebral, subdural, and epidural (Figure 14.2). Application of epidural tack-up stitches lets your examiner know that you are thinking of prevention. In each case, consider antiplatelet agents and anticoagulants as potential risk factors for the development of a postoperative hematoma. Patients will typically present with pain, new or worsening neurological deficit, or reduced level of consciousness. Confirmation of the diagnosis is done with a computed tomography (CT) scan of the brain, if time permits, and prompt evacuation is the typical trajectory.

Postoperative spinal hematomas can occur in an immediate or delayed fashion. Severe pain associated with worsening neurological symptoms is the typical presentation. An intended (e.g., intradural procedure) or inadvertent durotomy may increase the potential for development of a hematoma. Postoperative wound drains should theoretically reduce the risk for hematoma formation. Again, confirmation of the diagnosis with spinal MRI or CT and surgical evacuation of the hematoma are required.

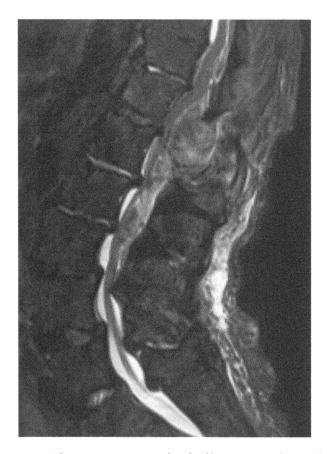

Figure 14.2 A large postoperative spinal epidural hematoma was diagnosed on day 2 postoperative after resection of a large intradural disc was resected after a T12 to L2 laminectomy. The hematoma can be seen to dissect under the caudal lamina and hence the laminectomy had to be extended.

HYPONATREMIA

Hyponatremia is one of the most commonly encountered neurosurgical complications. It can result in a decreased level of consciousness, as well as exacerbation of previously existing focal neurological deficits and, when severe (sodium level usually less than 120 mEq/L), can also result in seizures. We teach our residents a very simple scheme to work-up hyponatremia. Whenever hyponatremia develops, the urine sodium level and renal function (blood urea, nitrogen, and creatine) should be checked. If the urine sodium level is low (usually less than 10 mEq/L), sodium depletion should be suspected. This can be due to some diuretics, vomiting, diarrhea, ascites, pleural effusion, or nasogastric suction. If the urine sodium is high (usually more than 60 mEq/L) and renal function is impaired, pathologic sodium loss in the urine, such as occurs with chronic renal failure, or in the subacute phase of acute nephropathy, is the probable diagnosis. On the other hand, if renal function is normal, despite low serum sodium and high urinary sodium, the diagnosis is usually either a syndrome of inappropriate antidiuretic hormone (ADH) secretion or cerebral salt wasting secondary to excess natriuretic hormone as seen after subarachnoid hemorrhage (SAH). The basic difference between these two conditions is that in inappropriate ADH secretion, total extracellular volume and intravascular volume are increased, whereas in cerebral salt wasting, they are decreased. The problem is that it is difficult to tell this difference, and there are no quick and easy laboratory tests that can give us an answer. For practical purposes, if the patient has had a SAH, the diagnosis is almost certainly cerebral salt wasting. In the absence of SAH, the overwhelming likelihood is that the diagnosis is inappropriate ADH secretion. This difference is very important because, in the former condition, the treatment is replenishment of intravascular volume, which is best accomplished with colloid infusion, such as Albumisol. Replenishing the intravascular volume suppresses ADH secretion and gradually leads to restoration of sodium homeostasis.

With the syndrome of inappropriate ADH secretion, on the contrary, the treatment is volume restriction, which should be very strict (total fluids for 24 hours of less than 1 L/day and in severe cases of hyponatremia less than 600 mL/day). This can be accompanied by administration of sodium tablets when the patient is eating, and, when the hyponatremia is severe, hypertonic (3%) saline can be administered.

It is very important *not* to correct the sodium too rapidly or the patient can develop central pontine myelinolysis, especially when the sodium is corrected by more than 25 mEq/L in less than 48 hours. Patients will present with flaccid quadriplegia, locked-in syndrome, cranial nerve abnormalities, and mental status changes. Brainstem MRI will demonstrate high signal intensity within the pons, and possibly also in the thalamus. Many patients have a pre-existing history of alcoholism or malnutrition.

INTRAOPERATIVE BRAIN SWELLING

During a craniotomy, one may encounter uncontrolled brain swelling (Figure 14.3). Considerations include the development of an intracerebral hematoma, such as from a ruptured aneurysm, or a remote epidural or subdural hematoma, even potentially contralaterally situated; venous outflow obstruction (e.g., internal jugular vein); vasodilation of cerebral vessels from systemic hypercarbia due to anesthetic considerations; or progressive brain edema especially after trauma. A common example is uncontrolled brain swelling after removal of a subdural hematoma.

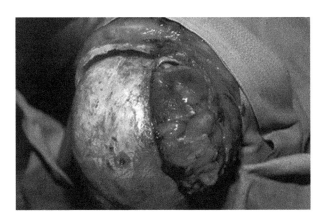

Figure 14.3 Massive brain swelling leads to brain herniation during a craniotomy for aneurysmal rupture and ultimately death despite the attempted ventriculostomy just to the midline of the dural opening.

Management pearls include elevating the head of the bed (anti-Trendelenburg position), making sure that neck rotation has not kinked the internal jugular vein, particularly in the park-bench position, ensuring that ventilatory pressures are not elevated by speaking to anesthesia, and measuring end-tidal P_{CO_2}. Employing measures to reduce intracranial pressure, including inducing hyperventilation to attain P_{CO_2} (30–35 mm Hg), giving mannitol (1 mg/kg IV bolus), and finally considering CSF drainage through a lumbar drain or ventriculostomy or draining CSF from an available operative cistern. All maneuvers are critical to avoid having herniated brain compress against the edge of the craniotomy wound and thereby lacerating the brain with further impairment of venous outflow. If all else fails, one may need to enlarge the craniotomy and consider aborting the procedure, and many times avoid replacing the bone flap until the swelling subsides.

A dramatic onset of brain swelling can occur when a large venous sinus is accidentally occluded during a craniotomy. This occasionally happens when the sinus is lacerated and vigorous bleeding develops, and in an attempt to stop the bleeding, the surgeon "packs" the area with Gelfoam or Surgicel. If this packing protrudes into the lumen of the sinus, it can occlude it, which may result in an immediate severe increase in venous pressure and progressive brain swelling. The correct way of handling a sinus laceration during craniotomy is first to elevate the head of the bed and then to place a strip of Gelfoam over the laceration, taking care to avoid any intraluminal obstruction by the Gelfoam. By placing a patty over the strip of Gelfoam, the bleeding almost always stops, particularly after some head elevation. At this point, under relaxed circumstances, the surgeon can proceed to repair the sinus in a variety of ways as necessary, although usually the bleeding simply stops and the Gelfoam strip can be left in place after removing the covering patty.

VASOSPASM

Vasospasm is, of course, a common sequela of SAH. Vasospasm (constriction of the large conductive arteries along the base of the brain) may be clinically asymptomatic or lead to severe neurological deficits and even death. One peculiarity of vasospasm is that it develops in a delayed fashion, and we can predict with relative accuracy, immediately after SAH, whether or not the patient is going to have severe vasospasm. A simple CT scan tells us how much blood there is in the subarachnoid space, and we have learned from Fisher and others[4] that there is a direct correlation with the thickness of the blood clot along the basal subarachnoid spaces and the development of vasospasm. This gives us a chance to treat the patient prophylactically. Essentially all SAH patients are treated with oral nimodipine, but this does not really prevent the development of vasospasm, although it does have a beneficial effect on outcome. For now, the only important prophylactic treatment in patients who have a high likelihood of developing vasospasm is to treat them with some degree of hypervolemia, or at the very minimum to avoid hypovolemia, which develops in these patient almost routinely for a variety of reasons (e.g., frequent blood drawing, supine diuresis, decreased red blood cell production). Certainly, hypotension should be avoided, and some degree of artificial hypertension can be safely induced if the aneurysm has been secured. When the clinical effects of vasospasm become manifest, the treatment with "the 3 Hs" (hemodilution, hypertension, and hypervolemia) is indicated and should be established early on. When the patient does not improve, repeat angiography and consideration of endovascular chemical vasodilation and mechanical angioplasty should be considered.

INTRAOPERATIVE ANEURYSM RUPTURE—OPEN OR ENDOVASCULAR

A key to open aneurysm surgery is proximal control. Ophthalmic artery aneurysm exposure will require prepping the neck for possible temporary internal carotid artery ligation. Proximal control is also key to more distal intracranial aneurysms. It is important to be prepared in advance with blood (2–4 units packed red blood cells) in the operating room, cell saver, and two large-bore suckers, so that you can clear the blood quickly to dissect around the bleeding aneurysm and identify the neck. When bleeding occurs, the goal is to achieve proximal and, if necessary, distal control with temporary clips and to control the bleeding with a strategically placed patty on the bleeding point and gentle pressure with a sucker while the neck is dissected. Avoid the temptation to put multiple large clips into the area of brisk bleeding, because you will likely injure the parent vessel. Consideration of adenosine administration to temporarily stop the heart can be considered as a last-ditch effort. Above all, the surgeon must remain cool and poised, which will ensure maximal efficiency of the entire surgical team.

MAJOR ARTERIAL INJURIES WITH CRANIAL AND SPINAL SURGERY

Some of the common scenarios in which large arterial vessels can be injured in neurosurgery include carotid artery injury with transsphenoidal surgery; vertebral artery injury with posterior cervical surgery, with instrumentation placed at C2 and with lateral dissection over the posterior arch of C1; and aortic injury and its branches with posterior lumbar spinal surgery.

The key elements are recognition, repair when possible, blood volume replacement, and follow-up angiography to diagnose and possibly treat endovascularly, usually with a stent, by embolizing the area of injury or sacrificing the parent vessel.

If there is an injury to the vertebral artery with C2 screw placement, it is important to place the screw to tamponade the vessel and *not* to put a screw on the other side because bilateral vertebral artery injuries can be lethal, whereas unilateral injuries are surprisingly well tolerated. Do not entertain drilling the bone of C2 to expose the artery and repairing it because the patient will bleed out before you accomplish this goal. Common error in judgment leading to vertebral artery injury with C2 pars screws placement is

lateral or low trajectory with the drill. A similar event can happen during an anterior cervical discectomy and fusion with a lateral bite within the foramen or during exposure of the longus colli. Postoperative angiography is important to confirm that the vessel is occluded, and not partially injured, which can lead to pseudoaneurysm formation, arteriovenous fistula, or a source of emboli (Figure 14.4).

In the case described in this chapter, the ipsilateral vertebral artery will need to be sacrificed by endovascular occlusion, provided there is good flow from the contralateral vertebral artery. When the vertebral artery is injured with open dissection over the arch of the atlas, arterial control can be quickly obtained with rapid dissection. When the injury is caused by sharp dissection, which we always recommend in this area, it can frequently be repaired primarily; however, blunt injuries and injuries caused by monopolar dissection usually cannot be repaired and require sacrifice of the artery.

Carotid artery injuries with transsphenoidal surgery are seen particularly when there is medial bowing of the carotid siphon into the sella or simply errors in judgment as to the location of the mid-line. Tamponade the vessel intraoperatively with a Cottonoid, and consider immediate angiography for possible repair or sacrifice of the vessel. Endovascular treatment options include vessel sacrifice, coil embolization (with or without stent assistance), and endoluminal reconstruction. Delayed complications such as pseudoaneurysm formation and rupture are common without treatment.

Finally, a simple lumbar laminectomy and discectomy can result in death after a ventral and lateral bite with the pituitary rongeurs that avulse a segmental branch from the aorta or iliac artery. Again, recognition is the most important issue. Intraoperative hypotension and tachycardia can signify a large retroperitoneal hematoma. When this is recognized intraoperatively, the best course of action is to

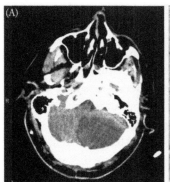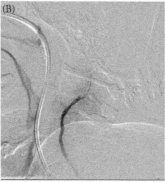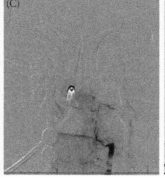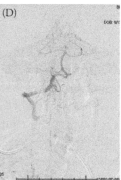

Figure 14.4 A-D. A large left cerebellar infarct is seen on day 2 post-op image after an occipital cervical fusion. Patient complained of nystagmus and left arm dysmetria. Postoperative angiography demonstrates complete occlusion of the left vertebral artery on lateral (B) and anterior–posterior (C) views with filling of the contralateral SCA, AICA, and PICA with right vertebral artery injection.

rapidly close the incision temporarily with 2 or 3 through-and-through stitches, turn the patient over, and start preparing the abdomen, while an emergency call to a vascular or general surgeon is placed. Prompt recognition in these cases can save a life. Postoperatively, the presence of abdominal bruising (Grey Turner sign), a low hemoglobin level, and signs of shock indicate the need to rush the patient back to the operating room to deal with bleeding arterial vessel through a retroperitoneal approach.

ESOPHAGEAL FISTULA

One has to be cognizant of the potential complication of an esophageal fistula after anterior cervical spinal surgery. Typically, these patients present with wound drainage, subcutaneous emphysema, pain, difficulty swallowing, and fever. The diagnosis can be confirmed with laboratory work, including white blood cell count, erythrocyte sedimentation rate, and C-reactive protein; further investigations may include barium swallow and rigid esophagoscopy. It is a very important diagnosis to make and treat early and aggressively because progression to mediastinitis can be lethal.

Patients require an otolaryngology consultation and exploration of the esophagus with these colleagues. Treatment options include simple repair of a small esophageal perforation or a more radical repair including the placement of a muscle flap, such as a sternocleidomastoid[5] or pectoralis major muscle. Part of the treatment often requires resting the esophagus, which would involve either a parentral or enterostomy feeding.

A rarer complication is a tracheoesophageal fistula. This is usually a delayed complication that frequently manifests as regurgitation and coughing up of food. The usual causes are excessive intraoperative pressure by a retractor on both the trachea and the esophagus or electrical burn to both structures, usually caused by a poorly insulated monopolar electrocoagulation tip.

REFERENCES

1. Levi AD, Dickman CA, Sonntag VK. Management of postoperative infections after spinal instrumentation. *J Neurosurg.* 1997;86(6):975–980.
2. McMahon P, Dididze M, Levi AD. Incidental durotomy after spinal surgery: a prospective study in an academic institution. *J Neurosurg.* 2012;17(1):30–36.
3. Farhat HI, Elhammady MS, Levi AD, Aziz-Sultan MA. Cervical subarachnoid catheter placement for continuous cerebrospinal fluid drainage: a safe and efficacious alternative to the classic lumbar cistern drain. *Neurosurgery.* 2011;68(1 Suppl Op):52–56; discussion 56.
4. Fisher CM, Kistler JP, Davis JM. Relation of cerebral vasospasm to subarachnoid hemorrhage visualized by computerized tomographic scanning. *Neurosurgery.* 1980;6(1):1–9.
5. Navarro R, Javahery R, Eismont F, et al. The role of the sternocleidomastoid muscle flap for esophageal fistula repair in anterior cervical spine surgery. *Spine.* 2005;30(20):E617–E622.

INDEX

Note: Tables and figures are indicated by *t* and *f* following the page number